Rheumatic Diseases: New Progress in Clinical Research and Pathogenesis

Rheumatic Diseases: New Progress in Clinical Research and Pathogenesis

Editors

**Ming-Chi Lu
Malcolm Koo**

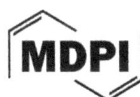

Basel • Beijing • Wuhan • Barcelona • Belgrade • Novi Sad • Cluj • Manchester

Editors

Ming-Chi Lu
Dalin Tzu Chi Hospital,
Buddhist Tzu Chi Medical
Foundation
Chiayi, Taiwan

Malcolm Koo
Tzu Chi University of Science
and Technology
Hualien, Taiwan

Editorial Office
MDPI
St. Alban-Anlage 66
4052 Basel, Switzerland

This is a reprint of articles from the Special Issue published online in the open access journal *Medicina* (ISSN 1648-9144) (available at: https://www.mdpi.com/journal/medicina/special_issues/ Rheumatic_Diseases_Pathogenesis).

For citation purposes, cite each article independently as indicated on the article page online and as indicated below:

Lastname, A.A.; Lastname, B.B. Article Title. *Journal Name* **Year**, *Volume Number*, Page Range.

ISBN 978-3-0365-8820-9 (Hbk)
ISBN 978-3-0365-8821-6 (PDF)
doi.org/10.3390/books978-3-0365-8821-6

© 2023 by the authors. Articles in this book are Open Access and distributed under the Creative Commons Attribution (CC BY) license. The book as a whole is distributed by MDPI under the terms and conditions of the Creative Commons Attribution-NonCommercial-NoDerivs (CC BY-NC-ND) license.

Contents

Malcolm Koo and Ming-Chi Lu
Rheumatic Diseases: New Progress in Clinical Research and Pathogenesis
Reprinted from: *Medicina* **2023**, *59*, 1581, doi:10.3390/medicina59091581 1

Angélica María Téllez Arévalo, Abraham Quaye, Luis Carlos Rojas-Rodríguez, Brian D. Poole, Daniela Baracaldo-Santamaría and Claudia M. Tellez Freitas
Synthetic Pharmacotherapy for Systemic Lupus Erythematosus: Potential Mechanisms of Action, Efficacy, and Safety
Reprinted from: *Medicina* **2023**, *59*, 56, doi:10.3390/medicina59010056 5

O. Capdevila, F. Mitjavila, G. Espinosa, L. Caminal-Montero, A. Marín-Ballvè, R. González León, et al.
Predictive Factors of the Use of Rituximab and Belimumab in Spanish Lupus Patients
Reprinted from: *Medicina* **2023**, *59*, 1362, doi:10.3390/medicina59081362 53

Hou-Hsun Liao, Hanoch Livneh, Miao-Chiu Lin, Ming-Chi Lu, Ning-Sheng Lai, Hung-Rong Yen and Tzung-Yi Tsai
Relationship between Chinese Herbal Medicine Use and Risk of Sjögren's Syndrome in Patients with Rheumatoid Arthritis: A Retrospective, Population-Based, Nested Case-Control Study
Reprinted from: *Medicina* **2023**, *59*, 683, doi:10.3390/medicina59040683 63

Ming-Chi Lu, Chia-Wen Hsu, Hui-Chin Lo, Hsiu-Hua Chang and Malcolm Koo
Association of Clinical Manifestations of Systemic Lupus Erythematosus and Complementary Therapy Use in Taiwanese Female Patients: A Cross-Sectional Study
Reprinted from: *Medicina* **2022**, *58*, 944, doi:10.3390/medicina58070944 75

Noha F. Mahmoud, Nashwa M. Allam, Islam I. Omara and Howida A. Fouda
Efficacy of Siwan Traditional Therapy on Erythrocyte Sedimentation Rate, Lipid Profile, and Atherogenic Index as Cardiac Risk Factors Related to Rheumatoid Arthritis
Reprinted from: *Medicina* **2023**, *59*, 54, doi:10.3390/medicina59010054 85

Dražen Bedeković, Ivica Bošnjak, Sandra Šarić, Damir Kirner and Srđan Novak
Role of Inflammatory Cytokines in Rheumatoid Arthritis and Development of Atherosclerosis: A Review
Reprinted from: *Medicina* **2023**, *59*, 1550, doi:10.3390/medicina59091550 99

Shomi Oka, Takashi Higuchi, Hiroshi Furukawa, Kota Shimada, Akira Okamoto, Atsushi Hashimoto, et al.
Antibodies against Serum Anti-Melanoma Differentiation- Associated Gene 5 in Rheumatoid Arthritis Patients with Chronic Lung Diseases
Reprinted from: *Medicina* **2023**, *59*, 363, doi:10.3390/medicina59020363 125

Chien-Han Chen, Chia-Wen Hsu and Ming-Chi Lu
Risk of Spine Surgery in Patients with Rheumatoid Arthritis: A Secondary Cohort Analysis of a Nationwide, Population-Based Health Claim Database
Reprinted from: *Medicina* **2022**, *58*, 777, doi:10.3390/medicina58060777 135

Min-Chih Hsieh, Malcolm Koo, Chia-Wen Hsu and Ming-Chi Lu
Increased Risk of Common Orthopedic Surgeries for Patients with Rheumatic Diseases in Taiwan
Reprinted from: *Medicina* **2022**, *58*, 1629, doi:10.3390/medicina58111629 145

Jolanta Dadonienė, Gabija Jasionytė, Julija Mironova, Karolina Staškuvienė and Dalia Miltinienė
How Did the Two Years of the COVID-19 Pandemic Affect the Outcomes of the Patients with Inflammatory Rheumatic Diseases in Lithuania?
Reprinted from: *Medicina* **2023**, *59*, 311, doi:10.3390/medicina59020311 . . . . **153**

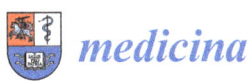

Editorial

Rheumatic Diseases: New Progress in Clinical Research and Pathogenesis

Malcolm Koo [1,2] and Ming-Chi Lu [3,4,*]

1 Department of Nursing, Tzu Chi University of Science and Technology, Hualien 970302, Taiwan; m.koo@utoronto.ca
2 Dalla Lana School of Public Health, University of Toronto, Toronto, ON M5T 3M7, Canada
3 Division of Allergy, Immunology and Rheumatology, Dalin Tzu Chi Hospital, Buddhist Tzu Chi Medical Foundation, Dalin, Chiayi 622401, Taiwan
4 School of Medicine, Tzu Chi University, Hualien 970374, Taiwan
* Correspondence: e360187@yahoo.com.tw

Rheumatic diseases encompass a group of disorders that primarily target the musculoskeletal system, including joints, bones, muscles, and connective tissue. Common rheumatic diseases, such as rheumatoid arthritis (RA), systemic lupus erythematosus (SLE), primary Sjögren's syndrome, and ankylosing spondylitis (AS), are chronic diseases that result in the dysregulation of the immune system [1]. These diseases often involve multiple organ systems, leading to significant morbidity and mortality among those diagnosed with rheumatic diseases [2,3]. Managing these diseases presents challenges not only for physicians but also for rheumatologists. The COVID-19 pandemic further complicated the management of patients with rheumatic diseases [4].

This Special Issue of *Medicina*, entitled "Rheumatic Diseases: New Progress in Clinical Research and Pathogenesis", features ten articles focusing on applying standard Western medications, Chinese medicine, and complementary therapies to patients with rheumatic diseases, increasing incidence of morbidity of these diseases, and changing mortality rates during the COVID-19 pandemic period, representing critical issues within the field.

Téllez Arévalo et al. [5] have provided us with a comprehensive review concerning the mechanism of action, efficacy, safety, and, most importantly, monitoring parameters of important synthetic drugs used in the treatment of SLE. SLE serves as a prototype for systemic autoimmune diseases. This article provided a valuable resource for physicians seeking to become familiar with SLE treatment. In addition to traditional immunosuppressants, biologic agents such as rituximab and belimumab are recommended for patients with SLE who demonstrate inadequate responses to standard therapies [6]. Capdevila et al. examined the characteristics and the predictive factors of rituximab and belimumab use in real-world practice among patients with SLE [7]. They found that rituximab was primarily used for conditions like hemolytic anemia or thrombocytopenia, lupus nephritis, and neuropsychiatric lupus, whereas belimumab was mainly used for arthritis. Currently, more biologic agents, such as anifrolumab, are available [8]. The integration of biologics could enhance the clinical outcomes for those with SLE.

Besides Western medicine, Chinese medicine and complementary therapies have been extensively investigated for their potential use in treating rheumatic diseases [9,10]. Liao et al. demonstrated that patients with RA using Chinese medicine could reduce the risk of developing Sjögren's Syndrome, a common extra-articular manifestation of RA [11]. Regarding complementary therapy usage, our previous study found that more than 85% of Taiwanese patients with SLE used complementary therapies on a regular basis [12]. We found that different clinical manifestations of SLE were associated with the use of specific complementary therapies. For example, Raynaud's phenomenon was significantly associated with fitness walking or strolling, and fish oil supplements. In contrast, photosensitivity was associated with probiotics and white renal involvement,

Citation: Koo, M.; Lu, M.-C. Rheumatic Diseases: New Progress in Clinical Research and Pathogenesis. *Medicina* **2023**, *59*, 1581. https://doi.org/10.3390/medicina59091581

Received: 8 August 2023
Revised: 26 August 2023
Accepted: 30 August 2023
Published: 31 August 2023

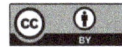

Copyright: © 2023 by the authors. Licensee MDPI, Basel, Switzerland. This article is an open access article distributed under the terms and conditions of the Creative Commons Attribution (CC BY) license (https://creativecommons.org/licenses/by/4.0/).

with both probiotics and visits to the Chinese medicine department in hospitals [13]. These associations might guide future research toward possible efficacious therapies for SLE.

Mahmoud et al. evaluated Siwan sand therapy, a traditional treatment in Egypt for alleviating joint pain. They found that five days of Siwan traditional therapy could reduce inflammation, improve the lipid profile, and enhance the quality of life in patients with RA compared to those receiving only three days of this therapy [14]. Although a systematic review indicated that limited evidence supports the therapeutic effect of hot sand baths on symptoms and functionality in patients with rheumatic diseases [15], the potential impact of hot sand baths on cardiovascular diseases and quality of life in patients with RA merits further study.

Cardiovascular disease is an important cause of death in patients with rheumatic diseases [16]. Bedeković et al. reviewed the effect of RA on the cardiovascular system [17]. They concluded that chronic inflammation and some medication for treating RA could accelerate atherosclerosis, and that maintaining long-term remission using novel therapeutic agents in RA may prevent cardiovascular events. Chronic lung disease is another leading cause of morbidity and mortality in patients with rheumatic diseases. Recently, the association between RA and the airway has been reported [18]. It is known that anti-melanoma differentiation-associated gene 5 (MDA5) antibodies (Abs) are linked with amyopathic dermatomyositis developing into rapidly progressive interstitial lung disease (ILD). Higher levels of anti-MDA5 Abs were found in RA patients with airway disease compared to those without [19]. Investigating the role of anti-MDA5 Abs in the pathogenesis of lung diseases in patients with rheumatic conditions can be a fruitful avenue of research.

Bones and joints are often the direct targets of rheumatic diseases, and it is unsurprising that patients with rheumatic diseases are seriously affected by joint deformity and bone damage. These individuals may experience a higher likelihood of undergoing orthopedic surgeries. Chen et al. revealed that patients with RA had an increased risk of receiving lumbar spine surgery, with older age and concurrent osteoporosis as risk factors [20]. Our group has been investigating this issue for years, summarizing the risks associated with four common orthopedic surgeries, including total knee replacement, total hip replacement, cervical spine surgery, and lumbar spine surgery, in prevalent rheumatic diseases including RA, SLE, AS, and psoriasis [21]. Given that joint deformity and bone damage in rheumatic patients take time to develop, we hope that the implementation of biologic agents and a treat-to-target strategy could minimize the need for orthopedic surgeries.

The recent COVID-19 pandemic has significantly impacted global health, including those with rheumatic diseases who have impaired immunity. Therefore, COVID-19 infections undoubtedly affect their clinical outcomes. Dadonienė et al. found that patients with rheumatic diseases had a lower mortality rate than expected in Lithuania [22]. Stringent lockdown measures, social distancing, and early vaccination can reduce the incidence of influenza and other infectious respiratory diseases. Though most restrictions have lifted with the end of the COVID-19 pandemic, continuing personal protective behaviors like handwashing, wearing masks, and regular vaccination is vital to prevent infections that could be fatal for those with weakened immunity.

The articles published in this Special Issue offer fresh perspectives on the clinical care of patients with rheumatic diseases. Rheumatologists can benefit from these insights, leveraging them to reduce patient morbidity and mortality.

Author Contributions: Conceptualization, M.K. and M.-C.L.; methodology, M.-C.L.; writing—original. preparation, M.-C.L.; writing—review and editing, M.K. and M.-C.L.; funding acquisition, M.-C.L. All authors have read and agreed to the published version of the manuscript.

Conflicts of Interest: The authors declare no conflict of interest.

References

1. Goldblatt, F.; O'Neill, S.G. Clinical aspects of autoimmune rheumatic diseases. *Lancet* **2013**, *382*, 797–808. [CrossRef]
2. Baillet, A.; Gossec, L.; Carmona, L.; Wit, M.D.; van Eijk-Hustings, Y.; Bertheussen, H.; Alison, K.; Toft, M.; Kouloumas, M.; Ferreira, R.J.; et al. Points to consider for reporting, screening for and preventing selected comorbidities in chronic inflammatory rheumatic diseases in daily practice: A EULAR initiative. *Ann. Rheum. Dis.* **2016**, *75*, 965–973. [CrossRef] [PubMed]
3. Salaffi, F.; Di Carlo, M.; Carotti, M.; Farah, S.; Ciapetti, A.; Gutierrez, M. The impact of different rheumatic diseases on health-related quality of life: A comparison with a selected sample of healthy individuals using SF-36 questionnaire, EQ-5D and SF-6D utility values. *Acta Biomed.* **2019**, *89*, 541–557.
4. Grainger, R.; Kim, A.H.J.; Conway, R.; Yazdany, J.; Robinson, P.C. COVID-19 in people with rheumatic diseases: Risks, outcomes, treatment considerations. *Nat. Rev. Rheumatol.* **2022**, *18*, 191–204. [CrossRef]
5. Téllez Arévalo, A.M.; Quaye, A.; Rojas-Rodríguez, L.C.; Poole, B.D.; Baracaldo-Santamaría, D.; Tellez Freitas, C.M. Synthetic pharmacotherapy for systemic lupus erythematosus: Potential mechanisms of action, efficacy, and safety. *Medicina* **2022**, *59*, 56. [CrossRef]
6. Fanouriakis, A.; Kostopoulou, M.; Alunno, A.; Aringer, M.; Bajema, I.; Boletis, J.N.; Cervera, R.; Doria, A.; Gordon, C.; Govoni, M.; et al. 2019 update of the EULAR recommendations for the management of systemic lupus erythematosus. *Ann. Rheum. Dis.* **2019**, *78*, 736–745. [CrossRef] [PubMed]
7. Capdevila, O.; Mitjavila, F.; Espinosa, G.; Caminal-Montero, L.; Marín-Ballvè, A.; González León, R.; Castro, A.; Canora, J.; Pinilla, B.; Fonseca, E.; et al. Predictive factors of the use of Rituximab and Belimumab in Spanish lupus patients. *Medicina* **2023**, *59*, 1362. [CrossRef] [PubMed]
8. Steiger, S.; Ehreiser, L.; Anders, J.; Anders, H.J. Biological drugs for systemic lupus erythematosus or active lupus nephritis and rates of infectious complications. Evidence from large clinical trials. *Front. Immunol.* **2022**, *13*, 999704. [CrossRef]
9. Greco, C.M.; Nakajima, C.; Manzi, S. Updated review of complementary and alternative medicine treatments for systemic lupus erythematosus. *Curr. Rheumatol. Rep.* **2013**, *15*, 378. [CrossRef]
10. Wang, Y.; Chen, S.; Du, K.; Liang, C.; Wang, S.; Owusu Boadi, E.; Li, J.; Pang, X.; He, J.; Chang, Y.X. Traditional herbal medicine: Therapeutic potential in rheumatoid arthritis. *J. Ethnopharmacol.* **2021**, *279*, 114368. [CrossRef]
11. Liao, H.-H.; Livneh, H.; Lin, M.-C.; Lu, M.-C.; Lai, N.-S.; Yen, H.-R.; Tsai, T.-Y. Relationship between Chinese herbal medicine use and risk of Sjögren's syndrome in patients with rheumatoid arthritis: A retrospective, population-based, nested case-control study. *Medicina* **2023**, *59*, 683. [CrossRef] [PubMed]
12. Lu, M.C.; Lo, H.C.; Chang, H.H.; Hsu, C.W.; Koo, M. Factors associated with the use of complementary therapies in Taiwanese patients with systemic lupus erythematosus: A cross-sectional study. *BMC Complement. Med. Ther.* **2021**, *21*, 247. [CrossRef]
13. Lu, M.C.; Hsu, C.W.; Lo, H.C.; Chang, H.H.; Koo, M. Association of clinical manifestations of systemic lupus erythematosus and complementary therapy use in Taiwanese female patients: A cross-sectional study. *Medicina* **2022**, *58*, 944. [CrossRef] [PubMed]
14. Mahmoud, N.F.; Allam, N.M.; Omara, I.I.; Fouda, H.A. Efficacy of Siwan traditional therapy on erythrocyte sedimentation rate, lipid profile, and atherogenic index as cardiac risk factors related to rheumatoid arthritis. *Medicina* **2022**, *59*, 54. [CrossRef] [PubMed]
15. Antonelli, M.; Donelli, D. Hot sand baths (psammotherapy): A systematic review. *Complement. Ther. Med.* **2019**, *42*, 1–6. [CrossRef]
16. Avina-Zubieta, J.A.; Thomas, J.; Sadatsafavi, M.; Lehman, A.J.; Lacaille, D. Risk of incident cardiovascular events in patients with rheumatoid arthritis: A meta-analysis of observational studies. *Ann. Rheum. Dis.* **2012**, *71*, 1524–1529. [CrossRef]
17. Bedeković, D.; Bošnjak, I.; Šarić, S.; Kirner, D.; Novak, S. Role of Inflammatory cytokines in rheumatoid arthritis and development of atherosclerosis: A review. *Medicina* **2023**, *59*, 1550. [CrossRef]
18. Matson, S.M.; Demoruelle, M.K.; Castro, M. Airway disease in rheumatoid arthritis. *Ann. Am. Thorac. Soc.* **2022**, *19*, 343–352. [CrossRef]
19. Oka, S.; Higuchi, T.; Furukawa, H.; Shimada, K.; Okamoto, A.; Hashimoto, A.; Komiya, A.; Saisho, K.; Yoshikawa, N.; Katayama, M.; et al. Antibodies against serum anti-melanoma differentiation-associated gene 5 in rheumatoid arthritis patients with chronic lung diseases. *Medicina* **2023**, *59*, 363. [CrossRef]
20. Chen, C.H.; Hsu, C.W.; Lu, M.C. Risk of spine surgery in patients with rheumatoid arthritis: A secondary cohort analysis of a nationwide, population-based health claim database. *Medicina* **2022**, *58*, 777. [CrossRef]
21. Hsieh, M.C.; Koo, M.; Hsu, C.W.; Lu, M.C. Increased risk of common orthopedic surgeries for patients with rheumatic diseases in Taiwan. *Medicina* **2022**, *58*, 1629. [CrossRef] [PubMed]
22. Dadonienė, J.; Jasionytė, G.; Mironova, J.; Staškuvienė, K.; Miltinienė, D. How did the two years of the COVID-19 pandemic affect the outcomes of the patients with inflammatory rheumatic diseases in Lithuania? *Medicina* **2023**, *59*, 311. [CrossRef] [PubMed]

Disclaimer/Publisher's Note: The statements, opinions and data contained in all publications are solely those of the individual author(s) and contributor(s) and not of MDPI and/or the editor(s). MDPI and/or the editor(s) disclaim responsibility for any injury to people or property resulting from any ideas, methods, instructions or products referred to in the content.

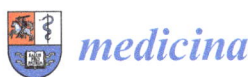

Review

Synthetic Pharmacotherapy for Systemic Lupus Erythematosus: Potential Mechanisms of Action, Efficacy, and Safety

Angélica María Téllez Arévalo [1], Abraham Quaye [2], Luis Carlos Rojas-Rodríguez [3], Brian D. Poole [2], Daniela Baracaldo-Santamaría [3] and Claudia M. Tellez Freitas [4,*]

1. Department of Physiological Sciences, School of Medicine, Pontificia Universidad Javeriana, Carrera 7 No. 40–62, Bogotá 110231, Colombia
2. Department of Microbiology and Molecular Biology, Brigham Young University, Provo, UT 84602, USA
3. Pharmacology Unit, Department of Biomedical Sciences, School of Medicine and Health Sciences, Universidad del Rosario, Bogotá 111221, Colombia
4. College of Dental Medicine, Roseman University of Health Sciences, South Jordan, UT 84095, USA
* Correspondence: cfreitas@roseman.edu; Tel.: +1-801-878-1269

Abstract: The pharmacological treatment of systemic lupus erythematosus (SLE) aims to decrease disease activity, progression, systemic compromise, and mortality. Among the pharmacological alternatives, there are chemically synthesized drugs whose efficacy has been evaluated, but which have the potential to generate adverse events that may compromise adherence and response to treatment. Therapy selection and monitoring will depend on patient characteristics and the safety profile of each drug. The aim of this review is to provide a comprehensive understanding of the most important synthetic drugs used in the treatment of SLE, including the current treatment options (mycophenolate mofetil, azathioprine, and cyclophosphamide), review their mechanism of action, efficacy, safety, and, most importantly, provide monitoring parameters that should be considered while the patient is receiving the pharmacotherapy.

Keywords: immunosuppressant agent; glucocorticoid; antimalarial drug; efficacy; safety; systemic lupus erythematosus

1. Introduction

The pharmacological treatment of systemic lupus erythematosus (SLE) aims to decrease disease activity, progression, systemic compromise, and mortality, thus improving patient quality of life [1]. However, all pharmacological alternatives can potentially precipitate adverse reactions, which is why risk management programs that evaluate the safety and efficacy of treatments must be an integral part of the selection and during therapy. A wide variety of drugs are available; therapy choice depends on many diverse factors, such as organ systems compromised, disease activity, previous therapy response, desire for parenthood, pregnancy or lactation, contraindications, and therapy adherence [2,3].

Non-adherence to drug therapy in SLE patients is a significant obstacle, as it ranges between 3–76% of patients and is associated with disease progression and increased morbimortality [4]. Education of all SLE patients at the time of diagnosis regarding the disease, the selected drugs, and non-adherence consequences is predicted to play a vital role in circumventing therapy non-adherence [3].

This section aims to provide a general description of chemically synthesized pharmacological agents for SLE treatment, emphasizing their safety margins and monitoring parameters.

2. Antimalarial Drugs

Chloroquine (CQ) and hydroxychloroquine (HCQ, a hydroxylated analog of CQ) are chemically synthesized disease-modifying drugs derived from alkaloids found in the cortex of *Chinchona officinalis* [5]. CQ and HCQ were synthesized in 1934 and 1950, respectively, and approved by the FDA for medical use in 1949 and 1955, respectively. Their anti-inflammatory and immunomodulatory effects underlie their effectiveness in treating SLE and other immunopathological diseases [6].

CQ and HCQ are lipophilic drugs that enter cells by simple diffusion. Their basic side chains concentrate in acidic organelles, such as endosomes, lysosomes, and Golgi vesicles, increasing the organelles' pH and interfering with multiple cellular processes involved in innate and adaptive immunity [7]. The pH changes in lysosomes—an increase from ~4.7 to ~6 [8]—destabilize its membrane and promote the loss of lysosomal enzymes in the cytosol. The pH changes also impede lysosomal enzyme function, which impairs endolysosome cargo degradation in autophagy, endocytosis, and phagocytosis pathways, essential in antigen processing for presentation [6] (See Figure 1).

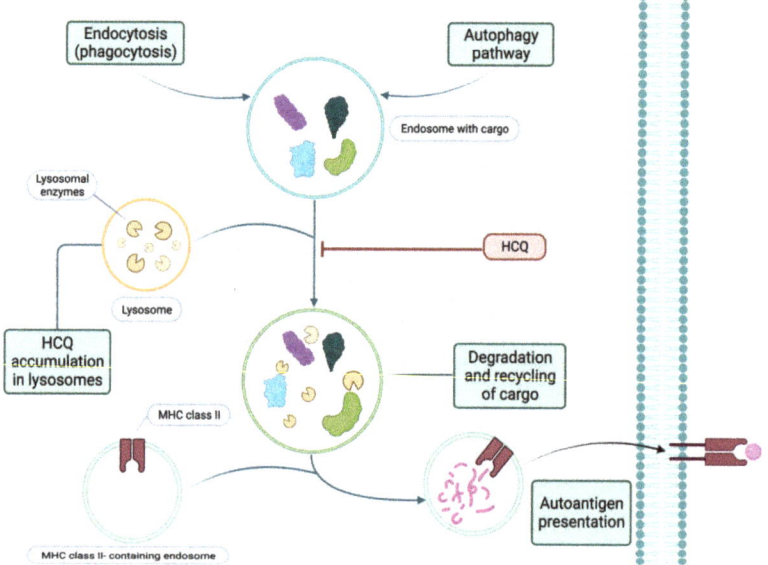

Figure 1. Mechanism of action of antimalarial immunomodulation during autoimmunity. HCQ accumulates in lysosomes and inhibits the degradation of cargo derived externally (via endocytosis or phagocytosis) or internally (via the autophagy pathway) in autolysosomes by increasing the pH to prevent the activity of lysosomal enzymes. Inhibition of lysosomal activity can prevent MHC class II-mediated autoantigen presentation. Adapted from Schrezenmeier et al. [6]. Created with BioRender.com (accessed on 17 October 2022).

Other immunomodulatory mechanisms of CQ and HCQ include: (1) Interference with the activation and signaling of Toll-like receptors 7 and 9 present on endosomal surfaces, which are involved in inflammatory responses and production of co-stimulatory molecules that participate in antigen presentation [6]. (2) Interference of cyclic GMP/AMP synthase, an essential enzyme in the function of type I interferon and IL-1. (3) Inhibition of Phospholipase A2 (PLA2) [7]. (4) Downregulation of the synthesis of proinflammatory cytokines, such as IL-1, IL-6, TNF, and IFN-γ in T and B cells [6]. (5) Enhancement of nitric oxide production by endothelial cells, inhibition of platelet aggregation [9,10], reduced formation of aPL-β2GPI complexes in phospholipid bilayers, and restoration of the anticoagulant function of annexin 5, collectively leading to vascular protective effects [8,11].

2.1. Efficacy

Antimalarials are most efficacious in treating mucocutaneous and musculoskeletal SLE [12]. They are effective in flare prevention and reduction of disease activity and mortality [13,14]. Accordingly, non-adherence to HCQ treatment was found to increase the patient's risk of flare-ups with lower complement C4 values, particularly those who only complied for less than a year [15]. CQ was shown in a randomized placebo-controlled trial of 24 patients to reduce disease progression rates, therapeutic glucocorticoid (GC) doses, and SLEDAI (Systemic Lupus Erythematosus Disease Activity Index) scores [16].

Antimalarials have also proved potent in managing lupus nephritis (LN), the commonest life-threatening complication of SLE [17]. A study showed that they improved the 12-month renal therapy response rates, reduced the risk of flares, and delayed the progression of renal insufficiency [18]. Additionally, they improve clinical outcomes in pregnant patients with SLE [18]. In a retrospective cohort study of 151 pregnant SLE patients, preeclampsia incidence was significantly lower, and neonatal weight was significantly greater, in patients treated with HCQ than control patients [19]. Furthermore, antimalarials reduced the risk of neonatal cardiac manifestations in pregnant SLE patients positive for anti-SSA/Ro antibodies [20].

Other benefits include a reduced risk of thromboembolism in patients with antiphospholipid antibodies [9], better glycemic control in SLE patients, and improved insulin sensitivity, thus decreasing the risk of developing diabetes [21,22]. The use of antimalarials leads to improved lipid profiles through reduced cholesterol synthesis and LDL receptor activity [7,22,23], improved bone density [24], and lower cancer risk [25].

2.2. Safety

HCQ and CQ have an established good safety profile and are usually well tolerated [7]. They are considered immunomodulatory, but not immunosuppressive, because their usage is not associated with an increased risk of infection or cancer [1]. Despite their ubiquitous clinical use in treating several inflammatory rheumatic diseases, antimalarials have an undetermined dose–response relationship and no defined minimum clinically efficacious dose. Hence, predicting dose-dependent side effects or toxicity is a challenge in clinical practice.

2.2.1. Gastrointestinal Adverse Reactions

The main adverse reactions associated with the antimalarials are gastrointestinal effects, including nausea, vomiting, abdominal pain, and diarrhea. For better tolerance, it is recommended to take them with meals. Cases of elevated liver enzymes in liver function tests and fulminant liver failure have been described. Hence, cautious use in patients with liver disease, alcoholism, or known use of hepatotoxic drugs is necessary [26].

2.2.2. Dermatologic Adverse Events

Generalized itching that responds poorly to antihistamine treatment, beginning a few hours after taking antimalarials, may occur. However, the itch usually resolves spontaneously within 72 h [8]. Furthermore, aquagenic pruritus has been described, but it is rare [27]. Another cutaneous manifestation is the loss of hair pigmentation [28] and hyperpigmentation; these are more frequent in patients with ecchymosis and those using antiplatelet agents or anticoagulants [29]. Still, other cutaneous reactions, such as DRESS (Drug Reaction with Eosinophilia and Systemic Symptoms), erythema multiforme, erythroderma, generalized exanthematous pustulosis, Stevens–Johnson syndrome, toxic epidermal necrolysis, or psoriasis exacerbations, may occur in the first days or weeks of treatment. These reactions strictly require treatment suspension [28].

2.2.3. Ocular Toxicity

CQ and HCQ have an affinity for melanin, whereby prolonged exposure causes concentration in melanin-rich tissues, such as the skin and retina [30]. When accumulated in these cells, they interfere with lysosome function, inhibiting autophagy and stimulating lipofuscin accumulation, which results in toxicity to the photoreceptors and the retinal epithelial cells [6,31]. HCQ also inhibits the activity of the OATP1A2 (Organic Anion Transporter Polypeptide 1A2), involved in the recycling of all-trans-retinol in the retinal epithelial cells, an essential step in the visual cycle [32]. This interference causes retinopathy, the most severe complication of antimalarial treatment [30,32]. Risk factors for ocular toxicity are described in Table 1.

Table 1. Risk factors for antimalarial-induced ocular toxicity [5,32].

1. Daily HCQ dose > 5 mg/kg (real weight)
2. CQ dose > 2.3 mg/kg (real weight)
3. Daily HCQ dose >6.5 mg/kg of ideal weight in obese patients
4. Use for >5 years
5. Cumulative dose > 600–1000 g
6. CKD stage 3, 4, or 5
7. Concomitant tamoxifen for >6 months
8. Macular degeneration, retinal dystrophy, cataracts

Clinical features include difficulty reading, scotomas, reduced visual acuity, altered color perception, and diminished peripheral and nocturnal vision [30–32]. In the fundoscopic examination, bulls-eye maculopathy can be visualized, a characteristic image caused by depigmentation of the retinal pigment epithelium of the macula with an unaffected central portion [31]. If exposure to the drug continues, retinal atrophy and retinitis pigmentosa may occur [33].

2.2.4. Cardiotoxicity

Antimalarial-induced cardiomyopathy (AICM) is a rare complication secondary to myocardial lysosomal dysfunction and cation (Na, K, and Ca) current alterations in the heart's electrical conduction system [34]. The features of AICM include hypertrophic and restrictive cardiomyopathy with or without conduction and rhythm abnormalities, bradycardia, tachycardia, T wave flattening, cQT interval prolongation [7,34], right bundle branch block, left anterior fascicular block, and complete atrioventricular block [35]. Due to cQT prolongation, pharmacological interactions that further increase the risk for ventricular arrhythmia must be avoided. Risk factors for AICM include advanced age, female sex, exposure for more than ten years, high daily dose per kg of body weight, high cumulative dose, preexistent cardiac disease, liver disease, renal disease, concurrent myopathy, and CYP2C8 polymorphisms [8].

2.2.5. Neuromuscular Adverse Events

In the central nervous system, headaches, dizziness, insomnia, vertigo, tinnitus, hearing loss, and lessened seizure threshold have been described [36]. Neuropsychiatric symptoms include psychosis, delirium, personality changes, and depression [8]. In the peripheral nervous system, reversible proximal myopathy and non-painful neuropathy with bilateral proximal limb involvement, associated with hyperreflexia, and respiratory muscle involvement may occur [8,37]. The induced myopathy is dose independent, detectable by various means. Creatine phosphokinase (CPK) levels may be normal or slightly elevated, but LDH (lactate dehydrogenase), being the most sensitive in detecting muscular damage, shows increased levels [38]. Electromyography can show a neuropathic, as well as a myopathic, component, but has a low diagnostic sensitivity [39]. Muscle biopsy can exhibit mitochondrial and vacuole alterations, as well as the presence of curvilinear bodies, atrophy, muscle fiber degeneration, and necrosis [38]. Risk factors include renal disease, use of myotoxic drugs, and Caucasian status [38–40]. Table 2 summarizes organ-specific side effects of antimalarial therapy.

Table 2. Summary of organ-specific side effects of antimalarial therapy.

Organ	Side Effects
Gastrointestinal tract	Nausea, vomiting, abdominal discomfort, diarrhea, hepatotoxicity
Skin	Pruritus (generalized, aquagenic), hyper- or depigmentation, ecchymosis, DRESS, erythema multiforme, erythroderma.
Eye	Retinopathy, diminished peripheral and nocturnal vision, bulls-eye maculopathy, difficulty reading, altered color perception.
Heart	Cardiomyopathy, bradycardia, tachycardia, T-wave flattening, left anterior fascicular block, complete atrioventricular block.
Neuromuscular system	Headaches, dizziness, insomnia, vertigo, tinnitus, hearing loss, psychosis, delirium, depression, reversible proximal myopathy, non-painful neuropathy.

2.3. Monitoring

Even though side effects of antimalarial use tend to be rare and less severe than some other immunomodulatory treatments, risk of these effects can be further minimized through proper administration and monitoring. Several references have established criteria for proper use, as follows.

1. Ensure the daily dose does not exceed 5 mg/kg [7,41].
2. In CKD patients with a GFR < 30 mL/min, the dosage must be adjusted to a maximum of 3 mg/kg of body weight [41].
3. Monitor complete blood count at the beginning and during prolonged therapy [8].
4. Surveillance of muscle strength and tendon reflexes [7].
5. Use CPK and LDH as a screening test for myopathy and cardiomyopathy at the beginning of treatment and 3 to 6 months later [41].
6. Monitor cQT prolongation in patients at risk [7].
7. During the first year of treatment, use fundoscopy with visual field and spectral-domain optical coherence tomography (SDOCT) or other objective tests as needed, according to the ophthalmologist criteria, such as multifocal electroretinogram and autofluorescence imaging (in case of maculopathy) to monitor ocular toxicity [5,41].
8. Ophthalmological control after five years of use or annually if the patient possesses risk factors [5,41].
9. Inform patients at the beginning of therapy about possible adverse events and the importance of early recognition.
10. Monitoring for the presence of new cardiac conduction abnormalities, biventricular and septal hypertrophy, or elevations in troponin, BNP, and CPK, can help identify patients at risk of cardiotoxicity to facilitate a diagnosis [35]. For this reason, an electrocardiogram could be performed at the start of treatment and annually.
11. Given its safety and benefits during pregnancy and lactation, treatment should continue if indicated.

3. Glucocorticoids (GCs)

After inflammation is induced to handle insults to the body, anti-inflammatory homeostatic mechanisms reverse the inflammatory processes as the insulting agent is removed. The hypothalamic–pituitary–adrenal axis, through the induction of endogenous GCs (cortisol, particularly), drives this anti-inflammatory process [42].

Endogenous GCs possess broad inhibitory effects on T- and B-cell-mediated functions, as well as a potent suppressive effect on the effector functions of monocytes/macrophages, dendritic cells, and neutrophils. Hence, the endogenous GCs are essential for the immune system's correct functioning, preventing tissue destruction and inflammatory diseases by obviating exaggerated and persistent responses to injury or infection [43–45]. A plethora of synthetic GCs, which mimic the potent effects of the endogenous GCs, have been developed to treat inflammatory disorders, such as asthma, allergies, sepsis, cancers, and autoimmune diseases, including rheumatoid arthritis and SLE [42,45,46]. The inhibitory effects of GCs on adaptive and innate immunologic functions, coupled with their rapid onset of action, account for their remarkable efficacy in managing the flare-ups of SLE [43,44].

The discovery of "Compound E" (hydrocortisone) in 1936 from animal adrenal gland extracts by Hench, Kendall, and Reichstein and its introduction as a clinical therapeutic agent for rheumatoid arthritis was a landmark in medical history, for which they received the Nobel Prize in Medicine and Physiology in 1950 [47–49]. Between 1954 and 1958, six synthetic steroids were developed for systemic anti-inflammatory therapy [49]. GCs have since become the cornerstone of SLE treatment [43]. GCs are used to treat such a wide range of inflammatory diseases that it is estimated that up to 2% of the population is receiving long-term GC therapy [50].

3.1. Mechanism of Action

Being highly lipophilic, GCs, after freely crossing the cell membrane, bind cytosolic GC receptors (GCRs), inducing an allosteric conformational change that results in the dissociation of the GCR from the heat shock proteins (HSPs) that chaperone the unbound GCRs to maintain their proper conformation for proper ligand binding [42,44,45,51,52]. The GC-GCR complex subsequently translocates to the nucleus in homodimeric or monomeric forms, where the immunomodulatory effects are exerted via several mechanisms [43] (see Figure 2). The first is termed transactivation. Homodimeric GC-GCR (hGC-GCR) complex binds to a specific DNA motif called glucocorticoid response element (GRE) on the promoter of glucocorticoid-responsive, anti-inflammatory genes, such as Ikβ, IL-1RII, Lipocortin-1, IL-10, and α2-macroglobulin. Binding of the GREs recruits chromatin-modifying co-factors and the transcriptional machinery to drive the anti-inflammatory genes [42–44,51–53]. In the second, termed transrepression, monomeric GC-GCR complex (mGC-GCR) binds to pro-inflammatory transcription factors, such as AP-1 and NF-kβ, inhibiting the expression of their target genes, including IL-1β, TNFα, and IL-2, cytokines, which are the major drivers of inflammation [42–44,51–53]. Additionally, prostaglandins, cytokine receptors, adhesion molecules, class II MHC molecules [43], and chemotactic proteins that play a crucial role in coordinating the inflammatory response are downregulated [54], and chemotactic proteins that play a crucial role in coordinating the inflammatory response are downregulated [55–57]. Another form of transrepression occurs through the GC-GCR complex binding directly to DNA sites (composite GREs), alongside AP-1 on its promoter, and hindering the expression of AP-1 target pro-inflammatory genes [44,45,52,53] (see Figure 2).

The mechanisms discussed above are collectively called genomic mechanisms because they all involve gene expression modulation. Several other mechanisms that preclude gene expression manipulations, termed non-genomic mechanisms, contribute significantly to the effects of GCs. They underlie the rapid onset of action of GCs, as they require no gene expression to impact the cell [54,58]. The best-elucidated non-genomic mechanism involves the activation of endothelial nitric oxide synthetase (eNOS) [59]. In this pathway, the GC-GCR complex activates phosphoinositide-3-kinase (PI3K) in endothelial cells, which activates Akt via phosphorylation. Phosphorylated Akt also activates eNOS via phosphorylation, resulting in nitric oxide production, which produces the physiological effects. This pathway was shown in mice to abate vascular inflammation and reduce myocardial infarct sizes following ischemia and reperfusion injury [46]. Other non-genomic mechanisms include: (1) activation of annexin I (lipocortin-1), an anti-inflammatory protein that inhibits phospholipase A_2 (PLA$_2$) and, therefore, arachidonic acid synthesis [54]; and (2) induction of the anti-inflammatory protein MAPK phosphatase 1, which inactivates all members of the MAPK protein family, including Jun N-terminal kinase and kinases 1, 2, and p38. As these MAPKs promote inflammatory pathways, their inactivation boosts the control of inflammation. Consequently, MAPK phosphatase 1 can indirectly inhibit the activity of PLA$_2$ by blocking the MAPKs required for its activation and reduce the activity of lymphocytes through the p38 MAPK inhibition [42,54,58].

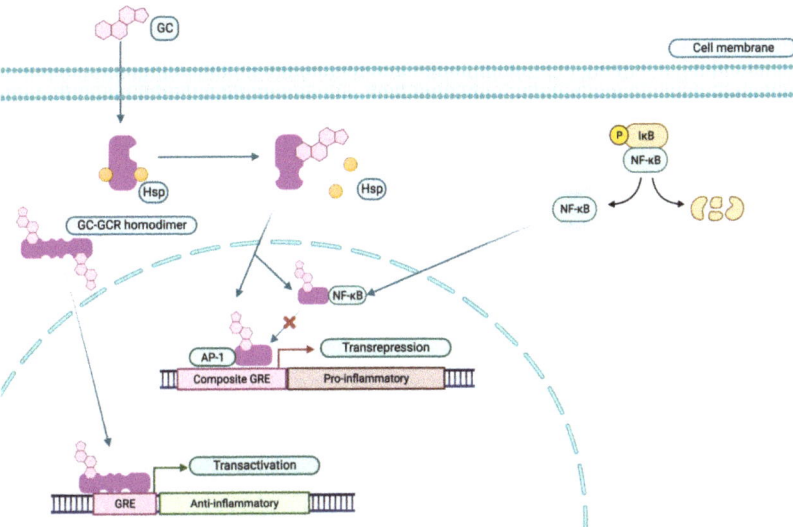

Figure 2. Genomic mechanisms of glucocorticoid-induced anti-inflammation. GCs bind to their cytosolic glucocorticoid receptor (GCR), which subsequently loses its chaperoning proteins, such as heat shock proteins (Hsp). Homodimers are formed, travel to the nucleus, bind to the glucocorticoid response element (GRE), and upregulate the expression of certain genes (e.g., lipocortin-1 and genes involved in metabolism), a mechanism called transactivation. Monomeric GC–GCR complex (mGC-GCR) can bind to transcription factors as AP-1 and NF-kβ, inhibiting the transcription of their target genes (e.g., IL-2 and TNFα) by a mechanism called transrepression. Further, direct binding of mGC-GCR alongside AP-1 on composite GREs lead to transrepression. Created with BioRender.com (accessed on 17 October 2022).

GCs also affect blood cell numbers; they increase the circulating neutrophil count, but decrease lymphocyte, eosinophil, basophil, and monocyte counts. The increased neutrophil count is secondary to their increased release from the bone marrow and the inhibition of their emigration [54]. The diminished circulating T cell numbers result from promoting apoptosis and migration to the bone marrow or secondary lymphoid tissues [47]. Furthermore, GCs can decrease fibroblast proliferation, fibronectin production [54], and dendritic cell maturation, survival, and migration, inhibiting their immunogenic functions, including stimulation of T cells [57].

3.2. Dosage

The dosage of GCs is more art than science. Albeit several organizations have published dosage guidelines, there are discrepancies between them, and standardization of GC dosage has proved challenging even till now. Consequently, physicians manage patients on a case-by-case basis, based on patient factors and their experience, guided by published recommendations [43,51,58,60]. The dosage of GC therapy determines the extent of GCR saturation. Low GC doses—i.e., prednisone doses—(up to 7.5 mg/day) are associated with up to 50% GCR saturation. Intermediate doses (>7.5–30 mg/day) achieve progressively higher saturation, with high doses (>30–100 mg/day) reaching 100% GCR saturation [43,54,58].

At very high doses (>100 mg/day), the rapid-onset non-genomic GC mechanisms are invoked [58]. Methylprednisolone (MP) and dexamethasone have non-genomic effects up to five times more potent than their genomic effects. Therefore, they act rapidly and are effectively used for intravenous (IV) pulse therapy, employed to manage severe organ and life-threatening manifestations [55,61].

SLE can be vaguely categorized as mild, moderate, or severe. The treatment of moderate to severe SLE comprises an initial phase of intensive immunosuppressive treatment called induction therapy, of which GCs (oral or IV) are central [62,63]. Induction therapy is purposed to halt active systemic inflammation and induce remission, followed by a less aggressive 'maintenance therapy' to consolidate remission and reduce the risk of flares [62,63]. The choice of GC dose, administration route, and duration of therapy, therefore, varies based on several factors [64]. In general, low prednisone doses are used as maintenance therapy and intermediate doses in moderate disease (fever, fatigue, weight loss, lymphadenopathy) or after MP pulses in severe SLE [43]. For instance, lymphadenopathy, arthritis, arthralgia, and myalgia can be controlled with doses of up to 20 mg/day of prednisone; however, lupus myositis cases will require higher doses of ≤60 mg/day coupled with cyclophosphamide (CYC) IV pulses [43,65,66]. In addition, Zhou et al. found that doses of ≤100 mg/day can suppress SLE-induced fever in 80.6% of patients [59]. High doses are indicated in severe manifestations [67], such as moderate cytopenia or some types of serositis. Moreover, very high doses or pulses of MP are used in life-threatening situations involving vital organs [55,56,61]. Such cases include lupus nephritis (LN), severe leukopenia or thrombocytopenia, and hemolytic or aplastic anemia. Others include gastrointestinal (autoimmune hepatitis, pancreatitis, enteritis), pulmonary (alveolar hemorrhage, shrinking lung syndrome), cardiac, and central nervous system (neuromyelitis optica, seizures, coma, peripheral neuropathy, optic neuritis, transverse myelitis) involvement [64].

In LN, the combination of medium-dose prednisone with IV pulses of MP, CYC, and HCQ is as effective as high-dose prednisone regimens, which are fraught with several adverse effects [51,68]. Ruiz-Arruza et al. compared the efficacy and safety of prednisone regimens at doses ≤30 mg/day versus >30 mg/day as initial treatment in recently diagnosed SLE patients with highly active disease without renal involvement. They found that the prednisone doses ≤30 mg/day were as effective as the higher doses for SLE treatment, but safer [69]. Accordingly, the lowest effective GC doses are increasingly preferred for treatment to reduce the risk of adverse events [64]. For this reason, the 2019 EULAR/ERA–EDTA (Joint European League Against Rheumatism and European Renal Association–European Dialysis and Transplant Association) guidelines for managing LN recommends a total intravenous MP dose of 500–2500 mg as induction therapy, then followed by oral prednisone maintenance therapy doses of 0.3–0.5 mg/kg/day for up to 4 weeks, and then reduced to ≤7.5 mg/day by 3–6 months [52,53].The current recommended doses are less than previous ones [70].

Once an SLE flare is diagnosed, the goal is to achieve remission as soon as possible and prevent new flare-ups, usually using GCs in combination with other drugs [51,63]. As the disease activity is controlled, less toxic immunosuppressive therapy is favored while the GC dose is tapered after 4–6 weeks of therapy initiation. A typical tapering starts with lowering the GC dose by 5–10 mg every 2–4 weeks until a daily dose of 20 mg, after which a reduction of 2.5–5 mg every 2–4 weeks is adopted until a maintenance dose of 2.5–10 mg/day is achieved [43]. A study showed that tapering GC doses below 5 mg have increased since 2000, probably due to a better understanding of long-term GC side effects even at low doses. The positive predictors of successful GC tapering in a cohort of SLE patients in the study were the absence of sustained skin and joint lupus activity [71].

3.3. Corticosteroid Resistance

In general, GC resistance is defined as the total or partial inability of cells to elicit GC responses or the absence of overt Cushing's syndrome signs with biological hypercortisolism [45,72]. Resistance to the therapeutic effects of GCs is a considerable problem in managing inflammatory diseases [45]. In fact, up to a third of SLE patients have a partial response to GCs [51]. This underlies the marked variability of patient response to GC treatment, leading to inadequate therapy in some patients, which indicates higher doses or the addition of immunosuppressive drugs [45]. Several molecular mechanisms underlie resistance to GCs: (a) GCR loss-of-function mutations [72]; (b) decreased expression of GCRα, the GCR isoform mediating GC's molecular effects [55]; (c) overexpression of GCRβ, a GCR isoform, functioning as a negative inhibitor of GCRα, hence, the action of GCs [43]; (d) post-translational modifications of GCR, altering its function [73]; (e) overexpression of pro-inflammatory transcription factors, such as AP-1 or NFκβ; (f) overexpression of macrophage migration inhibitory factor [74]; and (g) overexpression of P-gp (P-glycoprotein), a GC efflux pump that removes GCs from cells [43].

3.4. Safety

Although GCs are very potent quick-acting drugs, the concomitant damages of their use are substantial, especially with prolonged use at high doses [58,67]. Some side effects, including hyperglycemia, Cushing's syndrome, and psychosis, are reversible. These are ameliorated by decreasing doses or therapy suspension. Others, such as cataracts, avascular osteonecrosis, and growth retardation, are irreversible [67,75]. The severity of side effects correlates with the administered doses [58]. For instance, sustained prednisone doses >7.5 mg/day were associated with increased adverse events, correlating with increased patient morbidity and permanent damage [76,77]. Moreover, a study with a cohort of 747 SLE patients linked high cumulative prednisone doses to osteoporotic fractures, coronary artery disease, and cataracts; twice-monthly high-dose prednisone to avascular necrosis and stroke; and MP IV pulses to cognitive impairment [78]. The side effects of GCs are summarized in Table 3.

Table 3. Summary of Organ-Specific Side Effects of High-Dose or Prolonged GC Therapy.

Organ	Side Effects
Kidney	Increased sodium retention and potassium excretion
Musculoskeletal system	Osteoporosis, osteonecrosis, myopathy and atrophy, and growth retardation,
Cardiovascular system	Dyslipidemia, hypertension, hyperglycemia, lipodystrophy and weight gain, thrombosis, and vasculitis
Adrenal gland	Adrenal atrophy and Cushing's syndrome
Skin	Atrophy, delayed wound healing, erythema, hypertrichosis, perioral dermatitis, petechiae, glucocorticoid-induced acne, striae rubrae distensae, and telangiectasia
Eyes	Cataracts, glaucoma, myopia, exophthalmos, papilledema, chorioretinopathy, and subconjunctival hemorrhages.
Central nervous system	Depression, psychosis, bipolar disorders, delirium, panic attacks, obsessive–compulsive disorder, anxiety, insomnia, catatonia, and cognitive impairment
Gastrointestinal tract	Bleeding, pancreatitis, and peptic ulcer
Immune system	Broad immunosuppression; activation of latent viruses; increased risk of bacterial, fungal, and viral infections.
Reproductive system	Delayed puberty, fetal growth retardation, hypogonadism, gestational diabetes, hypertension, preeclampsia, premature rupture of membranes, and risk of cleft palate

Adapted from Rhen et al. [42].

3.4.1. Musculoskeletal Side Effects

Osteoporosis

GCs have been linked to bone diseases since 1932. Due to their wide usage, GC-induced osteoporosis is the most common cause of iatrogenic osteoporosis today and, in fact, the commonest cause of osteoporosis in adults 20 to 45 years old [50,51].

Within 12 months of therapy, GCs stimulate osteoclastic activity, decreasing bone density via excessive resorption—mediated by overexpression of the receptor activator of NFκβ ligand and macrophage colony-stimulating factor—and suppressing osteoprotegerin production, which promotes osteoclastogenesis. These osteoclast-mediated effects occur first, but transiently [79].

The slower, long-lasting impact of GCs is exerted via suppression of osteoblast activity, mediated via multiple mechanisms: (a) decreased expression of Insulin-like Growth

Factor-1, involved in osteoblastogenesis; (b) increased levels of the Dickkopf protein that negatively regulates the Wnt pathway involved with the differentiation, proliferation, and maturation of osteoblasts; (c) coaxing of osteoblast progenitor cells toward adipogenesis, hence, reducing osteoblast numbers; and (d) caspase 3 stimulation, which promotes apoptosis of osteoblasts and osteocytes [80,81].

Bone loss is more prominent in trabecular bone-rich areas, posing a higher risk of hip and vertebral fractures than forearm fractures. Loss of bone mass can become evident within three months of starting treatment and is correlated with high doses and longer treatment durations [82,83]. No GC dose eliminates the risk of osteoporosis. Even <2.5 mg prednisolone doses confer a higher risk of hip and vertebral fractures relative to controls [82].

Osteonecrosis

Osteonecrosis (ON) can result from significant reduction or interruption of the blood supply to bone, including intraluminal obstruction, vascular compression, or trauma to the vessels [84]. Several other conditions can cause ON, including SLE, sickle cell disease, pancreatitis, Gaucher's disease, and exogenous or endogenous hypercortisolism (GC medications, Cushing's disease) [84]. According to a meta-analysis published in 2017, the prevalence of symptomatic and asymptomatic avascular osteonecrosis (AO) in SLE patients is 9% and 29%, respectively. The most frequent site of AO is the femoral head because a terminal arterial system supplies it and it has no collateral blood supply, which renders it more susceptible to ischemia when occluded [85]. GCs induce an increase in the marrow fatty mass and fat cell sizes, resulting in intraosseous hypertension. Consequently, microvasculature occlusion by fatty emboli or impedance of sinusoidal blood flow occurs, leading to ischemia [84]. If ischemia is prolonged, necrosis progresses to sequestra formation, which results in a subchondral stress fracture, and then collapse and degenerative arthritis [84,86].

The mean daily dose and duration of GC exposure do not seem to be related to ON. Pharmacological interventions include low molecular weight heparin, lipid-lowering drugs, acetylsalicylic acid, and iloprost; however, it is not clear whether these treatments delay or reverse the disease progression. MRI is pivotal in diagnosis. The most useful MRI applications in ON diagnosis include (a) detecting early or small lesions, (b) differentiating ON from other bone diseases, and (c) predicting the likelihood of subchondral collapse. ON shows a characteristic MRI appearance for conclusive diagnosis [86].

Myopathy

Long-term use of GCs is associated with muscle atrophy, with decreased muscle strength mediated by two main mechanisms: reduced synthesis and increased degradation of proteins [87,88]. GC-induced myopathy primarily affects proximal muscles (e.g., the pelvic girdle muscles) [87]; yet, less frequently, distal muscles, sphincters, or facial muscles may be compromised [89]. Serum levels of CPK and aldolase are often normal, but LDH may be elevated [90]. Electromyography may present a myopathic pattern in the late stages. Muscle biopsy may show an increased number of central sarcolemma nuclei and loss of the crossed striae of type IIb muscle fibers without necrosis or inflammation, differentiating it from inflammatory myopathies [87,90].

Myopathy is uncommon in patients treated with prednisone doses of 10 mg/day, but with doses >40–60 mg/day, it can occur within the first 2 weeks of treatment [90]. Treatment suspension, physical therapy, and adequate protein intake have been shown to improve muscle strength between 3–4 weeks, although recovery may be slower [91].

Growth Retardation

GC-induced growth retardation is frequent in children receiving long-term GC treatment, averagely delaying skeletal maturation by 3.1 years and growth rates to only 3 cm/year [92]. GCs decrease growth hormone (GH) secretion, insulin-like growth factor

I (IGF-I) bioactivity, collagen synthesis, nitrogen and mineral retention, and chondrocyte proliferation [92]. They can also induce gonadotropin, testosterone, androstenedione, and estrogen deficiency [93]. For this reason, they have been associated with delayed growth and puberty. In a cohort of 25 GC-treated children with SLE, Abdalla et al. recorded 32% growth retardation [94]. Furthermore, in the PRINTO study with juvenile SLE patients, children with early-onset disease treated with cumulative doses of GCs > 400 mg/kg had a higher risk of growth disturbances and delayed puberty [94].

Given the significant degree of growth failure in many GC-treated children, there is great interest in the potential reversal of GC-induced growth failure with GH therapy [92]. In their study, Allen et al. showed that GH therapy counterbalances the effects of GCs effectively, albeit its effectiveness was negatively correlated with GC dose. They also showed that IGF-I, IGF-binding protein-3, osteocalcin, and procollagen were appropriate markers for monitoring growth retardation and GH therapy effectiveness [92].

3.4.2. Metabolic Side Effects

Hyperglycemia/Diabetes Mellitus (DM)

Along with chronic inflammation and obesity, GC therapy causes or exacerbates insulin resistance in non-diabetics or known diabetics, respectively [95]. The prevalence of GC-induced DM ranges between 5% and 45%; however, most studies agree that it is approximately 10–20% [96]. GC therapy increases the risk of DM by 2–3 times, the risk increasing in a dose-dependent manner [97]. In diabetics, administration of MP pulses increases the need for insulin therapy in up to 64% of patients [98]. GC-induced DM is mediated by complex mechanisms that are not well understood [99]. The effect of GCs on glucose metabolism likely results from the impairment of multiple pathways [99]. Excess GCs stimulate gluconeogenesis and glycogenolysis [100], alters insulin secretion and sensitivity in tissues [98], reduces β-cell mass [99], reduces GLUT-2 expression, inhibits GLUT4 translocation to the plasma membrane in skeletal muscle [101], and potentiates the effects of insulin-counteracting hormones, such as glucagon and epinephrine [102].

The main risk factors for developing DM include higher dosages, type of GC, longer duration of treatment, advanced age, high body mass index, family history of DM, and concurrent use of MMF (Mycophenolate Mofetil) and calcineurin inhibitors [102].

In general, GC-induced hyperglycemia improves with dose reduction; however, an individualized approach must be taken for each patient, such as lifestyle modifications and the requirement to initiate hypoglycemic drugs [102].

Dyslipidemia

The prevalence of dyslipidemia in SLE patients ranges from 36% at the time of diagnosis to 60% after 3 years [103], even 75% being reported in a cohort from Indonesia [104]. Sajjad et al. reported that the frequency of an altered lipid profile in SLE patients with LN of proteinuria > 1 g is increased significantly [105]. Dyslipidemia in SLE patients is associated with cardiovascular events and aggravation of kidney and central nervous system damage [106]. Many factors influence dyslipidemia development in SLE patients, such as autoantibodies, cytokines, and GC and cyclosporine A treatment [98,104,107]. The effects of GC on lipid metabolism are not well understood. However, it is known that cortisol activates lipolysis; increases triglycerides (TG) hydrolysis in adipocytes, free fatty acid levels [98,102], lipoprotein lipase and adipokine activity, and insulin resistance; and inhibits beta-oxidation of lipids [103]. Additionally, GCs induce changes in lipoprotein metabolism, stimulating the production of very-low-density lipoproteins (VLDL) and HDL and inhibiting the uptake of LDL [108]. As such, the lipid profile should be monitored in all SLE patients. Lipid-lowering drugs, mainly statins, should be administered when necessary to reduce coronary heart disease, cerebrovascular disease, kidney disease, and mortality [105,109].

While low doses equivalent to prednisolone < 10 mg/day do not significantly affect the lipid profile [109], doses ≥30 mg/dL are associated with high levels of total cholesterol (TC) and TG [104], but have a weak influence on LDL and HDL [108].

Weight Gain and Lipodystrophy

During systemic GC therapy, weight gain and morphological changes secondary to adipose tissue accumulation are frequently observed. This fatty tissue accumulation is often seen in the face ("full moon face"), dorsal-cervical area ("buffalo hump"), supraclavicular, and abdominal regions. However, there is a decrease in the subcutaneous fat of the extremities [110]. In a cohort of 236 SLE adolescent patients, 90% had a normal BMI at the beginning of GC therapy, but by the end, approximately 20% had a BMI > 25, and 10% were obese. Overall, 60% gained less than 10 kg, 25% gained 10–20 kg, and 15% gained more than 20 kg after treatment [111].

Cushingoid features can develop within the first two months of therapy. As many as 15–40% of patients may present with "moon face" after just 8–12 weeks of prednisone treatment (doses of 10–30 mg/day) [110].

The risk of these complications appears to depend on both the dose and the duration of treatment. In a cohort of 88 patients put on long-term systemic GC treatment, incidence rates increased over time. The risk of lipodystrophy was higher in patients who were women, were under 50 years of age, had a high BMI at the beginning of treatment, or had high caloric intakes [110].

The pathophysiologic mechanisms are multifactorial. They include the mechanisms of dyslipidemia and hyperglycemia described above; induced hormonal changes in growth hormone, testosterone, estrogens, catecholamines, and cytokines [112]; as well as stimulation of orexigenic pathways in the hypothalamus [98].

3.4.3. Cardiovascular Side Effects

Arterial Hypertension

Overall, about 20–30% of patients undergoing long-term GC therapy suffer GC-induced hypertension [100,113], and the incidence rates increase with higher cumulative doses [114]. L Fardet suggests that there may be two forms of arterial hypertension associated with GC therapy—an early-onset type (within days to weeks of treatment) in patients without risk factors and a late-onset type in patients with drug-induced lipodystrophy and weight gain [98]. Proposed mechanisms include an increased transcription of genes (*sgk-1*, *α-ENaC*, and *GILZ*) responsible for sodium reabsorption in the renal tubules and a decreased expression of the endothelial nitric oxide synthase. Other mechanisms include increased oxidative stress [115], increased expression of type I angiotensin II receptors, and stimulation of Na^+ and Ca^{2+} entry into endothelial cells [116].

Cardiovascular Risk

Patients with SLE treated with GCs at a dose greater than 10 mg/day or those with a cumulative dose equivalent to more than 10 mg/day for more than 10 years have significantly higher rates of cardiovascular events [117]. The use of oral GC is associated with heart failure [118], explained by sodium retention, increased extracellular fluid, stimulation of cardiac remodeling and fibrosis, increased myocardial oxidative stress, and coronary vascular inflammation mediated by mineralocorticoid receptors [119].

3.4.4. Adrenal Insufficiency

Exogenous GC administration generates a negative regulation of the hypothalamic–pituitary–adrenal (HPA) axis [106]. Minutes after GC administration, the increase in cortisol levels inhibits the release of ACTH and CRH. Later on (2–20 h), the transcription of pro-opiomelanocortin transcription factors (POMC) is inhibited, which leads to decreased ACTH synthesis, consequently reducing endogenous cortisol secretion by the adrenal gland [120].

The mean prevalence of adrenal insufficiency associated with GC use is 37% [106]. It occurs in up to one third of patients treated with 5 mg prednisolone/day, and the prevalence increases in patients who receive topical, intramuscular, or intra-articular GCs concurrently [121]. It most often occurs when therapy is discontinued abruptly or in acutely stressful situations. Physicians, therefore, wean patients off GCs by tapering the doses. After stopping treatment, HPA axis suppression may occur, with or without clinical manifestations such as asthenia, adynamia, nausea, abdominal pain, headache, or dizziness [122].

There is a great variety of information regarding the axis recovery time after therapy discontinuation. The earliest recovery time is 4 weeks [120], but axis suppression can persist for 24 months [123].

3.4.5. Skin Disorders

GCs cause a reduction in the mitotic activity of keratinocytes; reduce the size of fibroblasts, cause thinning of the dermis; and increase the fragility of the skin. Additionally, they cause a decline in monocyte and macrophage count, diminish phagocytosis, and delay re-epithelialization and fibroblast response [89].

The reported dermatological conditions include rosacea, erythema, telangiectasias, acneiform eruptions, purpura, pruritus, atrophy, hirsutism, stretch marks, decreased healing, and dermatitis [123]. Atrophy and ecchymoses are often reversible with GC therapy suspension, but stretch marks persist [89]. Purpura generally affects sun-exposed areas, such as the neck, back of the hands and forearms, face, and lower legs [79].

3.4.6. Neuropsychiatric Disorders

GCs can induce neuropsychiatric manifestations, such as depression, hypomania, psychosis, bipolar disorders, delirium, panic attacks, agoraphobia, obsessive–compulsive disorder, anxiety, insomnia, restlessness, catatonia, and cognitive impairment [124]. Symptoms can become severe in 5% of the treated patients [125]. They can appear within the first 6 weeks of treatment; in fact, some cohorts have reported 86% of patients presenting symptoms in the first week [126].

Female gender, SLE, and high doses may be risk factors for the development of symptoms [125]. Dose reduction or gradual suspension of GC is the mainstay of management; up to 90% of patients improve within the first 6 weeks of recess [127].

Some of the proposed pathophysiological mechanisms are the downregulation of GCR, the induction of neuronal oxidative stress, decreased serotonin levels, increased dopamine, and decreased sex steroid production [127].

3.4.7. Ophthalmic Alterations

The administration of systemic GC can lead to the formation of cataracts, glaucoma, myopia, exophthalmos, papilledema, chorioretinopathy, and subconjunctival hemorrhages [89]. GC-induced glaucoma is a form of open-angle glaucoma generated by morphological alterations of the trabecular meshwork, an increase in extracellular matrix proteins, and a decrease in vasodilator prostaglandins, which results in a diminished net output of aqueous humor. Risk factors include myopia, a history of penetrating keratoplasty or refractive surgery, patients under 10 years of age or the elderly, a history of diabetes mellitus, and endogenous hypercortisolism [128,129].

The frequency of oral GC-induced cataracts varies between 11% and 15% [129]. The risk is dependent on the dose and duration of therapy, and accrued damage is irreversible, even with treatment withdrawal. The mechanisms involved include enzymatic and cellular modifications, oxidative stress, protein alteration, and the action of various growth factors [128].

Central serous chorioretinopathy is a disorder characterized by neurosensory retinal detachment associated with detachment of the retinal pigment epithelium that can occur in patients with SLE [130], GC therapy being one of the main risk factors [131].

3.5. Safety in Pregnancy

GCs are one of the main treatments for lupus flares during gestation, as many other drugs are incompatible with pregnancy. They retain their potent anti-inflammatory effects without any significant teratogenicity [18]. The GC of choice depends on whether the goal is to treat the mother or the fetus [132,133]. Non-fluorinated GCs, such as prednisone, prednisolone, and MP, are the suitable GCs for treating the mother as they are inactivated by placental hydroxylases. Fluorinated GCs, such as betamethasone and dexamethasone, are less metabolized by the placenta. Hence, they are preferred if the fetus is the target of the treatment, especially in patients at risk of preterm birth, between 24 and 34 weeks of gestation, where induction of fetal lung maturation would be required [132,133].

The use of high GC doses during pregnancy is associated with an increased risk of complications, including infections, gestational diabetes, hypertension, preeclampsia, premature rupture of membranes, and the risk of cleft palate. For this reason, it is recommended to use the lowest possible dose for the shortest time, ideally a dose <20 mg/day. Hydrocortisone administration is recommended at delivery in patients on long-term GC therapy to reduce the risk of adrenal insufficiency [133].

During lactation, moderate doses are recommended, and at least a 4 h gap is to elapse after drug intake before breastfeeding [132].

3.6. Monitoring

As GCs have devastating effects, patients on GC treatment must be carefully monitored as follows:

1. Determine anthropometric measurements, blood pressure, metabolic profile (glucose, glycosylated hemoglobin, LDL, HDL, TC, TG, apoB), and densitometry at the beginning of treatment [79].
2. Guidelines for a healthier lifestyle, such as diet, regular physical activity, avoiding smoking, and reducing alcohol consumption [79].
3. Monitor blood glucose at least 48 h after the start of therapy, then every 3–6 months during the first year, and then annually [134].
4. Patients receiving prednisone doses >7.5 mg/day for more than 3 months should be prescribed calcium and vitamin D supplements [134].
5. Use FRAX scores to evaluate the risk of fractures at 10 years [79].
6. Determine anthropometric measurements in each consultation [134].
7. Perform bone densitometry at the start of therapy and annually if there is a decrease in bone mineral density or biannually if it remains stable [134].
8. X-ray of the lateral spine in patients ≥65 years for early detection of vertebral fractures [134].
9. Determine if the patient requires bisphosphonate therapy according to risk factors and bone mineral density [134].
10. Monitor lipid profile after 1 month of treatment, then every 6 to 12 months.
11. Assess cardiovascular risk periodically.
12. Perform bone densitometry and lateral column radiography in children receiving ≥3 months of GC therapy and repeat annually.
13. Monitor the growth rates of children and adolescents, and refer to endocrinology, if necessary, to ascertain if growth hormone therapy is needed [134].
14. Request an annual ophthalmological evaluation or earlier if there are risk factors or symptoms [134].
15. Monitor blood pressure, signs of fluid overload, and heart failure at each visit [134].
16. Watch for signs/symptoms of adverse reactions during therapy.
17. Patients treated with a GC concurrently with a nonsteroidal anti-inflammatory drug should receive gastroprotection with proton pump inhibitors or misoprostol. Alternatively, they could switch to a selective cyclooxygenase-2 inhibitor (taking into account increased cardiovascular risk) [134].

18. In patients requiring more than 10 mg prednisone/day, other less toxic immunosuppressants should be combined with GCs to accomplish quick tapering of prednisone and ultimately reduce GC-associated organ damage [58,62,135]. The immunosuppressants play an essential role in managing severe SLE manifestations, minimizing the risk of organ damage, reducing the cumulative dose of GCs, and preventing new flares of the disease [135]. Among the agents used are CYC (Cyclophosphamide), AZA (azathioprine), MMF (Mycophenolate Mofetil), Tacrolimus (TAC), and Methotrexate (MTX) [135].

4. Cyclophosphamide (CYC)

Developed by the German chemist Norbert Brock in 1958, CYC is an alkylating immunosuppressant derived from nitrogen mustard [136]. CYC was first used to treat SLE in the 1970s when Donadio et al. demonstrated that patients receiving prednisolone with oral CYC were more likely to have better renal preservation than GC monotherapy [137]. As with all other immunosuppressants, CYC is used in combination with GCs as oral or IV formulations [63,99].

4.1. Mechanism of Action

CYC is a prodrug predominantly (70–80%) hydroxylated by hepatic cytochrome P450 enzymes (CYP2B6, CYP2C9, CYP2C19, CYP3A4, CYP3A5, or CYP2J2) to 4-hydroxycyclophosphamide and its tautomer aldophosphamide. These metabolites enter target cells by simple diffusion [138], where 4-hydroxycyclophosphamide is inactivated. Aldophosphamide undergoes spontaneous non-enzymatic β-elimination, generating the active metabolite phosphoramide mustard and acrolein as a by-product. The former mediates the pharmacological effect of CYC, but the latter is urotoxic [136].

Phosphoramide mustard is a potent DNA alkylating agent that readily forms irreversible covalent bonds with N7 of guanine, leading to interstrand cross-links [139]. It can also bind other purine and pyrimidine atoms, blocking DNA replication and leading to apoptosis [140]. These actions exert a cytotoxic effect on actively proliferating cells, including mainly the less mature B lymphocytes, reducing antibody production by these lymphocytes [140]. Additionally, CYC dwindles the number of circulating effector T cells CD8+ CD44+ CD62L− and CD8+ CD44+ CD62L− [140].

4.2. Efficacy

CYC is a potent, but aggressive, drug; hence, it is only indicated for severe organ-threatening disease, especially neuropsychiatric SLE (NPSLE), cardiopulmonary, and renal compromise, where the toxicity-to-benefit ratio is justifiable [135]. It may also be indicated as rescue therapy in refractory manifestations of non-major organs [135].

A retrospective study that included 50 cases of CYC-treated patients with neuropsychiatric manifestations, such as psychosis, polyneuropathy, cerebrovascular disease, seizures, or cranial neuropathy, observed a partial or complete response in 84% of cases [141]. In a systematic review published by Cochrane in 2013 that compared CYC versus MP as NPSLE treatment, 94.7% of CYC-treated patients responded to treatment. Moreover, CYC was associated with a reduction in prednisone dose requirements [142].

GC monotherapy or in combination with CYC, MMF, or AZA is recommended in interstitial lung disease and constricted lung syndrome associated with SLE. However, this recommendation is mainly based on expert opinion as there is only tenuous evidence [142,143].

In the treatment of LN classes III, IV, and V, the combination of high-dose GC with low-dose CYC (500 mg IV bolus administered every 2 weeks for 3 months) or oral MMF (2 to 3 g/day for 6 months) is suggested [17]. High-dose CYC should be reserved for severe cases, such as rapidly progressive glomerulonephritis, where serum creatinine is >3 mg/dL with crescents or fibrinoid necrosis, or in those irresponsive to treatment [144]. However, in patients with a creatinine clearance of less than 30 mL/min, the dose should be reduced by about 30% [135]. The caution taken with high-dose CYC is due to its association with cervical neoplasms and ovarian failure [137] without superior efficacy than low doses, as evidenced by the multicenter prospective clinical trial (Euro-Lupus Nephritis Trial, ELNT). The ELNT trial compared high-dose and low-dose CYC IV regimens in patients with LN, followed by maintenance therapy with AZA. Treatment failure occurred in 16% and 20% of the low-dose and high-dose groups, respectively. In addition, renal remission was achieved in 71% and 54% of the low-dose and high-dose groups, respectively. While the efficacies were similar, episodes of severe infection occurred more frequently in the high-dose group [145].

CYC may be taken orally or intravenously, but IV pulse is preferred due to its superior efficacy-to-toxicity ratio [2]. Daily oral CYC as induction therapy may be more effective than intravenous pulses; however, its greater ovarian toxicity makes it justified only in high-risk or refractory LN [2]. Moreover, some studies suggest that CYC may have efficacy differences between different races of people [135]. For example, Dooley et al. [146] found a poorer renal survival in African Americans during the initial period of monthly IV CYC administration, with many of them rapidly progressing to renal failure. Further disparity was observed in long-term follow-up studies, with renal survival after 5 years at 94.5% for Caucasians and 57% for African Americans [146].

4.3. Safety

Notwithstanding its significant toxicity, CYC remains a mainstay of treatment for severe SLE. Its clinical effects (therapeutic or toxic) vary, depending on the dose, route of administration, duration of administration, and cumulative dose [135]. In the past two decades, minimizing the use of CYC for even the most severe SLE manifestations (particularly in LN) has assumed utmost importance. The main approaches for achieving this goal include: (1) using sequential therapy with CYC for induction of remission, followed by maintenance therapy with MMF or AZA; (2) shortening the period of induction with CYC; and (3) substituting MMF for CYC as induction therapy in LN [135]. The main side effects of CYC are compiled in Table 4.

Table 4. Summary of Organ-Specific Side Effects of Cyclophosphamide Therapy.

Organ	Side Effect
Gastrointestinal tract	Nausea, gastrointestinal dysmotility, emesis, and hepatotoxicity
Reproductive system	Ovarian failure (reduced estradiol, progesterone, maturation of oocytes, and number of ovarian follicles), amenorrhea, azoospermia, spontaneous abortions, congenital malformation, growth retardation, anatomical abnormalities, and cervical atypia
Urinary tract	Necrosis of bladder mucosa, hematuria, hemorrhagic cystitis, and bladder carcinoma
Immune system	Hematologic malignancies, neutropenia, lymphopenia, thrombocytopenia, anemia, and increased risk of infections.
Lung	Interstitial pneumonitis and fibrosis
Cardiovascular system	Hypertrophy, myocardial fibrosis, tachyarrhythmias, hypotension, heart failure, myocarditis, and perimyocarditis

4.3.1. Gastrointestinal Events

The most frequent CYC adverse effects are gastrointestinal-related, such as nausea, GI dysmotility, and emesis shortly after administration, especially with the dose ranges used for SLE treatment [147]. CYC is strongly emetic; hence, the American Society of Clinical Oncology recommends antiemetics, such as Ondansetron, a potent 5-hydroxytryptamine receptor antagonist, to alleviate emesis [147]. Furthermore, serious hepatotoxicity may occasionally occur with the doses used for autoimmune diseases [135].

4.3.2. Gonadal Insufficiency

Gonadal insufficiency is a significant side effect of CYC in both men and women. Amenorrhea may occur after treatment in 25–77% of treated women. The risk of ovarian failure is higher among older women and lower in patients receiving low doses. Ovarian failure results from a reduction in the number of granulosa cells, follicle sizes, maturation of oocytes, and levels of estradiol and progesterone [148]. In men, prolonged or permanent oligospermia or azoospermia has been observed [149]. Due to the risk of gonadal insufficiency, therapeutic alternatives, such as biologics, are suggested in patients of childbearing age. However, if CYC must be used, gonadotropin-releasing hormone analogs (GNRHa) should be combined with treatment [2]. GnRHa can exert direct protective effects on the ovaries through peripheral GnRH receptors and significantly reduce the risk of ovarian failure in young women with severe SLE [149]. CYC treatment is strongly associated with azoospermia; therefore, sperm banking before therapy should be considered. Additionally, testosterone supplementation during treatment helps preserve testicular functions and fertility [150,151].

4.3.3. Urotoxicity

Acrolein is an extremely reactive CYC metabolite [152]. In the urogenital epithelium, it promotes the intracellular production of reactive oxygen species (ROS) and nitric oxide (RNOS), which cause oxidative stress, lipid peroxidation, and mitochondrial dysfunction. The ROS and RNOS also promote protein-DNA adducts formation that causes inflammation, necrosis of the bladder mucosa, and gross hematuria [153]. Hemorrhagic cystitis (HC) can occur in 4–36% of CYC-treated patients with autoimmune diseases [151], with the cumulative CYC dose being the most important predictor for its presentation [154]. HC is considered a premalignant lesion that can eventually progress to transitional cell carcinoma of the urinary tract or fibrosis of the bladder, requiring the definitive interruption of treatment [155]. Patients should be advised to consume copious fluids or be given intravenous fluids with CYC administration to dilute the toxic metabolites in the urine to avoid HC. Patients receiving pulsed cyclophosphamide may simultaneously receive oral or IV sodium 2-mercaptoethanesulfonate (MESNA) at 20–40% of CYC dose, which will slow down the metabolism of 4-hydroxymetabolites and help detoxify acrolein in urine [156]. CYC increases the risk of bladder carcinoma and cervical intraepithelial neoplasms [147]. Daily CYC intake is associated with a heightened risk of bladder carcinoma and is dependent on the dose and duration of exposure. IV CYC regimens have lower total doses than prolonged daily oral regimens, and their associated incidence of bladder cancer may be lower because it is typically coupled with MESNA [154,157].

Additionally, development of non-urinary tract cancers in CYC-treated patients with rheumatic diseases, such as rheumatoid arthritis, is not uncommon. Neoplastic complications, including skin and hematologic malignancies and cervical atypia, are probable, even in patient treated with cumulative doses less than 10 g [135].

4.3.4. Infections

CYC can induce neutropenia, lymphopenia, thrombocytopenia, and anemia [158]. After CYC IV therapy, the lymphocyte count nadir occurs within approximately 7–10 days and granulocytes between 10 and 14 days. These counts typically recuperate after 21 to 28 days [135]; however, severe hematologic toxicity may occur in patients with polymorphisms of CYP2B6, GSTA1, and GSTP1 [159].

The frequency of infections—bacterial, herpes zoster, fungi, and some opportunistic infections (e.g., *P. carinii*), being the most reported—is about 37% [158,160]. The prevalence of infection is similar between IV CYC (39%) and oral (40%), the risk factors including leukocyte nadir ≤3000 cells, sequential CYC regimens, and combination with high-dose GC [161].

4.3.5. Pulmonary Toxicity

Adverse events affecting the pulmonary system occur in less than 1% of treated patients. They manifest as early-onset interstitial pneumonitis (within six months of starting treatment) or as late fibrosis [162]. Acute interstitial pneumonitis may mimic new lupus pulmonary manifestations in a patient with active disease, making it difficult to diagnose, and late-onset fibrosis may insidiously develop after months to years of CYC therapy [135].

4.3.6. Cardiac Toxicity

Oxidative stress and activation of the inflammatory pathway via NFκβ, with the simultaneous release of pro-inflammatory cytokines (IL-2, IL-10, IL-6, and TNF-α) associated with acrolein, induces hypertrophy, myocardial fibrosis, and arrhythmogenesis [163]. The clinical manifestations include tachyarrhythmias, hypotension, heart failure, myocarditis, and perimyocarditis. Albeit cardiac toxicity is rare with CYC treatment regimens in SLE, it is more frequent in oncology regimens [158].

4.4. Safety in Pregnancy

Exposure to cyclophosphamide during the first trimester of pregnancy can lead to spontaneous abortion or congenital malformations, including growth restriction, ear and craniofacial abnormalities, absence of fingers, hypoplastic limbs, exophthalmos, cleft palate, and skeletal abnormalities [164].

4.5. Monitoring

Due to the potentially severe toxicity of cyclophosphamide, the following monitoring regimens are of the highest importance.

1. Rule out pregnancy in women of childbearing age before starting therapy [165].
2. Advise women of childbearing potential to use effective contraception during treatment with cyclophosphamide and for up to one year after the last dose [165].
3. Recommend male patients with female partners of reproductive potential to use effective contraception during CYC treatment and for four months after the last dose.
4. Inform patients about the possible risks of infertility with therapy [165].
5. Perform a baseline blood count weekly for the first four weeks, every two weeks until the second month, and monthly thereafter. Do not start treatment in patients with an absolute neutrophil count of <1500/mm^3 and platelets of <50,000/mm^3 [166].
6. Correct or exclude any type of urinary obstruction because this may increase the risk of urotoxicity [166].
7. Perform urinalysis to evaluate the presence of hematuria, proteinuria, or bacterial infections. This test is initially recommended weekly for the first four weeks, then twice weekly until the second month, and monthly thereafter.
8. Surveillance for signs/symptoms of infection.
9. Monitor for signs and symptoms of cardiotoxicity or pulmonary toxicity [167].

5. Azathioprine (AZA)

AZA is one of the oldest immunosuppressive agents in use, having been used for several decades [135,168]. It is a purine analog developed from the anti-cancer agent 6-mercaptopurine (6-MP), initially purported to be a long-lived pro-drug version of 6-MP for better chemotherapy [168,169]. It was soon found to possess a better therapeutic index and effectively induced remission in childhood acute leukemia [168]. Later, it was shown to have immunosuppressive properties, such as reducing antibody production, prolonging allograft survival in transplant patients, reducing the severity of experimental lupus nephritis, and showing efficacy in treating rheumatologic diseases [168,169]. AZA is currently a valuable immunosuppressant for managing multiple SLE manifestations and a myriad of hematologic malignancies, rheumatologic disorders, and solid organ transplantation [168,170,171]. AZA is the only drug in its class currently in wide use for SLE management [171].

5.1. Mechanism of Action

Although the immunomodulatory mechanism of AZA is not well elucidated, its generally accepted to be mediated by DNA synthesis inhibition [171]. After its absorption, AZA is first non-enzymatically reduced by glutathione to 6-MP and then enzymatically converted to 6-thioinosinic acid (6-TIA), 6-thiouric acid (6-TUA), 6-methyl-MP (6-MMP), and 6-thioguanine (6-TG), which are collectively called thioguanine nucleotides (TGNs) [135,168,172]. The TGNs (6-TG and 6-TIA) block the de novo purine synthesis pathway and, ultimately, DNA synthesis by incorporation. Blocking the de novo purine synthesis is thought to underlie AZA's relative specificity to lymphocytes as they lack a salvage purine synthesis pathway; however, the DNA synthesis blockade alone does not sufficiently explain all the clinical findings of AZA-induced immunosuppression [168]. For instance, AZA reduces the levels of T cells, B cells, and natural killer cells, inhibiting both cellular and humoral immunity, as well as suppressing autoantibody formation and prostaglandin synthesis [173].

Other mechanisms contributing to AZA-induced immunosuppression, such as the following. (1) Direct apoptosis of T cells and inhibition of cell migration: in vitro studies showed that AZA and its metabolite, 6-TG triphosphate, interact with and block RAC1, a GTPase functioning in T-cell activation pathways, survival, migration, and adhesion. By blocking RAC1, all RAC1 target genes crucial for inflammation, T-cell activation, and survival, such as NF-κβ, mitogen-activated protein kinase (MAPK), and bcl-X_L, a protein complex with antiapoptotic properties, are suppressed [174]. Therefore, AZA surges T-cell susceptibility to apoptosis [174]. (2) Decreased synthesis of inducible nitric oxide synthase (iNOS): another in vitro study has shown that AZA can block RAC1 action in macrophages, a function necessary for iNOS expression. This blockade reduces iNOS mRNA levels, which is associated with decreased expression of IRF-1 (interferon regulatory factor 1) and IFN-beta (beta-interferon) mRNA. Hence, the inhibition of iNOS might contribute to the anti-inflammatory properties of AZA [174,175].

5.2. Efficacy

Despite several decades of clinical use, AZA has not been established as a first-line drug in severe SLE treatment [135]. In LN, it is most effectively used as a maintenance or steroid-sparing agent (2–3 mg/kg/day) employed after induction of remission with more potent and faster-acting agents, such as CYC or MMF [171]. Following the MAINTAIN trial, MMF usurped AZA as the preferred treatment in LN. However, AZA has found its niche in predominantly female patient populations of child-bearing age, as it is one of the few immunosuppressants deemed safe during pregnancy [176]. Indeed, it is considered the first-choice drug in pregnant patients [171,176].

The remission-maintaining benefits of AZA are not restricted to LN SLE manifestations alone. It is generally prescribed in SLE cases without renal involvement, where recurrent flares occur, due to its ability to reduce the frequency of flares [171,176]. It is reported to be effective in managing severe cutaneous SLE, autoimmune hepatitis, inflammatory bowel disease (IBD), and organ transplantation [135,170,173]. AZA is also efficacious as maintenance therapy in neuropsychiatric SLE and rheumatoid arthritis; however, it is not well tolerated with arthritis [177].

5.3. Safety

5.3.1. Genetic Predispositions

In hematopoietic cells, the primary enzyme that metabolizes AZA to its final active metabolites (TGNs) is thiopurine methyltransferase (TPMT). It has been shown that TGN accumulation in cells, which is inversely related to TPMT activity, is a significant determinant of AZA's toxicity and efficacy [172,178]. Interestingly, population studies show that 1 in 300 patients lack TPMT activity, and 10% have partial activity. These patients have genetic polymorphisms of TPMT that make for poor AZA metabolism; thus, they have an increased risk of toxicity or failed treatment [62,172,178]. Hence, testing for TPMT is recommended to help predict efficacy and drug-induced toxicity in AZA-treated patients with such polymorphisms [62]. However, pre-treatment TPMT genotyping or phenotyping is not widely implemented in rheumatology because it lacks consistency and may not identify many patients who eventually develop myelotoxicity [170,178]. The side effects of AZA are summarized in Table 5.

Table 5. Summary of Organ-Specific Side Effects of Azathioprine Therapy.

Organ	Side Effect
Reproductive system	Developmental delays, pancytopenia, premature birth, mild malformations
Gastrointestinal tract	Anorexia, nausea, vomiting, and diarrhea, pancreatitis, hepatotoxicity
Immune system	Myelosuppression (leucopenia and thrombocytopenia), anemia, bleeding, increased risk of herpesvirus (CMV, VZV, HSV, EBV) and bacterial infection, non-Hodgkin's lymphoma

5.3.2. Hematological Effects

Myelosuppression is a significant complication of AZA treatment. Leucopenia and thrombocytopenia complications occur in up to 27% and 5% of AZA-treated patients, respectively. The risk of these myelosuppressive side effects is greatest in patients with low TPMT activity [170], although it also occurs in patients with normal TPMT activity [135,178]. Low or no TPMT function leads to the accrual of higher intracellular concentrations of TGNs, increasing the risk of severe myelosuppression [178,179]. The MAINTAIN study showed that AZA induces hematological cytopenias more frequently than other drugs, such as MMF [176], eliciting subsequent complications, including sepsis, severe anemia, and bleeding [180]. Yet, mild symptoms are usually reversible with treatment withdrawal and are dose-dependent [170,178]. Concurrent usage with allopurinol, febuxostat, xanthine oxidase inhibitors, or ACE inhibitors augments the risk of myelosuppression by altering the balance between active and inactive metabolite levels [178,181]. Some authors recommend a switch to a different medication or tapering the doses in severe cases [170,180].

Reports of AZA causing neoplasms remain controversial, as the many studies designed to answer this conundrum have generally been underpowered and only yielded conflicting results. The preponderance of reported cancers in the literature is non-Hodgkin's lymphoma. Many of these lymphomas have been associated with Epstein–Barr virus (EBV) and immunosuppression, and some lymphomas resolve after treatment cessation [178].

5.3.3. Increased Risk of Infections

Like all immunosuppressive regimens, AZA increases the risk of infections. An extensive comparative study of SLE patients taking immunosuppressants found no significant difference between the infection rates of AZA (17.8%) and MMF (17.4%) [182]. Due to its cytotoxic effects on lymphocytes, AZA has a propensity for causing viral infections, including EBV, cytomegalovirus (CMV), or varicella-zoster virus (VZV) [178]. However, some studies suggest that bacterial infections are more common [182]. In contrast, studies show that MMF-AZA combination therapy gives a very low risk of severe infections compared to CYC, GCs, or either of them alone, being matched only by TAC [183].

As there is potentially an enhanced risk of vaccine-preventable infections in AZA-treated patients with rheumatological diseases, such as SLE and IBD, a vaccination strategy is essential. The European Crohn's and Colitis Organization (ECCO) guidelines espouse an intensive screening and vaccination program for infections, including VZV, pneumococcal, hepatitis B, HPV, and influenza, at the time of diagnosis for such patients as a preventive strategy. However, they advise against the use of live vaccines [184].

5.3.4. Gastrointestinal Effects

Gastrointestinal (GI) intolerance is the most prevalent side effect with AZA therapy, accounting for about 10% of treatment discontinuation [180]. AZA instigates several well-documented GI symptoms, including anorexia, nausea, vomiting, and diarrhea, occasionally severe enough to warrant therapy cessation [62,185].

AZA-induced pancreatitis rarely occurs in SLE patients; however, it affects 2–7% of IBD patients. It appears in a dose-dependent but unpredictable manner. Risk factors associated with onset include GC treatment and cigarette smoking; however, no predictive clinical tests are available to identify at-risk patients [185,186]. Yet, a recent retrospective study involving 373 AZA-exposed IBD patients by Wilson et al. has revealed that predictability is possible after all [185]. They showed in their work that single nucleotide polymorphisms in the class II HLA gene region at rs2647087 mapped to the *HLA-DQA1*02:01-HLA-DRB1*07:01* haplotype was a useful marker and predictor of AZA-induced pancreatitis. Accordingly, they proposed that a genotype-guided treatment algorithm be implemented to obviate adverse reactions [185].

Another significant AZA-induced complication is hepatotoxicity [187]. It has long been associated with AZA therapy and demonstrated as a dose-dependent and reversible (when the inciting agent is removed) phenomenon [178]. Generally, AZA-mediated liver toxicity arises within 12 months of therapy initiation. The overall incidence ranges from <1–10%, and about 90% of cases occur in males [187]. Several markers on the liver function test panel, including the liver enzymes, are usually elevated, which can mimic cholestatic hepatitis [187].

5.4. Safety in Pregnancy and Lactation

Notwithstanding the United States food and drugs board's classification of AZA as a class D agent (potentially harmful to the fetus, hence should be prescribed during pregnancy only after careful evaluation of risk versus benefit), it is considered the first-choice immunosuppressant during pregnancy [135,178,188]. The teratogenicity of AZA has been established in mice and rabbits, but human fetuses lack the requisite enzymes to convert the pro-drug (AZA) into active metabolites, hence, deemed protected from the disfiguring effects [178,189]. Some studies have corroborated this claim; however, some studies show that some mild complications, such as developmental delays, pancytopenia, increased risk of premature birth, and mild malformations, may occur [178,189,190].

AZA and its metabolites are detectable in breast milk; therefore, breastfeeding is ill-advised. However, some later studies show that AZA levels in breast milk are diminished significantly within four hours of drug intake; hence AZA treatment is compatible with breastfeeding [178,191,192].

5.5. Considerations in Renal Insufficiency

AZA is principally eliminated through the kidneys, and it has a short elimination half-life between 60–120 min after its conversion to 6-MP [193]. Although it is very effective as maintenance therapy (comparable to MMF) in treating LN [176], patients with KDIGO 3 chronic kidney disease have a higher risk of developing adverse reactions [194]. Where adverse effects occur, it is recommended to cut the dose by 75% for patients with estimated glomerular filtration rates of <50 mL/min/m^2 calculated by the Cockcroft-Gault equation. For patients with renal replacement therapy, such as hemodialysis, 50% of the dose should be administered before the procedure and supplemented with 0.25 mg/kg afterwards [194,195].

5.6. Monitoring

To prevent or minimize potential side effects of azathioprine administration, the following monitoring mechanisms are useful.

1. Consider genotyping or phenotyping patients for TPMT deficiency and genotyping for NUDT15 deficiency in patients who develop severe myelosuppression [195].
2. Monitor hemogram, including platelet counts weekly during the first month, twice monthly for the second and third months of treatment, then monthly or more frequently if dosage alterations or other therapy changes are necessary [196].
3. Liver function tests should be monitored periodically during therapy for early detection of hepatotoxicity https://www-micromedexsolutions-com.roseman.idm.oclc.org/micromedex2/librarian/CS/7F44AE/ND_PR/evidencexpert/ND_P/evidencexpert/DUPLICATIONSHIELDSYNC/217C6E/ND_PG/evidencexpert/ND_B/evidencexpert/ND_AppProduct/evidencexpert/ND_T/evidencexpert/PFActionId/evidencexpert.DoIntegratedSearch?SearchTerm=Azathioprine&fromInterSaltBase=true&UserMdxSearchTerm=%24userMdxSearchTerm&false=null&=null-cite97_de, every two weeks for the first four weeks and monthly thereafter [196].
4. Surveillance for signs/symptoms of infection.

6. Mycophenolate

MMF, synthesized around 1990, is an ester prodrug derivative of mycophenolic acid (MPA), an immunosuppressant used initially to avert rejection in kidney, heart, and liver transplantation, later employed to treat rheumatic diseases. The first MMF clinical trial in SLE was undertaken around the year 2000, and it is now considered a standard treatment for LN [197]. There are also clinical trials demonstrating its efficacy in treating non-renal SLE manifestations, such as arthritis, skin, or hematological involvement [198]. MMF is usually administered at a fixed oral dosage, and side effect monitoring is not routinely performed. However, MMF administration is sometimes associated with tolerability problems due to gastrointestinal adverse effects, such as vomiting, diarrhea, abdominal pain, and gastritis [199]. Hence, another MPA derivative, mycophenolate sodium (MPS), has been developed to tackle the side effects of MMF. The enteric-coated formulation of MPS (EC-MPS) releases MPA in the small intestine instead of the stomach, therefore, reducing MPA-related upper gastrointestinal adverse events [2].

6.1. Mechanism of Action

MMF, being a prodrug, is metabolized to its active form, MPA, which inhibits inosine 5-monophosphate dehydrogenase (IMPDH), an essential enzyme for guanine nucleotide synthesis. Thus, MMF causes the dwindling of B cell, T cell, and fibroblast numbers by inhibiting guanine synthesis. In addition, MMF has antifibrotic effects by reducing serum concentrations of transforming growth factor β (TGFβ), fibronectin synthesis, and proliferation of mesangial cells involved in the pathogenesis of renal fibrosis [173].

MPA has also been shown to inhibit the expression and function of cell adhesion molecules, thereby hindering the recruitment of lymphocytes and monocytes to sites of inflammation. It also induces apoptosis of activated T lymphocytes and suppresses nitric oxide production by reducing inducible nitric oxide synthase activity [200].

6.2. Efficacy

MMF or CYC combined with high dose GC are used as the induction and maintenance regimens for LN classes III, IV, and V. The ALMS study (Aspreva Lupus Management Study), involving 370 patients with LN classes III-V, compared MMF (3 g/day) with CYC (0.5–1.0 g/m^2 in monthly pulses) as induction therapy and showed that MMF and CYC had similar efficacies at 6 months and after 3.5 years. No significant differences were detected between the groups concerning the rates of serious adverse events or infections [201]. However, race, ethnicity, and geographic region were shown to affect response to treatment—more black and Hispanic patients responded to MMF than to CYC [201].

Rathi et al. compared MMF (1.5–3 g/day for 24 weeks) with low CYC doses (6 infusions of 500 mg every 15 days) as induction therapy in LN. All patients also received GC therapy. The complete remission rates were 50% and 54% in the CYC and MMF groups, respectively. Gastrointestinal symptoms were significantly more frequent in the MMF-treated patients, but other adverse events were similar [202]. Although gastrointestinal symptoms can occur with MMF and CYC, MMF symptoms tend to be mild and self-limiting, while in the CYC group, the risk of dehydration, hospitalizations, and discontinuation of therapy is higher. MMF is preferred in young men and women due to the high risk of sperm abnormalities and gonadal failure associated with CYC [203,204]. In a retrospective analysis of 63 patients, the ALMS and AURA clinical trials compared high- and low-dose MMF treatment combined with GCs in LN. The low-dose regimen showed no decrease in efficacy, but reduced the risk of lymphoproliferative disorders, skin cancer, and GC-related side effects [205].

As maintenance therapies, MMF and AZA are more effective and less toxic than CYC [17]. In a clinical trial that included 227 patients, treatment failure rates were 16.4% and 32.4% in the MMF and AZA groups, respectively. While minor side effects, such as infections and gastrointestinal disorders, occurred in more than 95% of patients in both groups, serious adverse effects occurred in 33.3% and 23.5% of the AZA and MMF groups, respectively [206]. MMF is the most widely used agent in maintenance treatment. However, MMF's superiority over AZA was neither affirmed in the MAINTAIN study that compared them in the long term [207], nor in a meta-analysis study that included seven controlled clinical trials, where no significant differences were found between groups in terms of mortality, relapse, exacerbation of renal disease, doubling of serum creatinine, infection, or gastrointestinal symptoms. Nonetheless, the MMF group had a lower risk of leukopenia and amenorrhea [203].

MMF's efficacy in managing non-renal SLE manifestations has only been published in case reports and uncontrolled clinical trials. In a retrospective study where a cohort of patients with vasculitis and SLE were treated with MMF and GC, the therapeutic GC doses were significantly lower when combined with MMF, and 46% of the patients responded well to therapy [208]. In their systematic review published in 2017, Fong et al. suggested that MMF may be efficacious in managing refractory SLE manifestations, such as hemolytic anemia, thrombocytopenia, and cutaneous lupus, and patients with low-grade disease activity that is irresponsive to other immunosuppressive agents, such as AZA and MTX [209]. There are reports of the use of MMF in treating pulmonary hemorrhage, interstitial lung disease, pericarditis, and myocarditis [210]. However, it is not possible to definitively determine the optimal dose or duration of treatment, as more compelling studies are required to make recommendations.

6.3. Safety

Patients treated with MMF have a lower risk of ovarian failure, alopecia, leukopenia, and serious infections compared to CYC, but diarrhea is more common with MMF [211]. Gastrointestinal symptoms, such as diarrhea, nausea, and vomiting, are more frequent with peak plasma concentrations of MPA. For better tolerance, it is advisable to subdivide the daily MMF dose into two or three administrations [139]. MPS has a lower peak plasma concentration and may decrease the incidence of gastrointestinal events compared to MMF [139].

The risk of leukopenia is low with the doses used in treating SLE [2]; hence, serious infections occur in less than 12%, and herpes zoster infection occurs in 4–18% of patients exposed to MMF [212]. Cases of progressive multifocal leukoencephalopathy (PML) have been reported in MMF-treated SLE patients [213], with hemiparesis, apathy, confusion, cognitive alterations, and ataxia being the most frequent manifestations [213].

6.4. Safety in Pregnancy

MMF is contraindicated in pregnancy because about 45–49% of MMF-treated pregnant women go through spontaneous abortions, and 23–27% of babies show congenital malformations, such as cleft lip, cleft palate, microtia, external auditory canal atresia, micrognathia, coloboma, and hypertelorism. Other less frequently reported anomalies are abnormalities in the extremities, congenital heart defects, esophageal atresia, diaphragmatic hernia, vertebral defects, and renal anomalies [214]. Due to its speculated teratogenic potential, the European Medicines Agency recommends that sexually active men on MMF use a condom during sexual intercourse and for 90 days after therapy discontinuation. Additionally, it recommends that men donate sperm no earlier than 90 days after MMF treatment [214]. Furthermore, breastfeeding is not recommended during MMF treatment; however, there is only tenuous evidence for this recommendation. Rats secrete MPA in their breast milk, but there is no data for human breast milk [214,215].

6.5. Monitoring

The following recommendations have been found to maximize effectiveness, while minimizing side effects using MPAs.

1. There is pharmacokinetic variability with MPA metabolism, and side effects are more probable with higher plasma concentrations in SLE patients. Hence, ascertaining the MPA concentration per patient can help reduce the risk of adverse reactions and improve effectiveness. Plasma MPA levels can be requested before and after any modification in MPA therapy, or when initiating or stopping concomitant medications [212].
2. Monitor patients with previous hepatitis B virus (HBV) or hepatitis C virus (HCV) infection for signs of reactivation [216].
3. Complete Blood Count weekly for the first month, twice a month for the second and third months, and then monthly for the first year of therapy [216].
4. Watch for signs/symptoms of infection [216].
5. Perform a pregnancy test 8 to 10 days before starting MMF, another immediately before starting the drug, and periodically with controls [217].
6. Women must use two effective contraception methods simultaneously before starting and during treatment and for six weeks after treatment [217].
7. Sexually active men (including vasectomized ones) taking MMF are advised to use condoms for intercourse during treatment and for 90 days after cessation. Their partners of childbearing potential should also use contraception during the same period [217].
8. Patients should be advised not to donate blood during therapy or within six weeks of stopping treatment [217].
9. Men should not donate sperm during therapy or for 90 days after discontinuation [217].

7. Calcineurin Inhibitors

7.1. Tacrolimus

Tacrolimus (TAC, FK506) is an immunosuppressant macrolide isolated from *Streptomyces tsukubaensis* in a soil sample obtained from Tsukuba, Japan, in 1984 [173,218,219]. It is categorized as a calcineurin inhibitor (CNI), along with its predecessor, cyclosporin A (CSA). However, TAC is more potent (about 30–100 times) and less toxic than CSA [220,221]. It was initially employed in preventing allograft rejection in transplant patients with very satisfactory outcomes [219]. Later, several studies demonstrated its efficacy in managing autoimmune diseases, such as SLE, rheumatoid arthritis, and psoriasis [222–224]. TAC is currently used in treating SLE, particularly recalcitrant LN, severe cutaneous and discoid manifestations [62,188,218].

7.1.1. Mechanism of Action

Calcineurin is a calcium/calmodulin-dependent serine/threonine protein phosphatase involved in T-cell activation. When activated, calcineurin dephosphorylates and activates target transcription factors, chiefly, nuclear factor of activated T-lymphocytes (NFATs), crucial in IL-2 expression and T-cell activation. TAC complexes FK506 binding protein 12 (FKBP12) and inhibits calcineurin's function by binding it tightly in the cytosol. Consequently, NFAT is left inactive and unable to upregulate IL-2 transcription. Hence, T-cell activation and subsequent secretion of cytokines, such as IL-2, IL-1β, IFN-γ, TNF-α, IL-6, and IL-10, as well as B-cell activation and antibody class-switching, is impaired [188,218,225,226].

Also, IL-2 production can be attenuated by inhibiting nuclear factor κβ (NF-κβ). TAC favors Iκβ/NF-κβ complex formation (the inactive state of NF-κβ), which leads to modulation of pro-inflammatory gene expression [227,228]. TAC has also been associated with other actions in vitro, such as promoting the expression of transforming growth factor-beta 1 (TGF-β1), which could underly the nephrotoxicity and pulmonary fibrosis associated with this drug [229].

7.1.2. Efficacy

Tacrolimus is available in injection, capsules, or ointment formulations for intravenous, oral, or topical administration, respectively [230]. TAC is strongly recommended for treating SLE, especially recalcitrant LN and severe cutaneous manifestations, due to its top-grade efficacy and safety profile [188,227,231]. Topical formulations of TAC have excellent effectiveness in treating a wide range of cutaneous autoimmune disease manifestations, such as atopic dermatitis, psoriasis, perineal Crohn disease, uveitis, and SLE [222–224,227]. Cutaneous autoimmune lesions are widespread and often mar its victims [231]. These cutaneous diseases are mainly treated with systemic immunosuppressants, such as HCQ, MMF, CYC, AZA, or methotrexate, with some good outcomes. However, this approach is fraught with systemic side effects stemming from the generalized immunosuppression [231,232]. Better results are achieved when topical TAC is employed, and the systemic side effects are circumvented [231]. Lampropoulos et al. showed that even 0.1% topical TAC was efficacious in treating cutaneous SLE resistant to other treatments [231].

In LN mouse models, TAC diminished proteinuria and preserved their renal function by stabilizing podocyte cytoskeleton and preventing podocyte apoptosis [218]. In these models, TAC also suppressed the progression of glomerular hypercellularity, crescent formation, and serum anti-dsDNA antibody levels [188]. Thus, it has been used in humans as both induction and maintenance therapy for LN, usually in combination with GCs ("duo therapy") or with MMF added ("triple therapy") [188]. Some small randomized clinical trials (RCTs) show that TAC is as potent as intravenous CYC in treating proliferative LN, but a meta-analysis study suggests that it is superior to CYC as induction therapy in LN. However, some of these reports should be taken with some reservations as their sample sizes were small [218]. RCTs comparing TAC with MMF and CYC as induction therapy in proliferative and membranous LN or with AZA as maintenance therapy showed equal efficacies in all cases [218]. Even in LN classes III, IV, and V, TAC (0.06–0.1 mg/kg/day) was shown to be non-inferior to MMF (2–3 g/day) over 6 months in an RCT involving 150 patients [218].

TAC combined with MMF (triple therapy) is even more potent. Low-dose MMF-TAC combination was shown in an RCT to be superior to IV CYC pulses over 24 weeks (45.9% versus 25.6%; $p < 0.001$) [233]. The same regimen was successfully used to treat recalcitrant LN and patients from diverse backgrounds (African Americans and Caucasians) with proliferative LN partially responsive to MMF treatment [218].

However, it is noteworthy that long-term evidence about the effectiveness of TAC is lacking, as most RCTs only extend to six months [188,218]. Secondly, the CNIs (TAC and CSA) exhibit inter- and intra-individual pharmacokinetic variability due to inherent high variability in absorption, distribution, metabolism, and clearance [234]. Lastly, TAC shows superior efficacy in Asians with LN than in other subgroups [188].

7.1.3. Safety
Drug–Drug Interactions

TAC undergoes substantial first-pass metabolism, mediated by hepatic cytochrome P450 enzymes, CYP3A4, and CYP3A5. Certain CYP3A5 polymorphisms are associated with increased TAC clearance and others with slower clearance. Hence, for optimal efficacy, the CYP3A5 genotyping of TAC-treated patients should be determined, as it would have dosage and toxicity implications [173,230,235]. TAC is also metabolized by P-glycoprotein (P-gp), whose expression levels are thought to be a good predictor of the dose requirements, especially within the first week of transplant [173,230,235]. TAC is often used concurrently with other drugs that are essential for transplant patients. Some of these drugs, including ketoconazole, cyclosporine A, diltiazem, erythromycin, and fluconazole, are also metabolized by P-gp and the CYP3A enzymes; hence, they affect the metabolism of TAC, decreasing its clearance [230,236]. Conversely, Rifampicin potentiates the elimination of TAC, reducing its bioavailability. Therefore, these drug-drug interactions should be considered in TAC dosage determination [230,236].

Renal Effects

Nephrotoxicity associated with CNIs is the primary concern with their usage; hence, it is dubbed their "Achilles heel" [237]. CNIs induce vasoconstriction of the afferent renal arteriole by elevating vasoconstrictors, such as endothelin and thromboxane, and activating the renin-angiotensin system, while suppressing vasodilator factors, such as prostaglandin E2, prostacyclin, and nitric oxide. In addition, CNIs inhibit COX-2, which contributes to the vasoconstriction, resulting in a reduced glomerular filtration rate [234,237]. This reversible, hemodynamically mediated renal dysfunction is known as "acute CNI nephrotoxicity" and is reversible [234,237]. Moreover, free radical formation plays a role in acute nephrotoxicity [237]. In addition to the hemodynamic effects, CNIs cause renal tubular functional alterations, leading to hypomagnesemia, hyperkalemia, hyperuricemia, and hyperchloremic metabolic acidosis [237]. Acute nephrotoxicity is associated with high systemic CNI doses [218].

In 1984, Myers et al. found that in addition to acute nephrotoxicity, long-term use of CSA in heart transplant recipients was associated with irreversible renal functional deterioration due to irreversible and progressive tubulointerstitial injury and glomerulosclerosis [238]. This irreversible injury was also found with TAC and termed "chronic CNI nephrotoxicity" [237,239]. Histological features, including arteriolar hyalinosis, tubular atrophy, interstitial fibrosis, and focal segmental or global glomerular sclerosis, are typical, but not pathognomonic of chronic CNI nephrotoxicity [218]. However, TAC appears to be less renotoxic than CSA because of its weaker vasoconstrictive effect and lower fibrogenic potential [218,237]. Risk factors for CNI nephrotoxicity include higher doses, concurrent use of other nephrotoxic drugs (e.g., NSAIDs), salt-depleting medicines and diuretics, and older kidney age. Others include genetic polymorphisms of the liver cytochrome enzymes (CYP3A4/5) and the multidrug efflux transporter P-gp and interactions with CYP3A4 and P-gp inhibitor drugs (e.g., ketoconazole) [218,234,237].

Neurological Effects

TAC-induced neurotoxicity occurs in approximately 25–31% of treated patients, of which 20% experience mild symptoms, such as tremors (most common), headaches, vertigo, photophobia, dysesthesia, paresthesia, mood disturbances, and insomnia [240]. Major neurotoxic symptoms, including confusion, seizures, cortical blindness, encephalopathy, and coma, occur in 5–8% of treated patients [240–242]. The major complications usually manifest within 30 days and are linked with high plasma TAC levels [241]. Rare complications, such as peripheral neuropathy and posterior cerebral edema syndrome, may occasionally occur [240,243]. These neurologic symptoms are reversible with cessation of TAC administration [240,241,243]. Some risk factors for developing TAC neurotoxicity include intravenous administration, high blood levels, and concurrent use with CYP3A4 inhibitor drugs (e.g., Nefazodone) [240].

Metabolic Abnormalities

Treatment with the CNIs is linked to metabolic disorders, including hyperglycemia, hyperuricemia, hypomagnesemia, and hyperkalemia, which are alterations that have been described in patients taking TAC; however, they tend to be less frequent compared to the other calcineurin inhibitors [244,245]. While hyperlipidemia (elevated LDL-cholesterol and triglyceride levels) is more uncommon with TAC treatment than CSA, diabetes mellitus (DM) is more frequent with TAC treatment [188,244]. TAC was shown to reversibly inhibit insulin mRNA transcription, insulin synthesis, and ergo insulin secretion in both in vitro and in vivo studies [244,246]. TAC-affected islet beta-cells show degranulation, vacuolation, and swelling of the mitochondria, Golgi apparatus, and rough endoplasmic reticulum [247]. These abnormalities usually resolve with dose reduction, although sometimes they require treatment suspension [244]. Consequently, all CNI-treated patients should have serum glucose, lipid profile, serum uric acid, and electrolyte monitoring [222].

Infections

Relative to other immunosuppressive regimens for SLE patients, TAC has a top-grade efficacy-to-toxicity ratio. In a comparative meta-analysis study of several immunosuppressive drugs for SLE, TAC was associated with a significantly lower risk of severe infections than AZA, MMF, GC, and CYC, only matched by MMF-AZA combination therapy [183]. Nevertheless, gram-negative sepsis and cytomegalovirus infection, as well as herpes simplex virus and chickenpox infections, have been described in transplant patients [183,248]. The risk of infections is linked with the concomitant use of other immunosuppressants, such as AZA, and hematological disorders, such as leukopenia [249]. Hence, clinical and laboratory monitoring is recommended for patients on CNIs [249].

7.1.4. Safety in Pregnancy and Lactation

Unlike CYC and MMF, TAC (along with AZA) is one of the few pregnancy-compatible immunosuppressants for SLE patients because it has no ill effects on fertility in women [214,250,251]. Albeit AZA is considered the first-choice medicine for pregnant LN patients, TAC is indicated in AZA-resistant or AZA-intolerant cases [188,218]. Further, only a negligible amount of TAC is detectable in breastmilk; hence, it is breastfeeding-safe and recommended for younger patients who want to preserve fertility [218]. Table 6 summarizes organ-specific side effects Tacrolimus therapy.

Table 6. Summary of Organ-Specific Side Effects of Tacrolimus Therapy.

Organ	Side Effect
Kidney	Acute nephrotoxicity (hypomagnesemia, hyperkalemia, hyperuricemia, hyperchloremic metabolic acidosis), chronic nephrotoxicity (arteriolar hyalinosis, tubular atrophy, interstitial fibrosis, glomerular sclerosis)
Central nervous system	Tremor, headache, vertigo, photophobia, dysesthesia, paresthesia, mood disturbances, insomnia, confusion, seizures, cortical blindness, encephalopathy, coma, peripheral neuropathy, posterior cerebral edema syndrome
Cardiovascular system	Hyperlipidemia (high LDL cholesterol and triglycerides), hyperglycemia
Immune system	Slightly increased risk of bacteria and herpesvirus infection

7.1.5. Recommendations in Drug Administration and Monitoring

There are two recommended administration forms: the conventional and modified release forms. The latter attempts to favor the drug's bioavailability and, therefore, reduces the dosage to once daily, increasing patient adherence to the treatment. Ideally, it should be taken on an empty stomach, and it is not recommended for the patient to chew the drug [173].

1. Monitor frequently: blood glucose, renal function, liver function, serum potassium levels (especially in patients receiving other medications associated with hyperkalemia), electrolytes (i.e., magnesium, potassium, calcium) [245,252].
2. Monitor ECGs periodically during treatment, especially in patients at risk for QT prolongation (concomitant use of other QT-prolonging drugs or CYP3A inhibitors, electrolyte disturbances, congestive heart failure, or bradyarrhythmia) [253].
3. Surveillance for signs/symptoms of opportunistic infections.
4. Surveillance for signs/symptoms of Neurologic abnormalities.

7.2. Cyclosporine

Cyclosporin A (CSA) was introduced as an alternative immunosuppressant in 1980 [254]. It is a calcineurin inhibitor that preferentially binds to cyclophilin, unlike tacrolimus, which has an effect on FKBP12. Cyclosporine is generally considered to have a lower potency (up to 100-fold less) than TAC [250].

Inhibition of calcineurin prevents the translocation of cytokine-related transcription factors (such as those responsive to IL-2), with subsequent inactivation of T cells achieving modulation of autoimmune activity [255]. In addition, cyclosporine has been shown to have effects on podocytes that may reduce proteinuria [250,254,256].

CSA is a lipophilic drug, with a narrow therapeutic range. It is metabolized mainly through CYP3A4 and is a substrate of P-glycoprotein. Its pharmacokinetics can be altered by food intake or even in situations such as hypoalbuminemia or hepatic failure [254,256].

7.2.1. Safety

In general, calcineurin inhibitors have been associated with metabolic, hematological, renal, and neurological effects. Monitoring of cyclosporine levels is recommended to avoid toxicity-associated effects [256]. Adverse effects usually improve after discontinuation of the drug. Currently, in different consensuses, the use of TAC is preferred over CSA due to its better safety profile and better control of the disease during maintenance therapy [17,256].

Nephrotoxicity

Acute and chronic nephrotoxicity have been described with cyclosporine. The drug's own vasoconstriction and fibrogenic potential were considered as factors associated with the development of this adverse reaction. The reduction in glomerular filtration rate associated with these drugs has not been associated only with elevated levels—it appears that other associated pathological or genetic conditions could trigger renal injury. It is recommended to monitor serum electrolytes as cyclosporine may be associated with hyperkalemia [256].

Metabolic

Cyclosporine patients are at risk of developing dyslipidemia and hirsutism, as well as hypertension. Monitoring of blood pressure, lipid profile, and changes in body hair distribution is recommended [256].

8. Methotrexate (MTX)

MTX is an antifolate drug derived from aminopterin. It is indicated as a disease-modifying drug in RA [257,258], inflammatory polyarthritis [259], severe psoriasis [260,261], psoriatic arthritis [261], juvenile idiopathic arthritis [257], ankylosing spondylitis [262], dermatomyositis [263], polymyositis [263], Crohn's disease [264], and SLE [258,265]. In

SLE, its use is indicated in patients who respond inadequately to antimalarials [266] and in patients with moderate SLE with skin, joint, and serous involvement, but without kidney involvement [258,265].

8.1. Mechanism of Action

MTX enters cells through the folate transporter type [257] and the reduced folate carrier type 1 (RFC1) [267]. At the intracellular level, MTX in the form of monoglutamate undergoes glutamic acid additions, forming polyglutamates, a more active and potent form of drug [267]. These polyglutamates inhibit several enzymes: (a) 5-aminoimidazole-4-carboxamide ribonucleotide (AICAR) transformylase (ATIC), an enzyme that participates in the de novo biosynthesis of purines [267]—when this enzyme is inhibited, levels of adenosine, a molecule with anti-inflammatory effects, increase [262]; (b) thymidylate synthase (TYMS), an enzyme that participates in the synthesis of pyridimines; (c) enzymes involved in polyamine transmethylation and synthesis reactions, thus decreasing the production of ammonium and H_2O_2, harmful agents for cells and joint tissues [267]; (d) dihydrofolate reductase (DHFR) and methylenetetrahydrofolate reductase (MTHFR), folate-dependent enzymes involved in the synthesis of purines, thymidylate, serine, methionine, and DNA [257,262].

Inhibition of DHFR further inhibits the production of tetrahydrobiopterin (BH4), a cofactor of nitric oxide synthase. By decreasing the activity of this enzyme, the formation of nitric oxide is decreased and the production of ROS that activate JUN N-terminal kinases (JNKs) increases. This activation increases the activity of the transcription factors AP-1 and NF-κB, promoting apoptosis of inflammatory cells [267].

8.2. Efficacy

In rheumatic diseases, MTX is administered once a week, orally, subcutaneously or intramuscularly [268]. It can be considered in moderate or severe SLE [268], which responds sub-optimally to antimalarials and in those cases where it is not possible to reduce the GC dose [269]. It is administered in doses of 7.5 to 25 mg per week, and favorable responses can be observed in 4 to 12 weeks [268]. Parenteral MTX seems to be useful in general, especially in those patients with insufficient response to oral MTX [270]. The parenteral route does not seem to increase the rate or severity of adverse events compared to the oral route and could reduce costs in those patients with an inadequate response to oral MTX [270].

Sakthiswary et al. evaluated the evidence for the use of MTX in SLE in a systematic review that included three controlled trials [258,271,272] and five observational studies [273–277], finding a significant reduction in the SLEDAI score and reduction in the mean dose of GC among patients treated with MTX [269]. MTX also reduces the average use time of prednisone [258], and this GC-sparing effect is relevant in light of the risk of adverse reactions associated with its use [258].

Patients with SLE where there is evidence of benefit are those with joint, cutaneous, and serous involvement [268,272,274]. In contrast, it seems to be effective in improving the serological alterations that are frequently observed during a lupus flare, observing increased levels of C3 and C4 and a decrease in the levels of anti-dsDNA, IgG, IgA, and IgM antibodies [277]. It is not recommended for interstitial lung disease, hepatitis, or cytopenias [268], and clinical trials where its efficacy has been studied have excluded patients with LN and NPSLE [278].

8.3. Safety

Although it is generally well tolerated, the use of MTX can cause pancytopenia, hepatotoxicity, pulmonary toxicity, nephrotoxicity, gastrointestinal adverse events, and skin rashes [279]. The most frequently reported adverse events are gastrointestinal [67,280] and leukopenia [67]. The prevalence of adverse events varies between 10–70% of patients with SLE [220,278,280], leading to the suspension of treatment in 19–33% of cases [67,280].

8.3.1. Gastrointestinal Side Effects

The prevalence of gastrointestinal symptoms varies between 20% and 40% in patients taking MTX [221]. The most frequent manifestations are nausea, vomiting, abdominal pain, and mucositis [281]. Risk factors for its presentation include doses greater than 8 mg/week [221]; concomitant drugs, such as NSAIDs; bisphosphonates and GC [221]; the absence of folic acid supplementation [282]; and kidney disease [279].

To reduce the risk of gastrointestinal reactions, it is recommended: (a) consider the administration of MTX as a relative contraindication in patients with active gastric ulcer; (b) supplement with folic or folinic acid at a dose greater than 5 mg/week [282,283]; (c) start with doses of 12.5 to 20 mg/week and slowly titrate [283]; (d) administer divided oral doses of MTX [284]; and (e) if gastrointestinal symptoms persist, consider changing the route of administration of MTX from oral to parenteral [270,283,284].

8.3.2. Hepatotoxicity

MTX can cause elevation in liver function tests in 10–43% of patients [285]. Temporary suspension of the drug or dose adjustment in general produces resolution of these alterations; however, the evolution to chronic disease due to fibrosis has been described [281,285]. Risk factors associated with hepatotoxicity include alcohol consumption, obesity, hypercholesterolemia, elevation of liver function tests before starting treatment with MTX, use of biological agents, absence of folic acid [286], advanced age, hypoalbuminemia, diabetes mellitus, kidney failure, and viral hepatitis [285].

Pathological changes found in liver biopsies include hepatic steatosis, focal necrosis, liver fibrosis, chronic inflammatory infiltrate in portal tracts, and nuclear pleomorphism [287].

8.3.3. Hematological Side Effects

Between 1–12% of patients treated with MTX present cytopenias [285,288], and in up to 1.4%, pancytopenia [288]. Risk factors for the development of pancytopenia include: advanced age, renal failure, hypoalbuminaemia, daily intake of MTX due to medication error, absence of folic acid substitution, polypharmacy [288], and being a carrier of the C677T polymorphism of methylenetetrahydrofolate reductase (MTHFR) [289].

The temporary suspension of the drug recovers the moderate suppression of the bone marrow within two weeks after withdrawal. However, a mortality rate between 17% and 44% can occur in patients with pancytopenia secondary to sepsis [288].

In contrast, MTX treatment has also been associated with lymphoproliferative disorders. Associated risk factors include intense immunosuppression, genetic predisposition, and increased frequency of latent infections with pro-oncogenic viruses [285,290,291].

8.3.4. Pulmonary Side Effects

Approximately 1% to 8% of patients receiving treatment with MTX may present with pulmonary alterations, such as interstitial pneumonitis [285,291]. Its presentation is independent of the accumulated dose and the duration of treatment [285]. Risk factors for the presence of MTX-induced pneumonitis include age older than 60 years, diabetes mellitus, hypoalbuminemia, previous use of DMARDs, kidney dysfunction, male gender, and pre-existing lung disease [292].

The proposed mechanism, although not clear, include hypersensitivity, direct toxicity of the drug, and repeated viral infections [292]. Within the paraclinical findings, it is possible to find a restrictive pattern in pulmonary function tests; a diffuse interstitial pattern on chest radiograph; ground glass opacities, with or without consolidation foci [291]; and basal fibrosis on CT in more advanced stages [292].

8.3.5. Renal Side Effects

The etiology of MTX-induced renal dysfunction is mediated by a direct toxic effect or by precipitation of MTX and its metabolites in the renal tubules at acidic urinary pH [293]. This crystallization generates infiltration of inflammatory cells and oxidative stress at the level of the renal tubules, which manifests with an increase in renal function tests and greater deterioration in the excretion of MTX [294].

Nephrotoxicity with low doses of MTX can be precipitated by doses not adjusted to renal function or by concomitant treatment with drugs that interfere with the excretion of MTX, such as probenecid, salicylates, sulfisoxazole, penicillins, and non-steroidal anti-inflammatory agents [293].

8.3.6. Neurotoxicity

The neurotoxicity induced by MTX is described mainly in patients who receive the drug at high doses or intrathecally [295]. The manifestations described include acute, subacute, or chronic neurotoxicity [296]. Acute neurotoxicity occurs after hours of administration of the drug and includes drowsiness, disorientation, seizures, headache, and dizziness. Subacute toxicity presents after days to weeks of treatment and includes findings of encephalopathy or myelopathy. Finally, chronic neurotoxicity, which occurs months to years of treatment, can manifest with cognitive alterations, dementia, and leukoencephalopathy [295].

At low doses, neurological symptoms are infrequent, mainly dizziness, vertigo, or headache [297].

8.4. Safety in Pregnancy

Associated abnormalities include spontaneous abortions, preterm delivery, metatarsal varus, palpebral angioma, growth deficiency, dysmorphic facies, multiple skeletal abnormalities of the skull and extremities, and less frequently, central nervous system abnormalities and congenital heart defects [298].

8.5. Monitoring

The following recommendations should be followed to ensure minimal side effects and optimal selection of candidates for MTX therapy.

1. Evaluate risk factors for serious adverse events due to MTX, such as alcohol intake, age over 70 years, and acute or chronic infections [299]. Avoid starting the drug in these patients [299].
2. Perform a complete blood count before the start of treatment and at least once a month during the first 3 months. It should then be done every 4 to 12 weeks during therapy [283,285].
3. Perform liver function tests before the start of treatment, every month for the first 3 months, and then every 2 to 4 months [283,285].
4. If liver function tests are elevated less than three times the upper normal value, a dose reduction is recommended. If they are persistently elevated more than three times the upper normal value despite dose reduction, it will be necessary to suspend the drug [299] and carry out complementary studies with evaluation by hepatology if the elevation of transaminases persists despite suspension [299].
5. It is recommended to take hepatitis B and C serology and measure serum albumin before starting treatment and repeat it in those patients who persist with altered liver function tests despite suspension of treatment [285].
6. The patient should receive simultaneous treatment with folic acid to reduce the adverse events associated with treatment with MTX [282,284,285].
7. Perform a pregnancy test before the start of treatment and periodically during treatment. Discuss with the patient the importance of contraception during treatment and the need to discontinue treatment with MTX 3 months before conception [299].

8. Determine the glomerular filtration rate before starting treatment, every month for the first 3 months, and then every 4–12 weeks during treatment [285]. The dose of MTX should be adjusted to renal function: Glomerular filtration rates (GFR) between 30 and 60 mL/min, require a reduction of the MTX dose of 30–50%, and perform renal function tests during therapy, initially twice a week and then every 4 weeks. The administration of MTX with a GFR <30 mL/min is not recommended [294].
9. Evaluation of respiratory symptoms and history in patients with suspected parenchymal lung disease, perform pulmonary function tests and chest radiography. Consider more frequent monitoring of respiratory symptoms and pulmonary function tests during therapy in this type of patient [299].

9. Dapsone

Dapsone, or 4,4-diaminodiphenylsulfone, is currently considered second-line therapy in bullous systemic lupus erythematosus (BSLE), either in monotherapy or in combination with GC [300–302]. Additionally, it is a treatment option in some refractory types of cutaneous lupus erythematosus (CLE), such as discoid lupus erythematosus (DEL) and subacute cutaneous lupus erythematosus (SCLE) [303].

After oral administration, it has a bioavailability of 70–80% [304]. It is hepatically metabolized by hydroxylation (CYP2E1, CYP2C9, CYP3A4) to dapsone hydroxylamine (DDS-NOH) or by N-acetylation to monoacetyldapsone (MADS) [305]. The parent molecule and its metabolites are conjugated with glucuronic acid or sulfate for renal elimination [304]. It has a volume of distribution of 1.5 L/kg, reaching most of the tissues, especially skin, kidney, liver, central nervous system, and placenta [305].

9.1. Mechanism of Action

The anti-inflammatory mechanism of action of dapsone involves multiple pathways: inhibition of pro-inflammatory cytokines, such as IL-8 [305,306]; alteration of chemotaxis and integrin-mediated neutrophil adhesion [307]; inhibition of leukocyte and eosinophil myeloperoxidases enzymes [308]; decrease in the generation of reactive oxygen species; and inhibition of the arachidonic acid cascade, thereby decreasing the generation of 5-lipoxygenase, prostaglandin E2, and thromboxane products [302].

9.2. Efficacy

EULAR recommends the use of dapsone at a dose of 100 mg per day in patients with BSLE who do not respond to or require high doses of GC [309]. However, it is common to start with a dose of 50 mg per day, which is titrated according to response and tolerance up to a maximum of 200 mg per day [300,309].

BSLE occurs in less than 5% of SLE cases [300] and may be the initial manifestation of the disease or be associated with lupus activity, in which case bullous lesions occur more frequently with lupus nephritis [300]. Most of the evidence for the use of dapsone, due to the frequency of the disease, results from case reports and retrospective analyses [300,310–312].

Hall et al. reported four patients with GC-resistant BSLE who, within the first day of dapsone therapy, had improvement of the lesions [310].

Lourenço et al. report 3 cases of BSLE in children aged 5 to 10 years. Two were treated with dapsone with improvement of the lesions on average between four weeks and four months of treatment. No adverse reactions were reported [313].

In a retrospective analysis of 181 cases of patients with BSLE, 91% of patients treated with dapsone improved partially or completely; however, treatment was discontinued in 23% of patients due to adverse reactions, mainly anemia, hypersensitivity reactions, and hepatitis [314]. Discontinuation of dapsone therapy before one year may result in recurrence of lesions, but they respond to reintroduction of the drug [300].

9.3. Safety

Hematological, cutaneous, and immunological, neuropsychiatric, gastrointestinal and hepatic alterations may occur [305].

9.3.1. Hematological Alterations

DDS-NOH, being a potent oxidizing agent, can submit the erythrocyte to oxidative stress, inducing hemolytic anemia, and can also oxidize the iron in hemoglobin, generating methemoglobinemia [305]. Some risk factors for these alterations include high doses, pre-existing hemoglobin abnormalities, low levels of cytochrome b5 reductase enzyme activity, glucose 6 phosphate dehydrogenase (G6PD) deficiency, and the use of other drugs that may induce methemoglobinemia [315]. Small amounts of DDS-NOH could be transported by the erythrocytes to the bone marrow, where it could possibly interact with neutrophils and induce agranulocytosis [305].

9.3.2. Cutaneous and Immunological Alterations

Dapsone has been associated with several cutaneous adverse reactions, such as fixed rash, exfoliative dermatitis, erythema nodosum, erythema multiforme, morbilliform and scarlatiniform rashes, Stevens–Johnson syndrome, toxic epidermal necrolysis, and DRESS [305,316].

Dapsone hypersensitivity syndrome (DHS), an idiosyncratic adverse reaction with multiorgan involvement, has been described [317], which develops within 1 to 6 weeks after the start of treatment [318], but it could occur even in the first 6 h of exposure in a previously sensitized individual [317], or after six months of therapy [319]. It has an incidence of 1.4% [320], and among the most frequent manifestations are fever, skin lesions, hepatosplenomegaly [317], hepatic lesion with a more frequent cholestatic than hepatocellular pattern, lymphadenopathy, nausea, vomiting, mucosal involvement, hematological alterations (hemolysis, agranulocytosis, leukocytosis, anemia, eosinophilia, reticulocytosis, atypical lymphocytosis, leukemoid reaction [317], interstitial pneumonitis, carditis, and nephritis [319].

Duration of DHS is about four weeks or more, usually self-limiting with drug discontinuation, but systemic GCs are often used as adjuvants [317]. A mortality rate of 11–13% has been described [315,318].

9.3.3. Neuropsychiatric

Ischemic optic neuropathy [315] and motor-predominant axonal degenerative peripheral neuropathy have been described. They may improve after one year of drug withdrawal, but recovery may be delayed and partial [302]. In addition, psychiatric symptoms, including irritability, insomnia, and confusion have been reported [321].

9.3.4. Gastrointestinal

Reactions at this level include nausea, vomiting, abdominal pain, liver injury, and pancreatitis [302,322,323]. The highly reactive metabolite DDS-NOH induces oxidative stress and lipid peroxidation in the liver, leading to hepatic necrosis, hepatitis, and cholestasis [322,323].

Cases of pancreatitis have been reported within 4 months after initiation of the drug, or weeks after dose increase in patients on prolonged therapy. All cases have resolved with discontinuation of the drug [323].

9.3.5. Safety in Pregnancy and Lactation

Dapsone is considered category C in pregnancy because it crosses the placental barrier, but no teratogenic effects have been observed in animals or humans [324].

It can be administered during lactation. However, because it is eliminated through breast milk, it should be avoided in infants with G6PD deficiency and/or hyperbilirubinemia [324].

9.4. Monitoring

1. Avoid use in patients with a history of allergy to sulfas and in patients with severe liver disease [302].
2. Determine glucose-6-phosphate dehydrogenase levels prior to initiating therapy [302,305].
3. Perform baseline CBC, then weekly for the first month, monthly for 6 months, and then semi-annually thereafter [305].
4. Request reticulocyte count at the beginning of treatment, and then periodically every 3–4 months [305].
5. Perform liver and renal function tests at the start of treatment, and then every 3–4 months thereafter [305].
6. Consider determining the methemoglobin level at the beginning of treatment and according to symptoms [302].
7. Monitor for clinical signs of jaundice, hemolysis, and blood dyscrasias during each visit [302,305], inquire about adverse reactions, monitor for neurological and psychiatric disorders [302].

10. Conclusions

SLE is one of the most common autoimmune diseases affecting our modern societies, hence, several immunomodulatory or immunosuppressive drugs, including antimalarials and glucocorticoids, have been developed to manage the disease. In this review article, we described current therapies and their possible side effects.

Having been in clinical use for several decades, the antimalarials have been rigorously studied. They are immunomodulatory rather than immunosuppressive; hence, their usage is associated with less risk of infection and cancer, and they are better tolerated than other treatment alternatives. Besides their high efficacy, antimalarials are also considerably safer than many other SLE drugs, as their side effects tend to be mild, few, and rare, and they are among the very few SLE drugs not contraindicated during pregnancy. However, they are generally employed in symptomatic management and not useful as induction therapy. Glucocorticoids are probably the most essential drug in treating autoimmune diseases, such as SLE. Owing to their efficacy as immunosuppressants, GCs are used to manage the most severe SLE manifestations as induction therapy, but are also commonly used as maintenance therapy, usually in combination with other treatments. Albeit effective, GCs engender significant dose-dependent side effects; hence, it is good practice to taper their dosage over the shortest amount of time possible. Antimalarials and GCs are both essential drugs in the doctor's cabinet for managing SLE. Multiple other drugs, such as cyclosporine, methotrexate, mycophenolate, azathioprine, and cyclophosphamide, are also useful in specific cases, especially when monitored carefully.

Author Contributions: Conceptualization: A.M.T.A., A.Q., L.C.R.-R., B.D.P. and C.M.T.F.; methodology: A.M.T.A., A.Q., L.C.R.-R., B.D.P. and C.M.T.F.; investigation: A.M.T.A., A.Q., L.C.R.-R., B.D.P., D.B.-S. and C.M.T.F., writing—original draft preparation, A.M.T.A., A.Q., L.C.R.-R., B.D.P., D.B.-S. and C.M.T.F.; writing—review and editing: A.M.T.A., A.Q., L.C.R.-R., B.D.P., D.B.-S. and C.M.T.F.; visualization: A.M.T.A., A.Q., L.C.R.-R., B.D.P., D.B.-S. and C.M.T.F.; supervision: A.M.T.A. and L.C.R.-R. All authors have read and agreed to the published version of the manuscript.

Funding: This research was funded by Roseman University of Health Sciences, College of Dental Medicine.

Institutional Review Board Statement: Not applicable.

Informed Consent Statement: Not applicable.

Data Availability Statement: Not applicable.

Conflicts of Interest: The authors declare no conflict of interest.

References

1. Basta, F.; Fasola, F.; Triantafyllias, K.; Schwarting, A. Systemic Lupus Erythematosus (SLE) Therapy: The Old and the New. *Rheumatol. Ther.* **2020**, *7*, 433–446. [CrossRef] [PubMed]
2. Velo-García, A.; Ntatsaki, E.; Isenberg, D. The Safety of Pharmacological Treatment Options for Lupus Nephritis. *Expert. Opin. Drug. Saf.* **2016**, *15*, 1041–1054. [CrossRef] [PubMed]
3. Gossec, L.; Molto, A.; Romand, X.; Puyraimond-Zemmour, D.; Lavielle, M.; Beauvais, C.; Senbel, E.; Flipo, R.M.; Pouplin, S.; Richez, C.; et al. Recommandations Pour l'évaluation et l'optimisation de l'adhésion Aux Traitements de Fond Médicamenteux Des Rhumatismes Inflammatoires Chroniques: Un Processus Basé Sur Des Revues de La Littérature et Un Consensus d'experts. *Rev. Du Rhum.* **2019**, *86*, 555–562. [CrossRef]
4. Costedoat-Chalumeau, N.; Pouchot, J.; Guettrot-Imbert, G.; le Guern, V.; Leroux, G.; Marra, D.; Morel, N.; Piette, J.-C. Adherence to Treatment in Systemic Lupus Erythematosus Patients. *Best. Pract. Res. Clin. Rheumatol.* **2013**, *27*, 329–340. [CrossRef] [PubMed]
5. Schwartzman, S.; Samson, C.M. Are the Current Recommendations for Chloroquine and Hydroxychloroquine Screening Appropriate? *Rheum. Dis. Clin. North Am.* **2019**, *45*, 359–367. [CrossRef] [PubMed]
6. Schrezenmeier, E.; Dörner, T. Mechanisms of Action of Hydroxychloroquine and Chloroquine: Implications for Rheumatology. *Nat. Rev. Rheumatol.* **2020**, *16*, 155–166. [CrossRef] [PubMed]
7. dos Reis Neto, E.T.; Kakehasi, A.M.; de Medeiros Pinheiro, M.; Ferreira, G.A.; Lopes Marques, C.D.; da Mota, L.M.H.; dos Santos Paiva, E.; Salviato Pileggi, G.C.; Sato, E.I.; Gomides Reis, A.P.M.; et al. Revisiting Hydroxychloroquine and Chloroquine for Patients with Chronic Immunity-Mediated Inflammatory Rheumatic Diseases. *Adv. Rheumatol.* **2020**, *60*, 32. [CrossRef]
8. Ponticelli, C.; Moroni, G. Hydroxychloroquine in Systemic Lupus Erythematosus (SLE). *Expert. Opin. Drug. Saf.* **2017**, *16*, 411–419. [CrossRef]
9. Nosál', R.; Jančinová, V.; Danihelová, E. Chloroquine: A Multipotent IInhibitor of Human Platelets in Vitro. *Thromb. Res.* **2000**, *98*, 411–421. [CrossRef]
10. Jancínová, V.; Nosál, R.; Petriková, M. On the Inhibitory Effect of Chloroquine on Blood Platelet Aggregation. *Thromb. Res.* **1994**, *74*, 495–504. [CrossRef]
11. Rand, J.H.; Wu, X.X.; Quinn, A.S.; Chen, P.P.; Hathcock, J.J.; Taatjes, D.J. Hydroxychloroquine Directly Reduces the Bindin of Antiphospholipid Antibody-B2-Glycoprotein I Complexes to Phospholipid Bilayers. *Blood* **2008**, *112*, 1687–1695. [CrossRef] [PubMed]
12. Yokogawa, N.; Eto, H.; Tanikawa, A.; Ikeda, T.; Yamamoto, K.; Takahashi, T.; Mizukami, T.; Sato, T.; Yokota, N.; Furukawa, F. Effects of Hydroxychloroquine in Patients with Cutaneous Lupus Erythematosus: A Multicenter, Double-Blind, Randomized, Parallel-Group Trial. *Arthritis Rheumatol.* **2017**, *69*, 791–799. [CrossRef] [PubMed]
13. Sharma, G.; Singh, J.A.; Khaleel, M.S.; Shrestha, S. Efficacy and Toxicity of Antimalarials in Systematic Lupus Erythematosus: A Systematic Review—ACR Meeting Abstracts. Available online: https://acrabstracts.org/abstract/efficacy-and-toxicity-of-antimalarials-in-systematic-lupus-erythematosus-a-systematic-review/ (accessed on 15 December 2020).
14. Shinjo, S.K.; Bonfá, E.; Wojdyla, D.; Borba, E.F.; Ramirez, L.A.; Scherbarth, H.R.; Brenol, J.C.T.; Chacón-Diaz, R.; Neira, O.J.; Berbotto, G.A.; et al. Antimalarial Treatment May Have a Time-Dependent Effect on Lupus Survival: Data from a Multinational Latin American Inception Cohort. *Arthritis. Rheum.* **2010**, *62*, 855–862. [CrossRef] [PubMed]
15. Aouhab, Z.; Hong, H.; Felicelli, C.; Tarplin, S.; Ostrowski, R.A. Outcomes of Systemic Lupus Erythematosus in Patients Who Discontinue Hydroxychloroquine. *ACR Open. Rheumatol.* **2019**, *1*, 593–599. [CrossRef]
16. Meinao, I.M.; Sato, E.I.; Andrade, L.E.C.; Ferraz, M.B.; Atra, E. Controlled Trial with Chloroquine Diphosphate in Systemic Lupus Erythematosus. *Lupus* **1996**, *5*, 237–241. [CrossRef]
17. Parikh, S.V.; Almaani, S.; Brodsky, S.; Rovin, B.H. Update on Lupus Nephritis: Core Curriculum 2020. *Am. J. Kidney Dis.* **2020**, *76*, 265–281. [CrossRef]
18. Shirley, E.; Chakravarty, E.F. Treatment of Systemic Lupus Erythematosus (SLE) in Pregnancy. *Curr. Treatm. Opt. Rheumatol.* **2018**, *4*, 110–118. [CrossRef]
19. Seo, M.R.; Chae, J.; Kim, Y.M.; Cha, H.S.; Choi, S.J.; Oh, S.; Roh, C.R. Hydroxychloroquine Treatment during Pregnancy in Lupus Patients Is Associated with Lower Risk of Preeclampsia. *Lupus* **2019**, *28*, 722–730. [CrossRef]
20. Izmirly, P.M.; Kim, M.Y.; Llanos, C.; Le, P.U.; Guerra, M.M.; Askanase, A.D.; Salmon, J.E.; Buyon, J.P. Evaluation of the Risk of Anti-SSA/Ro-SSB/La Antibody-Associated Cardiac Manifestations of Neonatal Lupus in Fetuses of Mothers with Systemic Lupus Erythosus Exposed to Hydroxychloroquine. *Ann. Rheum. Dis.* **2010**, *69*, 1827–1830. [CrossRef]
21. Kumar, D.M.; Kamath, L.; Reddy, N. Efficacy of Hydroxychloroquine as a Potential Antidiabetic Drug. *Int. J. Basic. Clin. Pharmacol.* **2017**, *6*, 895. [CrossRef]
22. Hage, M.P.; Al-Badri, M.R.; Azar, S.T. A Favorable Effect of Hydroxychloroquine on Glucose and Lipid Metabolism beyond Its Anti-Inflammatory Role. *Ther. Adv. Endocrinol. Metab.* **2014**, *5*, 77–85. [CrossRef] [PubMed]
23. Capell, H.A. Effect of Antimalarial Agents on Fasting Lipid Profile in Systemic Lupus Erythematosus. *J. Rheumatol.* **2001**, *28*, 1742. [PubMed]
24. Stapley, L. Bone Loss Prevention by an Antimalarial Drug. *Trends Endocrinol. Metab.* **2001**, *12*, 146. [CrossRef] [PubMed]
25. Ruiz-Irastorza, G.; Ugarte, A.; Egurbide, M.V.; Garmendia, M.; Pijoan, J.I.; Martinez-Berriotxoa, A.; Aguirre, C. Antimalarials May Influence the Risk of Malignancy in Systemic Lupus Erythematosus. *Ann. Rheum. Dis.* **2007**, *66*, 815–817. [CrossRef] [PubMed]

26. Abdel Galil, S.M. Hydroxychloroquine-Induced Toxic Hepatitis in a Patient with Systemic Lupus Erythematosus: A Case Report. *Lupus* **2015**, *24*, 638–640. [CrossRef]
27. Jimenez-Alonso, J.; Tercedor, J.; Jaimez, L.; Garcia-Lora, E. Antimalarial Drug-Induced Aquagenic-Type Pruritus in Patients with Lupus. *Arthritis. Rheum.* **1998**, *41*, 744–745. [CrossRef]
28. Marriott, P.; Borrie, P.F. Pigmentary Changes Following Chloroquine. *J. R. Soc. Med.* **1975**, *68*, 535–536. [CrossRef]
29. Jallouli, M.; Francès, C.; Piette, J.C.; Huong, D.L.T.; Moguelet, P.; Factor, C.; Zahr, N.; Miyara, M.; Saadoun, D.; Mathian, A.; et al. Hydroxychloroquine-Induced Pigmentation in Patients with Systemic Lupus Erythematosus a Case-Control Study. *JAMA Dermatol.* **2013**, *149*, 935–940. [CrossRef]
30. Bernstein, H.; Zvaifler, N.; Rubin, M.; Agnes Mary Mansour, A.M. The Ocular Deposition of Chloroquine. Available online: https://iovs.arvojournals.org/article.aspx?articleid=2160156 (accessed on 16 December 2020).
31. Garza-Leon, M.; Flores-Alvarado, D.E.; Muñoz-Bravo, J.M. Retinal Toxicity Induced by Antimalarial Drugs: Literature Review and Case Report. *Medwave* **2016**, *16*, e6471. [CrossRef]
32. Jorge, A.; Ung, C.; Young, L.H.; Melles, R.B.; Choi, H.K. Hydroxychloroquine Retinopathy—Implications of Research Advances for Rheumatology Care. *Nat. Rev. Rheumatol.* **2018**, *14*, 693–703. [CrossRef]
33. Costedoat-Chalumeau, N.; Dunogué, B.; Morel, N.; le Guern, V.; Guettrot-Imbert, G. Hydroxychloroquine: A Multifaceted Treatment in Lupus. *Presse. Med.* **2014**, *43*, e167–e180. [CrossRef] [PubMed]
34. Mubagwa, K. Cardiac Effects and Toxicity of Chloroquine: A Short Update. *Int. J. Antimicrob. Agents.* **2020**, *56*, 106057. [CrossRef] [PubMed]
35. Tselios, K.; Deeb, M.; Gladman, D.D.; Harvey, P.; Urowitz, M.B. Antimalarial-Induced Cardiomyopathy: A Systematic Review of the Literature. *Lupus* **2018**, *27*, 591–599. [CrossRef] [PubMed]
36. Hamm, B.S.; Rosenthal, L.J. Psychiatric Aspects of Chloroquine and Hydroxychloroquine Treatment in the Wake of Coronavirus Disease-2019: Psychopharmacological Interactions and Neuropsychiatric Sequelae. *Psychosomatics* **2020**, *61*, 597–606. [CrossRef]
37. Siddiqui, A.K.; Huberfeld, S.I.; Weidenheim, K.M.; Einberg, K.R.; Efferen, L.S. Hydroxychloroquine-Induced Toxic Myopathy Causing Respiratory Failure. *Chest* **2007**, *131*, 588–590. [CrossRef]
38. Khosa, S.; Khanlou, N.; Khosa, G.S.; Mishra, S.K. Hydroxychloroquine-Induced Autophagic Vacuolar Myopathy with Mitochondrial Abnormalities. *Neuropathology* **2018**, *38*, 646–652. [CrossRef]
39. Casado, E.; Graticós, J.; Tolosa, C.; Martínez, J.M.; Ojanguren, I.; Ariza, A.; Real, J.; Sanjuan, A.; Larrosa, M. Antimalarial Myopathy: An Underdiagnosed Complication? Prospective Longitudinal Study of 119 Patients. *Ann. Rheum. Dis.* **2006**, *65*, 385–390. [CrossRef] [PubMed]
40. Pillittere, J.; Mian, S.; Richardson, T.E.; Perl, A. Hydroxychloroquine-Induced Toxic Myopathy Causing Diaphragmatic Weakness and Lung Collapse Requiring Prolonged Mechanical Ventilation. *J. Investig. Med. High Impact. Case Rep.* **2020**, *8*, 1–5. [CrossRef]
41. Fiehn, C.; Ness, T.; Weseloh, C.; Specker, C.; Hadjiski, D.; Detert, J.; Krüger, K. Safety Management in Treatment with Antimalarials in Rheumatology. Interdisciplinary Recommendations on the Basis of a Systematic Literature Review. *Z. Rheumatol.* **2020**, *80*, 1–9. [CrossRef]
42. Rhen, T.; Cidlowski, J.A. Antiinflammatory Action of Glucocorticoids-New Mechanisms for Old Drugs. *N. Engl. J. Med.* **2005**, *353*, 1711–1723. [CrossRef]
43. Luijten, R.K.M.A.C.; Fritsch-Stork, R.D.; Bijlsma, J.W.J.; Derksen, R.H.W.M. The Use of Glucocorticoids in Systemic Lupus Erythematosus. After 60years Still More an Art than Science. *Autoimmun. Rev.* **2013**, *12*, 617–628. [CrossRef]
44. Chatham, W.W.; Kimberly, R.P. Treatment of Lupus with Corticosteroids. *Lupus* **2001**, *10*, 140–147. [CrossRef] [PubMed]
45. Ramamoorthy, S.; Cidlowski, J.A. Exploring the Molecular Mechanisms of Glucocorticoid Receptor Action from Sensitivity to Resistance. *Endocr. Dev.* **2013**, *24*, 41–56. [CrossRef] [PubMed]
46. Hafezi-Moghadam, A.; Simoncini, T.; Yang, Z.; Limbourg, F.P.; Plumier, J.C.; Rebsamen, M.C.; Hsieh, C.M.; Chui, D.S.; Thomas, K.L.; Prorock, A.J.; et al. Acute Cardiovascular Protective Effects of Corticosteroids Are Mediated by Non-Transcriptional Activation of Endothelial Nitric Oxide Synthase. *Nat. Med.* **2002**, *8*, 473–479. [CrossRef] [PubMed]
47. Burns, C.M. The History of Cortisone Discovery and Development. *Rheum. Dis. Clin. North Am.* **2016**, *42*, 1–14. [CrossRef]
48. Pasero, G.; Marson, P. Short History of Anti-Rheumatic Therapy. IV. Corticosteroids. *Reumatismo* **2011**, *62*, 292–299. [CrossRef]
49. Benedek, T.G. History of the Development of Corticosteroid Therapy. *Clin. Exp. Rheumatol.* **2011**, *29*, 5–12.
50. Compston, J. Glucocorticoid-Induced Osteoporosis: An Update. *Endocrine* **2018**, *61*, 7–16. [CrossRef]
51. Stojan, G.; Petri, M. The Risk Benefit Ratio of Glucocorticoids in SLE: Have Things Changed over the Past 40 Years? *Curr. Treatm. Opt. Rheumatol.* **2017**, *3*, 164–172. [CrossRef]
52. Biddie, S.C.; Conway-campbell, B.L.; Lightman, S.L. Dynamic Regulation of Glucocorticoid Signalling in Health and Disease. *Rheumatology* **2012**, *51*, 403–412. [CrossRef]
53. Surjit, M.; Ganti, K.P.; Mukherji, A.; Ye, T.; Hua, G.; Metzger, D.; Li, M.; Chambon, P. Widespread Negative Response Elements Mediate Direct Repression by Agonist-Liganded Glucocorticoid Receptor. *Cell* **2011**, *145*, 224–241. [CrossRef] [PubMed]
54. Buttgereit, F.; Saag, K.G.; Cutolo, M.; da Silva, J.A.P.; Bijlsma, J.W.J. The Molecular Basis for the Effectiveness, Toxicity, and Resistance to Glucocorticoids: Focus on the Treatment of Rheumatoid Arthritis. *Scand J. Rheumatol.* **2005**, *34*, 14–21. [CrossRef] [PubMed]
55. Strehl, C.; Ehlers, L.; Gaber, T.; Buttgereit, F. Glucocorticoids-All-Rounders Tackling the Versatile Players of the Immune System. *Front. Immunol.* **2019**, *10*, 1744. [CrossRef]

56. Kasturi, S.; Sammaritano, L.R. Corticosteroids in Lupus. *Rheum. Dis. Clin. North Am.* **2016**, *42*, 47–62. [CrossRef] [PubMed]
57. Liberman, A.C.; Budziński, M.L.; Sokn, C.; Gobbini, R.P.; Steininger, A.; Arzt, E. Regulatory and Mechanistic Actions of Glucocorticoids on T and Inflammatory Cells. *Front. Endocrinol.* **2018**, *9*, 1. [CrossRef]
58. Porta, S.; Danza, A.; Arias Saavedra, M.; Carlomagno, A.; Goizueta, M.C.; Vivero, F.; Ruiz-Irastorza, G. Glucocorticoids in Systemic Lupus Erythematosus. Ten Questions and Some Issues. *J. Clin. Med.* **2020**, *9*, 2709. [CrossRef]
59. Zhou, W.J.; Yang, C. de The Causes and Clinical Significance of Fever in Systemic Lupus Erythematosus: A Retrospective Study of 487 Hospitalised Patients. *Lupus* **2009**, *18*, 807–812. [CrossRef]
60. Liu, R.; Zhang, L.; Gao, S.; Chen, L.; Wang, L.; Zhu, Z.; Lu, W.; Zhu, H. Gastrointestinal Symptom Due to Lupus Peritonitis: A Rare Form of Onset of SLE. *Int. J. Clin. Exp. Med.* **2014**, *7*, 5917–5920.
61. Parker, B.J.; Bruce, I.N. High Dose Methylprednisolone Therapy for the Treatment of Severe Systemic Lupus Erythematosus. *Lupus* **2007**, *16*, 387–393. [CrossRef]
62. Amissah Arthur, M.B.; Gordon, C. Contemporary Treatment of Systemic Lupus Erythematosus: An Update for Clinicians. *Ther. Adv. Chronic. Dis.* **2010**, *1*, 163–175. [CrossRef]
63. Chan, T.M. Lupus Nephritis: Induction Therapy. *Lupus* **2005**, *14*, s27–s32. [CrossRef] [PubMed]
64. Barile-Fabris, L.; Ariza-Andraca, R.; Olguín-Ortega, L.; Jara, L.J.; Fraga-Mouret, A.; Miranda-Limón, J.M.; Fuentes De La Mata, J.; Clark, P.; Vargas, F.; Alcocer-Varela, J. Controlled Clinical Trial of IV Cyclophosphamide versus IV Methylprednisolone in Severe Neurological Manifestations in Systemic Lupus Erythematosus. *Ann. Rheum. Dis.* **2005**, *64*, 620–625. [CrossRef] [PubMed]
65. Afzal, W.; Arab, T.; Ullah, T.; Teller, K.; Doshi, K.J. Generalized Lymphadenopathy as Presenting Feature of Systemic Lupus Erythematosus: Case Report and Review of the Literature. *J. Clin. Med. Res.* **2016**, *8*, 819–823. [CrossRef] [PubMed]
66. Shapira, Y.; Weinberger, A.; Wysenbeek, A.J. Lymphadenopathy in Systemic Lupus Erythematosus. Prevalence and Relation to Disease Manifestations. *Clin. Rheumatol.* **1996**, *15*, 335–338. [CrossRef] [PubMed]
67. Tsang-A-Sjoe, M.W.P.; Bultink, I.E.M. Systemic Lupus Erythematosus: Review of Synthetic Drugs. *Expert. Opin. Pharmacother.* **2015**, *16*, 2793–2806. [CrossRef]
68. Ruiz-Irastorza, G.; Danza, A.; Perales, I.; Villar, I.; Garcia, M.; Delgado, S.; Khamashta, M. Prednisone in Lupus Nephritis: How Much Is Enough? *Autoimmun. Rev.* **2014**, *13*, 206–214. [CrossRef]
69. Ruiz-Arruza, I.; Barbosa, C.; Ugarte, A.; Ruiz-Irastorza, G. Comparison of High versus Low-Medium Prednisone Doses for the Treatment of Systemic Lupus Erythematosus Patients with High Activity at Diagnosis. *Autoimmun. Rev.* **2015**, *14*, 875–879. [CrossRef]
70. Fanouriakis, A.; Kostopoulou, M.; Alunno, A.; Aringer, M.; Bajema, I.; Boletis, J.N.; Cervera, R.; Doria, A.; Gordon, C.; Govoni, M.; et al. 2019 Update of the EULAR Recommendations for the Management of Systemic Lupus Erythematosus. *Ann. Rheum. Dis.* **2019**, *78*, 736–745. [CrossRef]
71. Zahr, Z.A.; Fang, H.; Magder, L.S.; Petri, M. Predictors of Corticosteroid Tapering in SLE Patients: The Hopkins Lupus Cohort. *Lupus* **2013**, *22*, 697–701. [CrossRef]
72. Vitellius, G.; Trabado, S.; Bouligand, J.; Delemer, B.; Lombès, M. Pathophysiology of Glucocorticoid Signaling. *Ann. Endocrinol.* **2018**, *79*, 98–106. [CrossRef]
73. Melo, A.; Melo, M.; Saramago, A.; Demartino, G.; Souza, B.; Longui, C. Persistent Glucocorticoid Resistance in Systemic Lupus Erythematosus Patients during Clinical Remission. *Genet. Mol. Res.* **2013**, *12*, 2010–2019. [CrossRef] [PubMed]
74. Wang, F.F.; Zhu, L.A.; Zou, Y.Q.; Zheng, H.; Wilson, A.; de Yang, C.; Shen, N.; Wallace, D.J.; Weisman, M.H.; Chen, S.-L.; et al. New Insights into the Role and Mechanism of Macrophage Migration Inhibitory Factor in Steroid-Resistant Patients with Systemic Lupus Erythematosus. *Arthritis. Res. Ther.* **2012**, *14*, R103. [CrossRef] [PubMed]
75. Nataraja, C.; Morand, E. Systemic Glucocorticoid Therapy for SLE. In *Dubois' Lupus Erythematosus and Related Syndromes*; Elsevier: Amsterdam, The Netherlands, 2018; pp. 661–672. ISBN 9780323479271.
76. Apostolopoulos, D.; Kandane-Rathnayake, R.; Raghunath, S.; Hoi, A.; Nikpour, M.; Morand, E.F. Independent Association of Glucocorticoids with Damage Accrual in SLE. *Lupus. Sci. Med.* **2016**, *3*, e000157. [CrossRef] [PubMed]
77. Ruiz-Arruza, I.; Ugarte, A.; Cabezas-Rodriguez, I.; Medina, J.A.; Moran, M.A.; Ruiz-Irastorza, G. Glucocorticoids and Irreversible Damage in Patients with Systemic Lupus Erythematosus. *Rheumatology* **2014**, *53*, 1470–1476. [CrossRef] [PubMed]
78. Zonana-Nacach, A.; Barr, S.G.; Magder, L.S.; Petri, M. Damage in Systemic Lupus Erythematosus and Its Association with Corticosteroids. *Arthritis. Rheum.* **2000**, *43*, 1801–1808. [CrossRef] [PubMed]
79. Liu, D.; Ahmet, A.; Ward, L.; Krishnamoorthy, P.; Mandelcorn, E.D.; Leigh, R.; Brown, J.P.; Cohen, A.; Kim, H. A Practical Guide to the Monitoring and Management of the Complications of Systemic Corticosteroid Therapy. *Allergy Asthma Clin. Immunol.* **2013**, *9*, 1–25. [CrossRef]
80. Weinstein, R.S.; Jilka, R.L.; Michael Parfitt, A.; Manolagas, S.C. Inhibition of Osteoblastogenesis and Promotion of Apoptosis of Osteoblasts End Osteocytes by Glucocorticoids Potential Mechanisms of Their Deleterious Effects on Bone. *J. Clin. Investig.* **1998**, *102*, 274–282. [CrossRef] [PubMed]
81. Mazziotti, G.; Angeli, A.; Bilezikian, J.P.; Canalis, E.; Giustina, A. Glucocorticoid-Induced Osteoporosis: An Update. *Trends Endocrinol. Metab.* **2006**, *17*, 144–149. [CrossRef]
82. van Staa, T.P.; Leufkens, H.G.M.; Abenhaim, L.; Zhang, B.; Cooper, C. Use of Oral Corticosteroids and Risk of Fractures. *J. Bone Miner. Res.* **2000**, *15*, 993–1000. [CrossRef]

83. Jagpal, A.; Saag, K.G. Glucocorticoid-Induced Osteoporosis: Update on Management. *Curr. Treatm. Opt. Rheumatol.* **2018**, *4*, 279–287. [CrossRef]
84. Mirzai, R.; Chang, C.; Greenspan, A.; Gershwin, M.E. The Pathogenesis of Osteonecrosis and the Relationships to Corticosteroids. *J. Asthma* **1999**, *36*, 77–95. [CrossRef] [PubMed]
85. Sayarlioglu, M.; Yuzbasioglu, N.; Inanc, M.; Kamali, S.; Cefle, A.; Karaman, O.; Onat, A.M.; Avan, R.; Cetin, G.Y.; Gul, A.; et al. Risk Factors for Avascular Bone Necrosis in Patients with Systemic Lupus Erythematosus. *Rheumatol. Int.* **2012**, *32*, 177–182. [CrossRef]
86. Lee, Y.J.; Cui, Q.; Koo, K.H. Is There a Role of Pharmacological Treatments in the Prevention or Treatment of Osteonecrosis of the Femoral Head?: A Systematic Review. *J. Bone Metab.* **2019**, *26*, 13–18. [CrossRef] [PubMed]
87. Gupta, Y.; Gupta, A. Glucocorticoid-Induced Myopathy: Pathophysiology, Diagnosis, and Treatment. *Indian J. Endocrinol. Metab.* **2013**, *17*, 913. [CrossRef]
88. Hardy, R.S.; Raza, K.; Cooper, M.S. Therapeutic Glucocorticoids: Mechanisms of Actions in Rheumatic Diseases. *Nat. Rev. Rheumatol.* **2020**, *16*, 133–144. [CrossRef] [PubMed]
89. Poetker, D.M.; Reh, D.D. A Comprehensive Review of the Adverse Effects of Systemic Corticosteroids. *Otolaryngol. Clin. North Am.* **2010**, *43*, 753–768. [CrossRef]
90. Silver, E.M.; Ochoa, W. Glucocorticoid-Induced Myopathy in a Patient with Systemic Lupus Erythematosus (SLE): A Case Report and Review of the Literature. *Am. J. Case Rep.* **2018**, *19*, 277–283. [CrossRef]
91. Nagpal, S.; Tierney, M. Corticosteroid-Induced Myopathy. *Can. J. Hosp. Pharm.* **1995**, *48*, 242–243. [CrossRef]
92. Allen, D.B.; Julius, J.R.; Breen, T.J.; Attie, K.M. Treatment of Glucocorticoid-Induced Growth Suppression with Growth Hormone. *J. Clin. Endocrinol. Metab.* **1998**, *83*, 2824–2829. [CrossRef]
93. Mushtaq, T.; Ahmed, S.F. The Impact of Corticosteroids on Growth and Bone Health. *Arch. Dis. Child.* **2002**, *87*, 93–96. [CrossRef]
94. Abdalla, E.; Jeyaseelan, L.; Ullah, I.; Abdwani, R. Growth Pattern in Children with Systemic Lupus Erythematosus. *Oman. Med. J.* **2017**, *32*, 284–290. [CrossRef] [PubMed]
95. Chung, C.P.; Oeser, A.; Solus, J.F.; Gebretsadik, T.; Shintani, A.; Avalos, I.; Sokka, T.; Raggi, P.; Pincus, T.; Stein, C.M. Inflammation-Associated Insulin Resistance: Differential Effects in Rheumatoid Arthritis and Systemic Lupus Erythematosus Define Potential Mechanisms. *Arthritis Rheum.* **2008**, *58*, 2105–2112. [CrossRef]
96. Angelopoulos, T.P.; Tentolouris, N.K.; Bertsias, G.K.; Boumpas, D.T. Steroid-Induced Diabetes in Rheumatologic Patients. *Clin. Exp. Rheumatol.* **2014**, *32*, 126–130. [PubMed]
97. Gurwitz, J.H. Glucocorticoids and the Risk for Initiation of Hypoglycemic Therapy. *Arch. Intern. Med.* **1994**, *154*, 97. [CrossRef] [PubMed]
98. Fardet, L. Effets Indésirables Métaboliques et Cardiovasculaires Des Corticothérapies Systémiques. *Rev. Med. Interne* **2013**, *34*, 303–309. [CrossRef]
99. Suh, S.; Park, M.K. Glucocorticoid-Induced Diabetes Mellitus: An Important but Overlooked Problem. *Endocrinol. Metab.* **2017**, *32*, 180–189. [CrossRef]
100. Rice, J.B.; White, A.G.; Scarpati, L.M.; Wan, G.; Nelson, W.W. Long-Term Systemic Corticosteroid Exposure: A Systematic Literature Review. *Clin. Ther.* **2017**, *39*, 2216–2229. [CrossRef] [PubMed]
101. Dimitriadis, G.; Leighton, B.; Parry-Billings, M.; Sasson, S.; Young, M.; Krause, U.; Bevan, S.; Piva, T.; Wegener, G.; Newsholme, E.A. Effects of Glucocorticoid Excess on the Sensitivity of Glucose Transport and Metabolism to Insulin in Rat Skeletal Muscle. *Biochem. J.* **1997**, *321*, 707–712. [CrossRef]
102. Tamez-Pérez, H.E. Steroid Hyperglycemia: Prevalence, Early Detection and Therapeutic Recommendations: A Narrative Review. *World J. Diabetes* **2015**, *6*, 1073. [CrossRef]
103. Tselios, K.; Koumaras, C.; Gladman, D.D.; Urowitz, M.B. Dyslipidemia in Systemic Lupus Erythematosus: Just Another Comorbidity? *Semin. Arthritis. Rheum.* **2016**, *45*, 604–610. [CrossRef]
104. Wijaya, L.K.; Kasjmir, Y.I.; Sukmana, N.; Subekti, I. The Proportion of Dyslipidemia in Systemic Lupus Erythematosus Patient and Distribution of Correlated Factors—PubMed. *Acta. Med. Indones.* **2005**, *37*, 132–144. [PubMed]
105. Sajjad, S.; Farman, S.; Saeed, M.A.; Ahmad, N.M.; Butt, B.A. Frequency of Dyslipidemia in Patients with Lupus Nephritis. *Pak. J. Med. Sci.* **2017**, *33*, 358–362. [CrossRef] [PubMed]
106. Joseph, R.M.; Hunter, A.L.; Ray, D.W.; Dixon, W.G. Systemic Glucocorticoid Therapy and Adrenal Insufficiency in Adults: A Systematic Review. *Semin. Arthritis Rheum.* **2016**, *46*, 133–141. [CrossRef] [PubMed]
107. Strohmayer, E.A.; Krakoff, L.R. Glucocorticoids and Cardiovascular Risk Factors. *Endocrinol. Metab. Clin. North Am.* **2011**, *40*, 409–417. [CrossRef]
108. Atik, N.; Hayati, R.U.; Hamijoyo, L. Correlation Between Steroid Therapy and Lipid Profile in Systemic Lupus Erythematosus Patients. *Open Access Rheumatol.* **2020**, *12*, 41–46. [CrossRef]
109. MacGregor, A.J.; Dhillon, V.B.; Binder, A.; Forte, C.A.; Knight, B.C.; Betteridge, D.J.; Isenberg, D.A. Fasting Lipids and Anticardiolipin Antibodies as Risk Factors for Vascular Disease in Systemic Lupus Erythematosus. *Ann. Rheum. Dis.* **1992**, *51*, 152–155. [CrossRef]
110. Fardet, L.; Cabane, J.; Lebbé, C.; Morel, P.; Flahault, A. Incidence and Risk Factors for Corticosteroid-Induced Lipodystrophy: A Prospective Study. *J. Am. Acad. Dermatol.* **2007**, *57*, 604–609. [CrossRef]

111. Manaboriboon, B.; Silverman, E.D.; Homsanit, M.; Chui, H.; Kaufman, M. Weight Change Associated with Corticosteroid Therapy in Adolescents with Systemic Lupus Erythematosus. *Lupus* **2013**, *22*, 164–170. [CrossRef]
112. Arnaldi, G.; Scandali, V.M.; Trementino, L.; Cardinaletti, M.; Appolloni, G.; Boscaro, M. Pathophysiology of Dyslipidemia in Cushing's Syndrome. *Neuroendocrinology* **2010**, *92*, 86–90. [CrossRef]
113. Mantero, F.; Boscaro, M. Glucocorticoid-Dependent Hypertension. *J. Steroid Biochem. Mol. Biol.* **1992**, *43*, 409–413. [CrossRef]
114. Mebrahtu, T.F.; Morgan, A.W.; West, R.M.; Stewart, P.M.; Pujades-Rodriguez, M. Oral Glucocorticoids and Incidence of Hypertension in People with Chronic Inflammatory Diseases: A Population-Based Cohort Study. *CMAJ* **2020**, *192*, E295–E301. [CrossRef] [PubMed]
115. Ong, S.L.H.; Zhang, Y.; Whitworth, J.A. Reactive Oxygen Species and Glucocorticoid-Induced Hypertension. In Proceedings of the Clinical and Experimental Pharmacology and Physiology. *Clin. Exp. Pharmacol. Physiol.* **2008**, *35*, 477–482. [CrossRef] [PubMed]
116. Goodwin, J.E.; Geller, D.S. Glucocorticoid-Induced Hypertension. *Pediatr. Nephrol.* **2012**, *27*, 1059–1066. [CrossRef]
117. Magder, L.S.; Petri, M. Incidence of and Risk Factors for Adverse Cardiovascular Events among Patients with Systemic Lupus Erythematosus. *Am. J. Epidemiol.* **2012**, *176*, 708–719. [CrossRef] [PubMed]
118. Souverein, P.C.; Berard, A.; van Staa, T.P.; Cooper, C.; Egberts, A.C.G.; Leufkens, H.G.M.; Walker, B.R. Use of Oral Glucocorticoids and Risk of Cardiovascular and Cerebrovascular Disease in a Population Based Case-Control Study. *Heart* **2004**, *90*, 859–865. [CrossRef]
119. Hattori, T.; Murase, T.; Iwase, E.; Takahashi, K.; Ohtake, M.; Tsuboi, K.; Ohtake, M.; Miyachi, M.; Murohara, T.; Nagata, K. Glucocorticoid-Induced Hypertension and Cardiac Injury: Effects of Mineralocorticoid and Glucocorticoid Receptor Antagonism. *Nagoya J. Med. Sci.* **2013**, *75*, 81–92. [CrossRef] [PubMed]
120. Younes, A.K.; Younes, N.K. Recovery of Steroid Induced Adrenal Insufficiency. *Transl. Pediatr.* **2017**, *6*, 269–273. [CrossRef]
121. Borresen, S.W.; Klose, M.; Baslund, B.; Rasmussen, Å.K.; Hilsted, L.; Friis-Hansen, L.; Locht, H.; Hansen, A.; Hetland, M.L.; Lydolph, M.C.; et al. Adrenal Insufficiency Is Seen in More than One-Third of Patients during Ongoing Low-Dose Prednisolone Treatment for Rheumatoid Arthritis. *Eur. J. Endocrinol.* **2017**, *177*, 287–295. [CrossRef]
122. Guerrero Pérez, F.; Marengo, A.P.; Villabona Artero, C. The Unresolved Riddle of Glucocorticoid Withdrawal. *J. Endocrinol. Investig.* **2017**, *40*, 1175–1181. [CrossRef]
123. Karangizi, A.H.K.; Al-Shaghana, M.; Logan, S.; Criseno, S.; Webster, R.; Boelaert, K.; Hewins, P.; Harper, L. Glucocorticoid Induced Adrenal Insufficiency Is Common in Steroid Treated Glomerular Diseases—Proposed Strategy for Screening and Management. *BMC Nephrol.* **2019**, *20*, 154. [CrossRef]
124. Bhangle, S.D.; Kramer, N.; Rosenstein, E.D. Corticosteroid-Induced Neuropsychiatric Disorders: Review and Contrast with Neuropsychiatric Lupus. *Rheumatol. Int.* **2013**, *33*, 1923–1932. [CrossRef] [PubMed]
125. Lewis, D.A.; Smith, R.E. Steroid-Induced Psychiatric Syndromes. A Report of 14 Cases and a Review of the Literature. *J. Affect. Disord.* **1983**, *5*, 319–332. [CrossRef] [PubMed]
126. Bostwick, J.M.; Warrington, T.P. *Psychiatric Adverse Effects of Corticosteroids*; Elsevier: Amsterdam, The Netherlands, 2006; Volume 81.
127. Moore, E.; Huang, M.W.; Putterman, C. Advances in the Diagnosis, Pathogenesis and Treatment of Neuropsychiatric Systemic Lupus Erythematosus. *Curr. Opin. Rheumatol.* **2020**, *32*, 152–158. [CrossRef] [PubMed]
128. Fel, A.; Aslangul, E.; le Jeunne, C. Indications et Complications Des Corticoïdes En Ophtalmologie. *Presse Med.* **2012**, *41*, 414–421. [CrossRef]
129. Sundmark, E. The Occurrence of Posterior Subcapsular Cataracts in Patients on Long-Term Systemic Cortcisteroid Therapy. *Acta Ophthalmol.* **2009**, *41*, 515–523. [CrossRef]
130. Cunningham, J.; Alfred, P.R.; Irvine, A.R. Central Serous Chorioretinopathy in Patients with Systemic Lupus Erythematosus. *Ophthalmology* **1996**, *103*, 2081–2090. [CrossRef]
131. Haimovici, R.; Koh, S.; Gagnon, D.R.; Lehrfeld, T.; Wellik, S. Risk Factors for Central Serous Chorioretinopathy: A Case-Control Study. *Ophthalmology* **2004**, *111*, 244–249. [CrossRef]
132. Øtensen, M.; Khamashta, M.; Lockshin, M.; Parke, A.; Brucato, A.; Carp, H.; Doria, A.; Rai, R.; Meroni, P.; Cetin, I.; et al. Anti-Inflammatory and Immunosuppressive Drugs and Reproduction. *Arthritis. Res. Ther.* **2006**, *8*, 209. [CrossRef]
133. Lateef, A.; Petri, M. Management of Pregnancy in Systemic Lupus Erythematosus. *Nat. Rev. Rheumatol.* **2012**, *8*, 710–718. [CrossRef]
134. Hoes, J.N.; Jacobs, J.W.G.; Boers, M.; Boumpas, D.; Buttgereit, F.; Caeyers, N.; Choy, E.H.; Cutolo, M.; da Silva, J.A.P.; Esselens, G.; et al. EULAR Evidence-Based Recommendations on the Management of Systemic Glucocorticoid Therapy in Rheumatic Diseases. *Ann. Rheum. Dis.* **2007**, *66*, 1560–1567. [CrossRef]
135. Litvin, I.; Dvorkina, O.; Ginzler, E.M. Immunosuppressive Drug Therapy. In *Dubois' Lupus Erythematosus and Related Syndromes.*; Elsevier: Amsterdam, The Netherlands, 2018; pp. 673–688. ISBN 9780323479271.
136. Veal, G.J.; Cole, M.; Chinnaswamy, G.; Sludden, J.; Jamieson, D.; Errington, J.; Malik, G.; Hill, C.R.; Chamberlain, T.; Boddy, A.V. Cyclophosphamide Pharmacokinetics and Pharmacogenetics in Children with B-Cell Non-Hodgkin's Lymphoma. *Eur. J. Cancer* **2016**, *55*, 56–64. [CrossRef] [PubMed]
137. Houssiau, F. Thirty Years of Cyclophosphamide: Assessing the Evidence. *Lupus* **2007**, *16*, 212–216. [CrossRef] [PubMed]

138. Helsby, N.A.; Yong, M.; van Kan, M.; de Zoysa, J.R.; Burns, K. E The Importance of Both CYP2C19 and CYP2B6 Germline Variations in Cyclophosphamide Pharmacokinetics and Clinical Outcomes. *Br. J. Clin. Pharmacol.* **2019**, *85*, 1925–1934. [CrossRef] [PubMed]
139. Moroni, G.; Ponticelli, C. Synthetic Pharmacotherapy for Lupus Nephritis. *Expert. Opin. Pharmacother.* **2017**, *18*, 175–186. [CrossRef] [PubMed]
140. Yap, D.Y.H.; Chan, T.M. B Cell Abnormalities in Systemic Lupus Erythematosus and Lupus Nephritis—Role in Pathogenesis and Effect of Immunosuppressive Treatments. *Int. J. Mol. Sci.* **2019**, *20*, 6231. [CrossRef]
141. Fanouriakis, A.; Pamfil, C.; Sidiropoulos, P.; Damian, L.; Flestea, A.; Gusetu, G.; Rednic, S.; Bertsias, G.; Boumpas, D.T. Cyclophosphamide in Combination with Glucocorticoids for Severe Neuropsychiatric Systemic Lupus Erythematosus: A Retrospective, Observational Two-Centre Study. *Lupus* **2016**, *25*, 627–636. [CrossRef]
142. Fernandes Moça Trevisani, V.; Castro, A.A.; Ferreira Neves Neto, J.; Atallah, Á.N. Cyclophosphamide versus Methylprednisolone for Treating Neuropsychiatric Involvement in Systemic Lupus Erythematosus. *Cochrane Database Syst. Rev.* **2013**, *2013*. [CrossRef]
143. Carmier, D.; Diot, E.; Diot, P. Shrinking Lung Syndrome: Recognition, Pathophysiology and Therapeutic Strategy. *Expert. Rev. Respir. Med.* **2011**, *5*, 33–39. [CrossRef]
144. Anders, H.J.; Saxena, R.; Zhao, M.H.; Parodis, I.; Salmon, J.E.; Mohan, C. Lupus Nephritis. *Nat. Rev. Dis. Primers* **2020**, *6*, 1–25. [CrossRef]
145. Houssiau, F.A.; Vasconcelos, C.; D'Cruz, D.; Sebastiani, G.D.; de Ramon Garrido, E.; Danieli, M.G.; Abramovicz, D.; Blockmans, D.; Mathieu, A.; Direskeneli, H.; et al. Immunosuppressive Therapy in Lupus Nephritis: The Euro-Lupus Nephritis Trial, a Randomized Trial of Low-Dose versus High-Dose Intravenous Cyclophosphamide. *Arthritis Rheum.* **2002**, *46*, 2121–2131. [CrossRef]
146. Dooley, M.A.; Hogan, S.; Jennette, C.; Falk, R. Cyclophosphamide Therapy for Lupus Nephritis: Poor Renal Survival in Black Americans. *Kidney. Int.* **1997**, *51*, 1188–1195. [CrossRef] [PubMed]
147. Ognenovski, V.M.; Marder, W.; Somers, E.C.; Johnston, C.M.; Farrehi, J.G.; Selvaggi, S.M.; McCune, W.J. Increased Incidence of Cervical Intraepithelial Neoplasia in Women with Systemic Lupus Erythematosus Treated with Intravenous Cyclophosphamide. *J. Rheumatol.* **2004**, *31*, 1763–1767. [PubMed]
148. Wang, C.L.; Wang, F.; Bosco, J.J. Ovarian Failure in Oral Cyclophosphamide Treatment for Systemic Lupus Erythematosus. *Lupus* **1995**, *4*, 11–14. [CrossRef] [PubMed]
149. Somers, E.C.; Marder, W.; Christman, G.M.; Ognenovski, V.; McCune, W.J. Use of a Gonadotropin-Releasing Hormone Analog for Protection against Premature Ovarian Failure during Cyclophosphamide Therapy in Women with Severe Lupus. *Arthritis Rheum.* **2005**, *52*, 2761–2767. [CrossRef]
150. Masala, A.; Faedda, R.; Alagna, S.; Satta, A.; Chiarelli, G.; Rovasio, P.P.; Ivaldi, R.; Taras, M.S.; Lai, E.; Bartoli, E. Use of Testosterone to Prevent Cyclophosphamide-Induced Azoospermia. *Ann. Intern. Med.* **1997**, *126*, 292–295. [CrossRef]
151. Wetzels, J.F.M. Cyclophosphamide-Induced Gonadal Toxicity: A Treatment Dilemma in Patients with Lupus Nephritis? *Neth. J. Med.* **2004**, *62*, 347–352.
152. Moghe, A.; Ghare, S.; Lamoreau, B.; Mohammad, M.; Barve, S.; McClain, C.; Joshi-Barve, S. Molecular Mechanisms of Acrolein Toxicity: Relevance to Human Disease. *Toxicological. Sci.* **2015**, *143*, 242–255. [CrossRef]
153. Korkmaz, A.; Topal, T.; Oter, S. Pathophysiological Aspects of Cyclophosphamide and Ifosfamide Induced Hemorrhagic Cystitis; Implication of Reactive Oxygen and Nitrogen Species as Well as PARP Activation. *Cell Biol. Toxicol.* **2007**, *23*, 303–312. [CrossRef]
154. Yilmaz, N.; Emmungil, H.; Gucenmez, S.; Ozen, G.; Yildiz, F.; Balkarli, A.; Kimyon, G.; Coskun, B.N.; Dogan, I.; Pamuk, O.N.; et al. Incidence of Cyclophosphamide-Induced Urotoxicity and Protective Effect of Mesna in Rheumatic Diseases. *J. Rheumatol.* **2015**, *42*, 1661–1666. [CrossRef]
155. Fu, D.; Ye, S.; Xiao, C.; Xie, Y.; Gao, J.; Liang, L.; Yang, X. Original Article Incidence of Cyclophosphamide-Induced Hemorrhagic Cystitis in Chinese Han Population with Autoimmune Disease. *Int. J. Clin. Exp. Med.* **2016**, *9*, 13160–13165.
156. Yates, M.; Watts, R.A.; Bajema, I.M.; Cid, M.C.; Crestani, B.; Hauser, T.; Hellmich, B.; Holle, J.U.; Laudien, M.; Little, M.A.; et al. EULAR/ERA-EDTA Recommendations for the Management of ANCA-Associated Vasculitis. *Ann. Rheum. Dis.* **2016**, *75*, 1583–1594. [CrossRef] [PubMed]
157. Santiago, M.G.; Ferreira, J.F.; Loio, M.; Santiago, T.; Serra, S.; Salvador, M.J.; Malcata, A.; da Silva, J.A.P. Bacterial Peritonitis: The Presentation of a Cyclophosphamide-Associated Bladder Carcinoma in a Long-Standing Systemic Lupus Erythematosus Patient. *Eur. J. Intern. Med.* **2013**, *24*, e136. [CrossRef]
158. Subramanian, R.; Pathak, H.; Ravindran, V. Safety of Cyclophosphamide Therapy in Autoimmune Rheumatic Diseases. *Indian J. Rheumatol.* **2019**, *14*, 127. [CrossRef]
159. Tran, A.; Bournerias, F.; le Beller, C.; Mir, O.; Rey, E.; Pons, G.; Delahousse, M.; Tréluyer, J.M. Serious Haematological Toxicity of Cyclophosphamide in Relation to CYP2B6, GSTA1 and GSTP1 Polymorphisms. *Br. J. Clin. Pharmacol.* **2008**, *65*, 279–280. [CrossRef] [PubMed]
160. Woytala, P.J.; Morgiel, E.; Luczak, A.; Czesak-Woytala, K.; Wiland, P. The Safety of Intravenous Cyclophosphamide in the Treatment of Rheumatic Diseases. *Adv. Clin. Exp. Med.* **2016**, *25*, 479–484. [CrossRef] [PubMed]
161. Pryor, B.D.; Bologna, S.G.; Kahl, L.E. Risk Factors for Serious Infection during Treatment with Cyclophosphamide and High-Dose Corticosteroids for Systemic Lupus Erythematosus. *Arthritis Rheum.* **1996**, *39*, 1475–1482. [CrossRef]

162. Pugh, D.; Farrah, T.E.; Gallacher, P.J.; Kluth, D.C.; Dhaun, N. Cyclophosphamide-Induced Lung Injury. *Kidney Int. Rep.* 2019, *4*, 484–486. [CrossRef]
163. Yang, X.; Li, X.; Yuan, M.; Tian, C.; Yang, Y.; Wang, X.; Zhang, X.; Sun, Y.; He, T.; Han, S.; et al. Anticancer Therapy-Induced Atrial Fibrillation: Electrophysiology and Related Mechanisms. *Front. Pharmacol.* 2018, *9*, 1058. [CrossRef]
164. Clowse, M.E.B.; Magder, L.; Petri, M. Cyclophosphamide for Lupus during Pregnancy. *Lupus* 2005, *14*, 593–597. [CrossRef]
165. Food and Drug Administration Cyclophosphamide for Injection; USP Cyclophosphamide Tablets, USP. Package Insert and Prescribing Information. Available online: https://www.accessdata.fda.gov/drugsatfda_docs/label/2012/012142s109lbl.pdf (accessed on 20 December 2022).
166. Ogino, M.; Tadi, P. NCBI Bookshelf: Cyclophosphamide. Available online: https://www.ncbi.nlm.nih.gov/books/NBK553087/ (accessed on 20 December 2022).
167. Fraiser, L.H.; Kanekal, S.; Kehrer, J.P. Cyclophosphamide Toxicity: Characterising and Avoiding the Problem. *Drugs* 1991, *42*, 781–795. [CrossRef]
168. Maltzman, J.S.; Koretzky, G.A. Azathioprine: Old Drug, New Actions. *J. Clin. Investig.* 2003, *111*, 1122–1124. [CrossRef] [PubMed]
169. Elion, G.B. The Purine Path to Chemotherapy. *Science* 1989, *244*, 41–47. [CrossRef]
170. Croyle, L.; Hoi, A.; Morand, E.F. Characteristics of Azathioprine Use and Cessation in a Longitudinal Lupus Cohort. *Lupus Sci. Med.* 2015, *2*, 1–6. [CrossRef] [PubMed]
171. Abu-Shakra, M.; Shoenfeld, Y. Azathioprine Therapy for Patients with Systemic Lupus Erythematosus. *Lupus* 2001, *10*, 152–153. [CrossRef] [PubMed]
172. Aarbakke, J.; Janka-Schaub, G.; Elion, G.B. Thiopurine Biology and Pharmacology. In Proceedings of the Trends in Pharmacological Sciences. *Trends Pharmacol. Sci.* 1997, *18*, 3–7. [CrossRef] [PubMed]
173. Broen, J.C.A.; Laar, J.M. Mycophenolate Mofetil, Azathioprine and Tacrolimus: Mechanisms in Rheumatology. *Nat. Rev. Rheumatol.* 2020, *16*, 167–178. [CrossRef]
174. Tiede, I.; Fritz, G.; Strand, S.; Poppe, D.; Dvorsky, R.; Strand, D.; Lehr, H.A.; Wirtz, S.; Becker, C.; Atreya, R.; et al. CD28-Dependent Rac1 Activation Is the Molecular Target of Azathioprine in Primary Human CD4+ T Lymphocytes. *J. Clin. Investig.* 2003, *111*, 1133–1145. [CrossRef]
175. Moeslinger, T.; Friedl, R.; Spieckermann, P.G. Inhibition of Inducible Nitric Oxide Synthesis by Azathioprine in a Macrophage Cell Line. *Life Sci.* 2006, *79*, 374–381. [CrossRef]
176. Houssiau, F.A.; D'Cruz, D.; Sangle, S.; Remy, P.; Vasconcelos, C.; Petrovic, R.; Fiehn, C.; Garrido, E.D.R.; Gilboe, I.M.; Tektonidou, M.; et al. Azathioprine versus Mycophenolate Mofetil for Long-Term Immunosuppression in Lupus Nephritis: Results from the MAINTAIN Nephritis Trial. *Ann. Rheum. Dis.* 2010, *69*, 2083–2089. [CrossRef]
177. Man, B.L.; Mok, C.C.; Fu, Y.P. Neuro-Ophthalmologic Manifestations of Systemic Lupus Erythematosus: A Systematic Review. *Int. J. Rheum. Dis.* 2014, *17*, 494–501. [CrossRef]
178. O'connor, A.; Qasim, A.; O'morain, C.A. The Long-Term Risk of Continuous Immunosuppression Using Thioguanides in Inflammatory Bowel Disease. *Ther. Adv. Chronic. Dis.* 2010, *1*, 7–16. [CrossRef] [PubMed]
179. Magro-Checa, C.; Zirkzee, E.J.; Huizinga, T.W.; Steup-Beekman, G.M. Management of Neuropsychiatric Systemic Lupus Erythematosus: Current Approaches and Future Perspectives. *Drugs* 2016, *76*, 459–483. [CrossRef] [PubMed]
180. Simms, R.W.; Kwoh, C.K.; Anderson, L.G.; Erlandson, D.M.; Greene, J.M.; Kelleher, M.; O'Dell, J.R.; Partridge, A.J.; Roberts, W.N.; Robbins, M.L.; et al. Guidelines for Monitoring Drug Therapy in Rheumatoid Arthritis. *Arthritis Rheum.* 1996, *39*, 723–731. [CrossRef]
181. Jordan, A.; Gresser, U. Side Effects and Interactions of the Xanthine Oxidase Inhibitor Febuxostat. *Pharmaceuticals* 2018, *11*, 51. [CrossRef] [PubMed]
182. Feldman, C.H.; Marty, F.M.; Winkelmayer, W.C.; Guan, H.; Franklin, J.M.; Solomon, D.H.; Costenbader, K.H.; Kim, S.C. Comparative Rates of Serious Infections Among Patients with Systemic Lupus Erythematosus Receiving Immunosuppressive Medications. *Arthritis Rheumatol.* 2017, *69*, 387–397. [CrossRef]
183. Singh, J.A.; Hossain, A.; Kotb, A.; Wells, G. Risk of Serious Infections with Immunosuppressive Drugs and Glucocorticoids for Lupus Nephritis: A Systematic Review and Network Meta-Analysis. *BMC Med.* 2016, *14*, 137. [CrossRef]
184. Rahier, J.F.; Magro, F.; Abreu, C.; Armuzzi, A.; Ben-Horin, S.; Chowers, Y.; Cottone, M.; de Ridder, L.; Doherty, G.; Ehehalt, R.; et al. Second European Evidence-Based Consensus on the Prevention, Diagnosis and Management of Opportunistic Infections in Inflammatory Bowel Disease. *J. Crohns. Colitis* 2014, *8*, 443–468. [CrossRef]
185. Wilson, A.; Jansen, L.E.; Rose, R.V.; Gregor, J.C.; Ponich, T.; Chande, N.; Khanna, R.; Yan, B.; Jairath, V.; Khanna, N.; et al. HLA-DQA1-HLA-DRB1 Polymorphism Is a Major Predictor of Azathioprine-Induced Pancreatitis in Patients with Inflammatory Bowel Disease. *Aliment. Pharmacol. Ther.* 2018, *47*, 615–620. [CrossRef]
186. Teich, N.; Mohl, W.; Bokemeyer, B.; Bündgens, B.; Büning, J.; Miehlke, S.; Hüppe, D.; Maaser, C.; Klugmann, T.; Kruis, W.; et al. Azathioprine-Induced Acute Pancreatitis in Patients with Inflammatory Bowel Diseases-a Prospective Study on Incidence and Severity. *J. Crohns. Colitis* 2016, *10*, 61–68. [CrossRef]
187. Horning, K.; Schmidt, C. Azathioprine-Induced Rapid Hepatotoxicity. *J. Pharm. Technol.* 2014, *30*, 18–20. [CrossRef]
188. Kraaij, T.; Bredewold, O.W.; Trompet, S.; Huizinga, T.W.J.; Rabelink, T.J.; de Craen, A.J.M.; Teng, Y.K.O. TAC-TIC Use of Tacrolimus-Based Regimens in Lupus Nephritis. *Lupus Sci. Med.* 2016, *3*, e000169. [CrossRef] [PubMed]

189. Alstead, E.M.; Ritchie, J.K.; Lennard-Jones, J.E.; Farthing, M.J.G.; Clark, M.L. Safety of Azathioprine in Pregnancy in Inflammatory Bowel Disease. *Gastroenterology* **1990**, *99*, 443–446. [CrossRef] [PubMed]
190. Cleary, B.J.; Källén, B. Early Pregnancy Azathioprine Use and Pregnancy Outcomes. *Birth. Defects Res. A Clin. Mol. Teratol.* **2009**, *85*, 647–654. [CrossRef] [PubMed]
191. Bitencourt, N.; Bermas, B.L. Pharmacological Approach to Managing Childhood-Onset Systemic Lupus Erythematosus During Conception, Pregnancy and Breastfeeding. *Pediatric. Drugs.* **2018**, *20*, 511–521. [CrossRef] [PubMed]
192. Cooper, W.C.; Cheetham, T.C.; Stein, C.M.; Callahan, S.T.; Morgan, T.M.; Shintani, A.K.; Chen, N.; Griffin, M.R.; Ray, W.A. Adverse Fetal Outcomes Associated with Immunosuppressive Medications for Chronic Immune Mediated Diseases in Pregnancy. *Arthritis Rheumatol.* **2014**, *66*, 444–450. [CrossRef]
193. van Scoik, K.G.; Johnson, C.A.; Porter, W.R. The Pharmacology and Metabolism of the Thiopurine Drugs 6-Mercaptopurine and Azathioprine. *Drug. Metab. Rev.* **1985**, *16*, 157–174. [CrossRef]
194. Weiner, S.M.; Bergner, R. Dosierung Und Toxizität von Antirheumatika Bei Niereninsuffizienz. *Z. Rheumatol.* **2015**, *74*, 300–309. [CrossRef]
195. Weiner, S.M. Treatment of Rheumatic Disease with Renal Insufficiency. *Orthopade* **2019**, *48*, 927–935. [CrossRef]
196. Gaffney, K.; Scott, D.G. Azathioprine and Cyclophosphamide in the Treatment of Rheumatoid Arthritis. *Rheumatology* **1998**, *37*, 824–836. [CrossRef]
197. Felten, R.; Scher, F.; Sibilia, J.; Ois Chasset, F.; Arnaud, L. Advances in the Treatment of Systemic Lupus Erythematosus: From Back to the Future, to the Future and Beyond. *Joint Bone Spine* **2019**, *86*, 429–436. [CrossRef]
198. Dall'Era, M. Mycophenolate Mofetil in the Treatment of Systemic Lupus Erythematosus. *Curr. Opin. Rheumatol.* **2011**, *23*, 454–458. [CrossRef] [PubMed]
199. Cattaneo, D.; Cortinovis, M.; Baldelli, S.; Bitto, A.; Gotti, E.; Remuzzi, G.; Perico, N. Pharmacokinetics of Mycophenolate Sodium and Comparison with the Mofetil Formulation in Stable Kidney Transplant Recipients. *Clin. J. Am. Soc. Nephrol.* **2007**, *2*, 1147–1155. [CrossRef] [PubMed]
200. Olech, E.; Merrill, J.T. Mycophenolate Mofetil for Lupus Nephritis. *Expert. Rev. Clin. Immunol.* **2008**, *4*, 313–319. [CrossRef] [PubMed]
201. Appel, G.B.; Contreras, G.; Dooley, M.A.; Ginzler, E.M.; Isenberg, D.; Jayne, D.; Li, L.S.; Mysler, E.; Sánchez-Guerrero, J.; Solomons, N.; et al. Mycophenolate Mofetil versus Cyclophosphamide for Induction Treatment of Lupus Nephritis. *J. Am. Soc. Nephrol.* **2009**, *20*, 1103–1112. [CrossRef]
202. Rathi, M.; Goyal, A.; Jaryal, A.; Sharma, A.; Gupta, P.K.; Ramachandran, R.; Kumar, V.; Kohli, H.S.; Sakhuja, V.; Jha, V.; et al. Comparison of Low-Dose Intravenous Cyclophosphamide with Oral Mycophenolate Mofetil in the Treatment of Lupus Nephritis. *Kidney Int.* **2016**, *89*, 235–242. [CrossRef]
203. Deng, J.; Xie, H.; Zhu, L.; Luo, L.; Xie, H. Maintenance Therapy for Lupus Nephritis with Mycophenolate Mofetil or Azathioprine. A Meta-Analysis. *Clin. Nephrol.* **2019**, *91*, 172–179. [CrossRef]
204. Soares, P.M.F.; Borba, E.F.; Bonfa, E.; Hallak, J.; Corrêa, A.L.; Silva, C.A.A. Gonad Evaluation in Male Systemic Lupus Erythematosus. *Arthritis Rheum.* **2007**, *56*, 2352–2361. [CrossRef]
205. Dall'Era, M.; Solomons, N.; Federico, R.; Truman, M. Comparison of Standard of Care Treatment with a Low Steroid and Mycophenolate Mofetil Regimen for Lupus Nephritis in the ALMS and AURA Studies. *Lupus* **2019**, *28*, 591–596. [CrossRef]
206. Dooley, M.A.; Jayne, D.; Ginzler, E.M.; Isenberg, D.; Olsen, N.J.; Wofsy, D.; Eitner, F.; Appel, G.B.; Contreras, G.; Lisk, L.; et al. Mycophenolate versus Azathioprine as Maintenance Therapy for Lupus Nephritis. *N. Engl. J. Med.* **2011**, *365*, 1886–1895. [CrossRef]
207. Tamirou, F.; D'Cruz, D.; Sangle, S.; Remy, P.; Vasconcelos, C.; Fiehn, C.; del Mar Ayala Guttierez, M.; Gilboe, I.M.; Tektonidou, M.; Blockmans, D.; et al. Long-Term Follow-up of the MAINTAIN Nephritis Trial, Comparing Azathioprine and Mycophenolate Mofetil as Maintenance Therapy of Lupus Nephritis. *Ann. Rheum. Dis.* **2016**, *75*, 526–531. [CrossRef]
208. Lourdudoss, C.; van Vollenhoven, R. Mycophenolate Mofetil in the Treatment of SLE and Systemic Vasculitis: Experience at a Single University Center. *Lupus* **2014**, *23*, 299–304. [CrossRef] [PubMed]
209. Mok, C.C. Mycophenolate Mofetil for Non-renal Manifestations of Systemic Lupus Erythematosus: A Systematic Review. *Scand. J. Rheumatol.* **2007**, *36*, 329–337. [CrossRef] [PubMed]
210. Fong, K.Y. Mycophenolate Mofetil in the Treatment of Non-Renal Manifestations of Systemic Lupus Erythematosus: A Review. *APLAR J. Rheumatol.* **2006**, *9*, 408–412. [CrossRef]
211. Henderson, L.K.; Masson, P.; Craig, J.C.; Roberts, M.A.; Flanc, R.S.; Strippoli, G.F.M.; Webster, A.C. Induction and Maintenance Treatment of Proliferative Lupus Nephritis: A Meta-Analysis of Randomized Controlled Trials. *Am. J. Kidney Dis.* **2013**, *61*, 74–87. [CrossRef] [PubMed]
212. Mok, C.C. Mycophenolate Mofetil for Lupus Nephritis: An Update. *Expert. Rev. Clin. Immunol.* **2015**, *11*, 1353–1364. [CrossRef] [PubMed]
213. Pavlovic, A.M.; Bonaci-Nikolic, B.; Kozic, D.; Ostojic, J.; Abinun, M.; Svabic-Medjedovic, T.; Nikolic, M.; Sternic, N. Progressive Multifocal Leukoencephalopathy Associated with Mycophenolate Mofetil Treatment in a Woman with Lupus and CD4+ T-Lymphocyte Deficiency. *Lupus* **2012**, *21*, 100–102. [CrossRef]

214. Le, H.L.; Francke, M.I.; Andrews, L.M.; de Winter, B.C.M.; van Gelder, T.; Hesselink, D.A. Usage of Tacrolimus and Mycophenolic Acid During Conception, Pregnancy, and Lactation, and Its Implications for Therapeutic Drug Monitoring: A Systematic Critical Review. *Ther. Drug. Monit.* **2020**, *42*, 518–531. [CrossRef]
215. Skorpen, C.G.; Hoeltzenbein, M.; Tincani, A.; Fischer-Betz, R.; Elefant, E.; Chambers, C.; da Silva, J.; Nelson-Piercy, C.; Cetin, I.; Costedoat-Chalumeau, N.; et al. The EULAR Points to Consider for Use of Antirheumatic Drugs before Pregnancy, and during Pregnancy and Lactation. *Ann. Rheum. Dis.* **2016**, *75*, 795–810. [CrossRef]
216. Food and Drug Administration. CellCept ®(Mycophenolate Mofetil Capsules) (Mycophenolate Mofetil Tablets), CellCept ®Oral Suspension (Mycophenolate Mofetil for Oral Suspension), CellCept ®Intravenous (Mycophenolate Mofetil Hydrochloride for Injection). Package Insert and Prescribing Information. Available online: https://www.accessdata.fda.gov/drugsatfda_docs/label/2013/050722s030s031,050723s029s030,050758s028s029,.pdf (accessed on 20 December 2022).
217. European Medicines Agency. EMA Recommends Additional Measures to Prevent Use of Mycophenolate in Pregnancy. London, UK. Available online: https://www.ema.europa.eu/en/news/ema-recommends-additional-measures-prevent-use-mycophenolate-pregnancy (accessed on 20 December 2022).
218. Mok, C.C. Pro: The Use of Calcineurin Inhibitors in the Treatment of Lupus Nephritis. *Nephrol. Dial. Transplant.* **2016**, *31*, 1561–1566. [CrossRef]
219. Gold, B.G. FK506 and the Role of Immunophilins in Nerve Regeneration. *Mol. Neurobiol.* **1997**, *15*, 285–306. [CrossRef]
220. Rothenberg, R.J.; Graziano, F.M.; Grandone, J.T.; Goldberg, J.W.; Bjarnason, D.F.; Finesilver, A.G. The Use of Methotrexate in Steroid-resistant Systemic Lupus Erythematosus. *Arthritis Rheum.* **1988**, *31*, 612–615. [CrossRef] [PubMed]
221. Asai, S.; Nagai, K.; Takahashi, N.; Watanabe, T.; Matsumoto, T.; Asai, N.; Sobue, Y.; Ishiguro, N.; Kojima, T. Influence of Methotrexate on Gastrointestinal Symptoms in Patients with Rheumatoid Arthritis. *Int. J. Rheum. Dis.* **2019**, *22*, 207–213. [CrossRef] [PubMed]
222. Jegasothy, B.V.; Ackerman, C.D.; Todo, S.; Fung, J.J.; Abu Elmagd, K.; Starzl, T.E. Tacrolimus (FK 506)—A New Therapeutic Agent for Severe Recalcitrant Psoriasis. *Arch. Dermatol.* **1992**, *128*, 781–785. [CrossRef] [PubMed]
223. Takabayashi, K.; Koike, T.; Kurasawa, K.; Matsumura, R.; Sato, T.; Tomioka, H.; Ito, I.; Yoshiki, T.; Yoshida, S. Effect of FK-506, a Novel Immunosuppressive Drug on Murine Systemic Lupus Erythematosus. *Clin. Immunol. Immunopathol.* **1989**, *51*, 110–117. [CrossRef]
224. Kondo, H.; Abe, T.; Hashimoto, H.; Uchida, S.; Irimajiri, S.; Hara, M.; Sugawara, S. Efficacy and Safety of Tacrolimus (FK506) in Treatment of Rheumatoid Arthritis: A Randomized, Double Blind, Placebo Controlled Dose-Finding Study. *J. Rheumatol.* **2004**, *31*, 243–251.
225. Tedesco, D.; Haragsim, L. Cyclosporine: A Review. *J. Transplant.* **2012**, *2012*, 1–7. [CrossRef]
226. Shaw, K.T.Y.; Ho, A.M.; Raghavan, A.; Kim, J.; Jain, J.; Park, J.; Sharma, S.; Rao, A.; Hogan, P.G. Immunosuppressive Drugs Prevent a Rapid Dephosphorylation of Transcription Factor NFAT1 in Stimulated Immune Cells. *Proc. Natl. Acad. Sci. USA* **1995**, *92*, 11205–11209. [CrossRef]
227. Lan, C.C.E.; Yu, H.S.; Wu, C.S.; Kuo, H.Y.; Chai, C.Y.; Chen, G.S. FK506 Inhibits Tumour Necrosis Factor-α Secretion in Human Keratinocytes via Regulation of Nuclear Factor-KB. *Br. J. Dermatol.* **2005**, *153*, 725–732. [CrossRef]
228. Hoyos, B.; Ballard, D.W.; Böhnlein, E.; Siekevitz, M.; Greene, W.C. Kappa B-Specific DNA Binding Proteins: Role in the Regulation of Human Interleukin-2 Gene Expression. *Science* **1989**, *244*, 457–460. [CrossRef]
229. Maluccio, M.; Sharma, V.; Lagman, M.; Vyas, S.; Yang, H.; Li, B.; Suthanthiran, M. Tacrolimus Enhances Transforming Growth Factor-B1 Expression and Promotes Tumor Progression. *Transplantation* **2003**, *76*, 597–602. [CrossRef]
230. Iwasaki, K. Metabolism of Tacrolimus (FK506) and Recent Topics in Clinical Pharmacokinetics. *Drug. Metab. Pharmacokinet.* **2007**, *22*, 328–335. [CrossRef] [PubMed]
231. Lampropoulos, C.E.; Sangle, S.; Harrison, P.; Hughes, G.R.V.; D'Cruz, D.P. Topical Tacrolimus Therapy of Resistant Cutaneous Lesions in Lupus Erythematosus: A Possible Alternative. *Rheumatology* **2004**, *43*, 1383–1385. [CrossRef] [PubMed]
232. Vesely, M.D. Getting under the Skin: Targeting Cutaneous Autoimmune Disease. *Yale J. Biol. Med.* **2020**, *93*, 197–206.
233. Liu, Z.; Zhang, H.; Liu, Z.; Xing, C.; Fu, P.; Ni, Z.; Chen, J.; Lin, H.; Liu, F.; He, Y.; et al. Multitarget Therapy for Induction Treatment of Lupus Nephritis: A Randomized Trial. *Ann. Intern. Med.* **2015**, *162*, 18–26. [CrossRef] [PubMed]
234. Issa, N.; Kukla, A.; Ibrahim, H.N. Calcineurin Inhibitor Nephrotoxicity: A Review and Perspective of the Evidence. *Am. J. Nephrol.* **2013**, *37*, 602–612. [CrossRef]
235. Macphee, I.; Fredericks, S.; Tai, T.; Syrris, P.; Carter, N.; Johnston, A.; Goldberg, L.; Holt, D. Tacrolimus Pharmacogenetics: Polymorphisms Associated with Expression of Cytochrome P4503A5 and P-Glycoprotein Correlate with Dose Requirement. *Transplantation* **2002**, *74*, 1486. [CrossRef] [PubMed]
236. Christians, U.; Jacobsen, W.; Benet, L.Z.; Lampen, A. Mechanisms of Clinically Relevant Drug Interactions Associated with Tacrolimus. *Clin. Pharmacokinet.* **2002**, *41*, 813–851. [CrossRef] [PubMed]
237. Naesens, M.; Kuypers, D.; Sarwal, M. Calcineurin Inhibitor Nephrotoxicity. *Clin. J. Am. Soc. Nephrol.* **2009**, *4*, 481. [CrossRef]
238. Myers, B.D.; Ross, J.; Newton, L.; Luetscher, J.; Perlroth, M. Cyclosporine-Associated Chronic Nephropathy. *N. Engl. J. Med.* **1984**, *311*, 699–705. [CrossRef]
239. Starzl, T.E.; Fung, J.; Jordan, M.; Shapiro, R.; Tzakis, A.; McCauley, J.; Johnston, J.; Iwaki, Y.; Jain, A.; Alessiani, M.; et al. Kidney Transplantation Under FK 506. *JAMA: J. Am. Med. Assoc.* **1990**, *264*, 63–67. [CrossRef]

240. Wu, G.; Weng, F.L.; Balaraman, V. Tacrolimus-Induced Encephalopathy and Polyneuropathy in a Renal Transplant Recipient. *BMJ Case Rep.* **2013**, *2013*, 1–4. [CrossRef] [PubMed]
241. Eidelman, B.; Abu-Elmagd, K.; Wilson, J.; Fung, J.; Alessiani, M.; Jain, A.; Takaya, S.; Todo, S.; Tzakis, A.; van Thiel, D. Neurologic Complications of FK 506. *Transplant Proc.* **1991**, *23*, 3175. [PubMed]
242. Hinchey, J.; Chaves, C.; Appignani, B.; Breen, J.; Pao, L.; Wang, A.; Pessin, M.; Lamy, C.; Mas, J.; Caplan, L. A Reversible Posterior Leukoencephalopathy Syndrome. *N. Engl. J. Med.* **1996**, *334*, 494. [CrossRef] [PubMed]
243. Oliverio, P.J.; Restrepo, L.; Mitchell, S.A.; Tornatore, C.S.; Frankel, S.R. Reversible Tacrolimus-Induced Neurotoxicity Isolated to the Brain Stem from the Departments of Radiology. *Am. J. Neuroradiol.* **2000**, *21*, 1251–1254. [PubMed]
244. Marchetti, P.; Navalesi, R. The Metabolic Effects of Cyclosporin and Tacrolimus. *J. Endocrinol. Investig.* **2000**, *23*, 482–490. [CrossRef]
245. Chang, H.L.; Kim, G.H. Electrolyte and Acid-Base Disturbances Induced by Clacineurin Inhibitors. *Electrolyte Blood Press.* **2007**, *5*, 126–130.
246. Redmon, J.B.; Olson, L.K.; Armstrong, M.B.; Greene, M.J.; Robertson, R.P. Effects of Tacrolimus (FK506) on Human Insulin Gene Expression, Insulin MRNA Levels, and Insulin Secretion in HIT-T15 Cells. *J. Clin. Investig.* **1996**, *98*, 2786–2793. [CrossRef]
247. Hirano, Y.; Fujihira, S.; Ohara, K.; Katsuki, S.; Noguchi, H. Morphological and Functional Changes of Islets of Langerhans in FK506-Treated Rats. *Transplantation* **1992**, *53*, 889–894. [CrossRef]
248. Malpica, L.; Moll, S. Practical Approach to Monitroing and Prevention of Infectious Complications Associated with Ssytemic Corticosteroids, Antimetabolites, Cyclosporina and Cyclophosphamide in Nonmalignant Hematologic Diseases. *Hematol. Am. Soc. Hematol. Educ. Program.* **2020**, *1*, 319–327. [CrossRef]
249. Barber, M.R.W.; Clarke, A.E. Systemic Lupus Erythematosus and Risk of Infection. *Expert. Rev. Clin. Immunol.* **2020**, *16*, 527–538. [CrossRef]
250. Mok, C.C. Calcineurin Inhibitors in Systemic Lupus Erythematosus. *Best. Pract. Res. Clin. Rheumatol.* **2017**, *31*, 429–438. [CrossRef] [PubMed]
251. Noviani, M.; Wasserman, S.; Clowse, M.E.B. Breastfeeding in Mothers with Systemic Lupus Erythematosus. *Lupus* **2016**, *25*, 973–979. [CrossRef] [PubMed]
252. Cheung, J.; Wentzell, J.; Trinacty, M.; Giguère, P.; Patel, P.; Kekre, N.; Nguyen, T. Efficacy, Safety, and Practicality of Tacrolimus Monitoring after Bone Marrow Transplant: Assessment of a Change in Practice. *Can J. Hosp. Pharm.* **2020**, *73*, 37–44. [CrossRef] [PubMed]
253. Cosansu, K.; Cakmak, H.A.; Karadag, B.; Aivazov, M.; Seyahi, N.; Vural, V.A. Impact of Different Immunosuppressive Drugs on QT Interval in Renal Transplant Patients. *Heart* **2011**, *97*, A186. [CrossRef]
254. Filler, G. Calcineurin Inhibitors in Pediatric Renal Transplant Recipients. *Pediatric. Drugs* **2007**, *9*, 165–174. [CrossRef]
255. Park, Y.J.; Yoo, S.A.; Kim, M.; Kim, W.U. The Role of Calcium–Calcineurin–NFAT Signaling Pathway in Health and Autoimmune Diseases. *Front. Immunol.* **2020**, *11*, 1–14. [CrossRef]
256. Ponticelli, C.; Reggiani, F.; Moroni, G. Old and New Calcineurin Inhibitors in Lupus Nephritis. *J. Clin. Med.* **2021**, *10*, 1–15. [CrossRef]
257. Betancourt, B.Y.; Biehl, A.; Katz, J.D.; Subedi, A. Pharmacotherapy Pearls in Rheumatology for the Care of Older Adult Patients: Focus on Oral Disease-Modifying Antirheumatic Drugs and the Newest Small Molecule Inhibitors. *Rheum. Dis. Clin. North Am.* **2018**, *44*, 371–391. [CrossRef]
258. Fortin, P.R.; Abrahamowicz, M.; Ferland, D.; Lacaille, D.; Smith, C.D.; Zummer, M. Steroid-Sparing Effects of Methotrexate in Systemic Lupus Erythematosus: A Double-Blind, Randomized, Placebo-Controlled Trial. *Arthritis Rheum.* **2008**, *59*, 1796–1804. [CrossRef]
259. Moutsopoulos, H.M.; Zampeli, E. Medications, Therapeutic Modalities, and Regimens Used in the Management of Rheumatic Diseases. In *Immunology and Rheumatology in Questions*; Springer International Publishing: Cham, Switzerland, 2021; pp. 205–243. ISBN 978-3-030-56669-2.
260. Haustein, U.F.; Rytter, M. Methotrexate in Psoriasis: 26 Years' Experience with Low-Dose Long-Term Treatment. *J. Eur. Acad. Dermatol. Venereol.* **2000**, *14*, 382–388. [CrossRef]
261. Ceponis, A.; Kavanaugh, A. Use of Methotrexate in Patients with Psoriatic Arthritis. *Clin. Exp. Rheumatol.* **2010**, *28*, 132–137.
262. Cipriani, P.; Ruscitti, P.; Carubbi, F.; Liakouli, V.; Giacomelli, R. Methotrexate: An Old New Drug in Autoimmune Disease. *Expert. Rev. Clin. Immunol.* **2014**, *10*, 1519–1530. [CrossRef] [PubMed]
263. Choy, E.H.; Hoogendijk, J.E.; Lecky, B.; Winer, J.B.; Gordon, P. Immunosuppressant and Immunomodulatory Treatment for Dermatomyositis and Polymyositis. *Cochrane Database Syst. Rev.* **2009**, *4*, 1465–1858. [CrossRef]
264. Lee, S.D.; Shivashankar, R.; Quirk, D.; Zhang, H.; Telliez, J.B.; Andrews, J.; Marren, A.; Mukherjee, A.; Loftus, E.V. Therapeutic Drug Monitoring for Current and Investigational Inflammatory Bowel Disease Treatments. *J. Clin. Gastroenterol.* **2021**, *55*, 195–206. [CrossRef] [PubMed]
265. Li, M.; Zhao, Y.; Zhang, Z.; Huang, C.; Liu, Y.; Gu, J.; Zhang, X.; Xu, H.; Li, X.; Wu, L.; et al. 2020 Chinese Guidelines for the Diagnosis and Treatment of Systemic Lupus Erythematosus. *Rheumatol. Immunol. Res.* **2020**, *1*, 5–23. [CrossRef] [PubMed]
266. Ruiz-Irastorza, G.; Bertsias, G. Treating Systemic Lupus Erythematosus in the 21st Century: New Drugs and New Perspectives on Old Drugs. *Rheumatology* **2020**, *59*, v69–v81. [CrossRef]

267. Cronstein, B.N.; Aune, T.M. Methotrexate and Its Mechanisms of Action in Inflammatory Arthritis. *Nat. Rev. Rheumatol.* **2020**, *16*, 145–154. [CrossRef]
268. Wallace, D.J. Systemic and Biologic Agents for Lupus Erythematosus. In *Biologic and Systemic Agents in Dermatology*; Springer International Publishing: Berlin/Heidelberg, Germany, 2018; pp. 377–390. ISBN 9783319668840.
269. Sakthiswary, R.; Suresh, E. Methotrexate in Systemic Lupus Erythematosus: A Systematic Review of Its Efficacy. *Lupus* **2014**, *23*, 225–235. [CrossRef]
270. Otón, T.; Carmona, L.; Loza, E.; Rosario, M.P.; Andreu, J.L. Use of Parenteral Methotrexate in Rheumatic Diseases: A Systematic Review. *Reumatol. Clin.* **2022**, *18*, 207–226. [CrossRef]
271. Carneiro, J.R.M.; Sato, E.I. Double Blind, Randomized, Placebo Controlled Clinical Trial of Methotrexate in Systemic Lupus Erythematosus. *J. Rheumatol.* **1999**, *26*, 1275–1279.
272. Islam, M.N.; Hossain, M.; Haq, S.A.; Alam, M.N.; ten Klooster, P.M.; Rasker, J.J. Efficacy and Safety of Methotrexate in Articular and Cutaneous Manifestations of Systemic Lupus Erythematosus. *Int. J. Rheum. Dis.* **2012**, *15*, 62–68. [CrossRef] [PubMed]
273. Wilson, K.; Abeles, M. A 2 Year, Open Ended Trial of Methotrexate in Systemic Lupus Erythematosus. *J. Rheumatol.* **1994**, *21*, 1674–1677. [PubMed]
274. Gansauge, S.; Breitbart, A.; Rinaldi, N.; Schwarz-Eywill, M. Methotrexate in Patients with Moderate Systemic Lupus Erythematosus (Exclusion of Renal and Central Nervous System Disease). *Ann. Rheum. Dis.* **1997**, *56*, 382–385. [CrossRef] [PubMed]
275. Kipen, Y.; Littlejohn, G.O.; Morand, E.F. Methotrexate Use in Systemic Lupus Erythematosus. *Lupus* **1997**, *6*, 385–389. [CrossRef] [PubMed]
276. Rahman, P.; Humphrey-Murto, S.; Gladman, D.D.; Urowitz, M.B. Efficacy and Tolerability of Methotrexate in Antimalarial Resistant Lupus Arthritis. *J. Rheumatol.* **1998**, *25*, 243–246.
277. Miyawaki, S.; Nishiyama, S.; Aita, T.; Yoshinaga, Y. The Effect of Methotrexate on Improving Serological Abnormalities of Patients with Systemic Lupus Erythematosus. *Mod. Rheumatol.* **2013**, *23*, 659–666. [CrossRef]
278. Wise, C.M.; Vuyyuru, S.; Roberts, W.N. Methotrexate in Nonrenal Lupus and Undifferentiated Connective Tissue Disease—A Review of 36 Patients. *J. Rheumatol.* **1996**, *23*, 1005–1010.
279. Wollina, U.; Ständer, K.; Barta, U. Toxicity of Methotrexate Treatment in Psoriasis Arthritis—Short- and Long-Term Toxicity in 104 Patients. *Clin. Rheumatol.* **2001**, *20*, 406–410. [CrossRef]
280. Wong, J.M.; Esdaile, J.M. Methotrexate in Systemic Lupus Erythematosus. *Lupus* **2005**, *14*, 101–105. [CrossRef]
281. Solomon, D.H.; Glynn, R.J.; Karlson, E.W.; Lu, F.; Corrigan, C.; Colls, J.; Xu, C.; MacFadyen, J.; Barbhaiya, M.; Berliner, N.; et al. Adverse Effects of Low-Dose Methotrexate: A Randomized Trial. *Ann. Intern. Med.* **2020**, *172*, 369–380. [CrossRef]
282. Shea, B.; Swinden, M.V.; Tanjong Ghogomu, E.; Ortiz, Z.; Katchamart, W.; Rader, T.; Bombardier, C.; Wells, G.A.; Tugwell, P. Folic Acid and Folinic Acid for Reducing Side Effects in Patients Receiving Methotrexate for Rheumatoid Arthritis. *Cochrane Database Syst. Rev.* **2013**, *2013*. [CrossRef] [PubMed]
283. Visser, K.; Katchamart, W.; Loza, E.; Martinez-Lopez, J.A.; Salliot, C.; Trudeau, J.; Bombardier, C.; Carmona, L.; van der Heijde, D.; Bijlsma, J.W.J.; et al. Multinational Evidence-Based Recommendations for the Use of Methotrexate in Rheumatic Disorders with a Focus on Rheumatoid Arthritis: Integrating Systematic Literature Research and Expert Opinion of a Broad International Panel of Rheumatologists in the 3E. *Ann. Rheum. Dis.* **2009**, *68*, 1086–1093. [CrossRef] [PubMed]
284. Katchamart, W.; Bourré-Tessier, J.; Donka, T.; Drouin, J.; Rohekar, G.; Bykerk, V.P.; Haraoui, B.; LeClerq, S.; Mosher, D.P.; Pope, J.E.; et al. Canadian Recommendations for Use of Methotrexate in Patients with Rheumatoid Arthritis. *J. Rheumatol.* **2010**, *37*, 1422–1430. [CrossRef]
285. Albrecht, K.; Müller-Ladner, U. Side Effects and Management of Side Effects of Methotrexate in Rheumatoid Arthritis. *Clin. Exp. Rheumatol.* **2010**, *28*, 502–516.
286. Conway, R.; Carey, J.J. Risk of Liver Disease in Methotrexate Treated Patients. *World J. Hepatol.* **2017**, *9*, 1092–1100. [CrossRef]
287. Kevat, S.; Ahern, M.; Hall, P. Hepatotoxicity of Methotrexate in Rheumatic Diseases. *Med. Toxicol. Adverse Drug. Exp.* **1988**, *3*, 197–208. [CrossRef]
288. Cansu, D.Ü.; Teke, H.Ü.; Bodakçi, E.; Korkmaz, C. How Should We Manage Low-Dose Methotrexate-Induced Pancytopenia in Patients with Rheumatoid Arthritis? *Clin. Rheumatol.* **2018**, *37*, 3419–3425. [CrossRef]
289. Berkun, Y.; Levartovsky, D.; Rubinow, A.; Orbach, H.; Aamar, S.; Grenader, T.; Abou Atta, I.; Mevorach, D.; Friedman, G.; Ben-Yehuda, A. Methotrexate Related Adverse Effects in Patients with Rheumatoid Arthritis Are Associated with the A1298C Polymorphism of the MTHFR Gene. *Ann. Rheum. Dis.* **2004**, *63*, 1227–1231. [CrossRef]
290. Al-Anazi, K.A.; Eltayeb, K.I.; Bakr, M.; Al-Mohareb, F.I. Methotrexate-Induced Acute Leukemia: Report of Three Cases and Review of the Literature. *Clin. Med. Case Rep.* **2009**, *2009*, 43–49. [CrossRef]
291. Jakubovic, B.D.; Donovan, A.; Webster, P.M.; Shear, N.H. Methotrexate-Induced Pulmonary Toxicity. *Can Respir. J.* **2013**, *20*, 153–155. [CrossRef]
292. Fragoulis, G.E.; Nikiphorou, E.; Larsen, J.; Korsten, P.; Conway, R. Methotrexate-Associated Pneumonitis and Rheumatoid Arthritis-Interstitial Lung Disease: Current Concepts for the Diagnosis and Treatment. *Front. Med.* **2019**, *6*, 1–10. [CrossRef] [PubMed]
293. Widemann, B.C.; Adamson, P.C. Understanding and Managing Methotrexate Nephrotoxicity. *Oncologist* **2006**, *11*, 694–703. [CrossRef] [PubMed]

294. Erdbrügger, U.; de Groot, K. Nierenschädigung Durch Methotrexat? Dosisabhängigkeit, Komorbidität Und Komedikation. *Z. Rheumatol.* **2011**, *70*, 549–552. [CrossRef] [PubMed]
295. Vezmar, S.; Becker, A.; Bode, U.; Jaehde, U. Biochemical and Clinical Aspects of Methotrexate Neurotoxicity. *Chemotherapy* **2003**, *49*, 92–104. [CrossRef]
296. Watanabe, K.; Arakawa, Y.; Oguma, E.; Uehara, T.; Yanagi, M.; Oyama, C.; Ikeda, Y.; Sasaki, K.; Isobe, K.; Mori, M.; et al. Characteristics of Methotrexate-Induced Stroke-like Neurotoxicity. *Int. J. Hematol.* **2018**, *108*, 630–636. [CrossRef] [PubMed]
297. Wernick, R.; Smith, D.L. Central Nervous System Toxicity Associated with Weekly Low-dose Methotrexate Treatment. *Arthritis Rheum.* **1989**, *32*, 770–775. [CrossRef]
298. Lewden, B.; Vial, T.; Elefant, E.; Nelva, A.; Carlier, P.; Descotes, J. Low Dose Methotrexate in the First Trimester of Pregnancy: Results of a French Collaborative Study. *J. Rheumatol.* **2004**, *31*, 2360–2365.
299. Valerio, V.; Kwok, M.; Loewen, H.; Winkler, J.; Mody, G.M.; Scuccimarri, R.; Meltzer, M.; Mengistu, Y.; Feldman, C.H.; Weinblatt, M.E.; et al. Systematic Review of Recommendations on the Use of Methotrexate in Rheumatoid Arthritis. *Clin. Rheumatol.* **2021**, *40*, 1259–1271. [CrossRef]
300. Contestable, J.J.; Edhegard, K.D.; Meyerle, J.H. Bullous Systemic Lupus Erythematosus: A Review and Update to Diagnosis and Treatment. *Am. J. Clin. Dermatol.* **2014**, *15*, 517–524. [CrossRef]
301. Fairley, J.L.; Oon, S.; Saracino, A.M.; Nikpour, M. Management of Cutaneous Manifestations of Lupus Erythematosus: A Systematic Review. *Semin. Arthritis. Rheum.* **2020**, *50*, 95–127. [CrossRef]
302. Wozel, V.E.G. Innovative Use of Dapsone. *Dermatol. Clin.* **2010**, *28*, 599–610. [CrossRef] [PubMed]
303. Lu, Q.; Long, H.; Chow, S.; Hidayat, S.; Danarti, R.; Listiawan, Y.; Deng, D.; Guo, Q.; Fang, H.; Tao, J.; et al. Guideline for the Diagnosis, Treatment and Long-Term Management of Cutaneous Lupus Erythematosus. *J. Autoimmun.* **2021**, *123*, 102707. [CrossRef] [PubMed]
304. Zuidema, J.; Hilbers-Modderman, E.S.M.; Merkus, F.W.H.M. Clinical Pharmacokinetics of Dapsone. *Clinical. Pharmacokinet.* **2012**, *11*, 299–315. [CrossRef] [PubMed]
305. Molinelli, E.; Paolinelli, M.; Campanati, A.; Brisigotti, V.; Offidani, A. Metabolic, Pharmacokinetic, and Toxicological Issues Surrounding Dapsone. 2019, *15*, 367–379. [CrossRef]
306. Schmidt, E.; Reimer, S.; Kruse, N.; Bröcker, E.B.; Zillikens, D. The IL-8 Release from Cultured Human Keratinocytes, Mediated by Antibodies to Bullous Pemphigoid Autoantigen 180, Is Inhibited by Dapsone. *Clin. Exp. Immunol.* **2001**, *124*, 157–162. [CrossRef] [PubMed]
307. Debol, S.M.; Herron, M.J.; Nelson, R.D. Anti-Inflammatory Action of Dapsone: Inhibition of Neutrophil Adherence Is Associated with Inhibition of Chemoattractant-Induced Signal Transduction. *J. Leukoc. Biol.* **1997**, *62*, 827–836. [CrossRef]
308. Bozeman, P.M.; Learn, D.B.; Thomas, E.L. Inhibition of the Human Leukocyte Enzymes Myeloperoxidase and Eosinophil Peroxidase by Dapsone. *Biochem. Pharmacol.* **1992**, *44*, 553–563. [CrossRef]
309. Verdelli, A.; Corrà, A.; Mariotti, E.B.; Aimo, C.; Ruffo di Calabria, V.; Volpi, W.; Quintarelli, L.; Caproni, M. An Update on the Management of Refractory Cutaneous Lupus Erythematosus. *Front. Med.* **2022**, *9*, 941003. [CrossRef]
310. Hall, R.P.; Lawley, T.J.; Smith, H.R.; Katz, S.I. Bullous Eruption of Systemic Lupus Erythematosus. Dramatic Response to Dapsone Therapy. *Ann. Intern. Med.* **1982**, *97*, 165–170. [CrossRef]
311. Lalova, A.; Pramatarov, K.; Vassileva, S. Facial Bullous Systemic Lupus Erythematosus. *Int. J. Dermatol.* **1997**, *36*, 369–371. [CrossRef]
312. Ludgate, M.W.; Greig, D.E. Bullous Systemic Lupus Erythematosus Responding to Dapsone. *Australas. J. Dermatol.* **2008**, *49*, 91–93. [CrossRef]
313. Lourenço, D.M.R.; Cunha Gomes, R.; Aikawa, N.E.; Campos, L.M.A.; Romiti, R.; Silva, C.A. Childhood-Onset Bullous Systemic Lupus Erythematosus. *Lupus* **2014**, *23*, 1422–1425. [CrossRef]
314. de Risi-Pugliese, T.; Cohen Aubart, F.; Haroche, J.; Moguelet, P.; Grootenboer-Mignot, S.; Mathian, A.; Ingen-Housz-Oro, S.; Hie, M.; Wendremaire, N.; Aucouturier, F.; et al. Clinical, Histological, Immunological Presentations and Outcomes of Bullous Systemic Lupus Erythematosus: 10 New Cases and a Literature Review of 118 Cases. *Semin. Arthritis. Rheum.* **2018**, *48*, 83–89. [CrossRef] [PubMed]
315. Hanuschk, D.; Kozyreff, A.; Tafzi, N.; Tennstedt, D.; Hantson, P.; Saint-Marcoux, F. Acute Visual Loss Following Dapsone-Induced Methemoglobinemia and Hemolysis. *Clin. Toxicol.* **2015**, *53*, 489–492. [CrossRef] [PubMed]
316. Satapornpong, P.; Pratoomwun, J.; Rerknimitr, P.; Klaewsongkram, J.; Nakkam, N.; Rungrotmongkol, T.; Konyoung, P.; Saksit, N.; Mahakkanukrauh, A.; Amornpinyo, W.; et al. HLA-B*13: 01 Is a Predictive Marker of Dapsone-Induced Severe Cutaneous Adverse Reactions in Thai Patients. *Front. Immunol.* **2021**, *12*, 661135. [CrossRef] [PubMed]
317. Agrawal, S.; Agarwalla, A. Dapsone Hypersensitivity Syndrome: A Clinico-Epidemiological Review. *J. Dermatol.* **2005**, *32*, 883–889. [CrossRef] [PubMed]
318. Sheen, Y.S.; Chu, C.Y.; Wang, S.H.; Tsai, T.F. Dapsone Hypersensitivity Syndrome in Non-Leprosy Patients: A Retrospective Study of Its Incidence in a Tertiary Referral Center in Taiwan. *J. Dermatol. Treat.* **2009**, *20*, 340–343. [CrossRef]
319. Pahadiya, H.R.; Lakhotia, M. Dapsone Hypersensitivity Syndrome with Leukemoid Reaction and Severe Thrombocytosis. *Cureus* **2021**, *13*, 1–4. [CrossRef]
320. Lorenz, M.; Wozel, G.; Schmit, J. Hypersensitivity Reactions to Dapsone: A Systematic Review. *Acta Derm. Venereol.* **2012**, *92*, 194–199. [CrossRef]

321. Fine, J.D.; Katz, S.I.; Donahue, M.J.; Hendricks, A.A. Psychiatric Reaction to Dapsone and Sulfapyridine. *J. Am. Acad. Dermatol.* **1983**, *9*, 274–275. [CrossRef]
322. Ezhilarasan, D. Dapsone-Induced Hepatic Complications: It's Time to Think beyond Methemoglobinemia. *Drug Chem. Toxicol.* **2019**, *44*, 330–333. [CrossRef]
323. Soliman, Y.Y.; Soliman, M.S.; Abbas, F. Why Now? Delayed Drug-Induced Pancreatitis Due to Dapsone for Dermatitis Herpetiformis. *J. Community Hosp. Intern. Med. Perspect.* **2018**, *8*, 156–157. [CrossRef] [PubMed]
324. Wan, J.; Imadojemu, S.; Werth, V.P. Management of Rheumatic and Autoimmune Blistering Disease in Pregnancy and Postpartum. *Clin. Dermatol.* **2016**, *34*, 344–352. [CrossRef] [PubMed]

Disclaimer/Publisher's Note: The statements, opinions and data contained in all publications are solely those of the individual author(s) and contributor(s) and not of MDPI and/or the editor(s). MDPI and/or the editor(s) disclaim responsibility for any injury to people or property resulting from any ideas, methods, instructions or products referred to in the content.

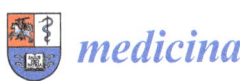

Article

Predictive Factors of the Use of Rituximab and Belimumab in Spanish Lupus Patients

O. Capdevila [1,*], F. Mitjavila [1,2], G. Espinosa [3], L. Caminal-Montero [4], A. Marín-Ballvè [5], R. González León [6], A. Castro [7], J. Canora [8], B. Pinilla [9], E. Fonseca [10] and G. Ruiz-Irastorza [11] on behalf of RELES, Autoimmune Diseases Study Group (GEAS), Spanish Society of Internal Medicine

1. Autoimmune Diseases Unit, Department of Internal Medicine, Hospital Universitari de Bellvitge, L'Hospitalet de Llobregat, 08907 Barcelona, Spain; fmitjavila@bellvitgehospital.cat
2. Bellvitge Biomedical Research Institute (IDIBELL), L'Hospitalet de Llobregat, 08907 Barcelona, Spain
3. Department of Autoimmune Diseases, Hospital Clinic, 08036 Barcelona, Spain; gespino@clinic.cat
4. Group of Basic and Translational Research in Inflammatory Diseases, Department of Internal Medicine, Hospital Universitario Central de Asturias, Instituto de Investigación Sanitaria del Principado de Asturias (ISPA), 33011 Oviedo, Spain; lcaminal@yahoo.es
5. Department of Internal Medicine, Hospital Clínico Universitario Lozano Blesa, 50009 Zaragoza, Spain
6. Department of Internal Medicine, Hospital Universitario Virgen del Rocío, 41013 Seville, Spain; pacolageno@gmail.com
7. Department of Internal Medicine, Hospital Universitari Sant Joan de Reus, 43204 Reus, Spain
8. Department of Internal Medicine, Hospital Universitario de Fuenlabrada, 28942 Madrid, Spain
9. Department of Internal Medicine, Hospital General Universitario Gregorio Marañón, 28007 Madrid, Spain; blancapinilla@telefonica.net
10. Department of Internal Medicine, Hospital de Cabueñes, 33394 Gijón, Spain; evamfonseca@yahoo.es
11. Autoimmune Diseases Research Unit, Department of Internal Medicine, BioCruces Bizkaia Health Research Institute, Hospital Universitario Cruces, UPV/EHU, 48903 Barakaldo, Spain
* Correspondence: ocapdevila@bellvitgehospital.cat

Abstract: *Objectives*: To analyze the characteristics and the predictive factors of the use of rituximab and belimumab in daily practice in patients from the inception cohort Registro Español de Lupus (RELES). *Material and methods*: The study included 518 patients. We considered patients treated with biologics who received at least one dose of rituximab or belimumab, and possible indications of those manifestations registered at the same time or in the previous 2 months of the start of the therapy. *Results*: In our cohort, 37 (7%) patients received at least one biological treatment. Rituximab was prescribed in 26 patients and belimumab in 11. Rituximab was mainly prescribed for hemolytic anemia or thrombocytopenia (11 patients, 42%), lupus nephritis and neuropsychiatric lupus (5 patients each, 19%). Belimumab was mostly used for arthritis (8 patients, 73%). In the univariate analysis, the predictive factors at diagnosis for the use of biologic therapy were younger age ($p = 0.022$), a higher SLEDAI ($p = 0.001$) and the presence of psychosis ($p = 0.011$), organic mental syndrome (SOCA) ($p = 0.006$), hemolytic anemia ($p = 0.001$), or thrombocytopenia ($p = 0.01$). In the multivariant model, only younger age, psychosis, and hemolytic anemia were independent predictors of the use of biologics. *Conclusions*: Rituximab is usually given to patients with hematological, neuropsychiatric and renal involvement and belimumab for arthritis. Psychosis, hemolytic anemia and age at the diagnosis of lupus were independent predictive factors of the use of biological agents. Their global effects are beneficial, with a significant reduction in SLE activity and a low rate of side effects.

Keywords: systemic lupus erythematosus; belimumab; rituximab

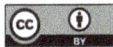

1. Introduction

Systemic lupus erythematosus (SLE) is a heterogeneous autoimmune multisystemic disease, with a complex pathogenesis in which immune dysregulation plays an important role [1].

Signs and symptoms of SLE can affect a single organ or several organ systems, making it a difficult disease to diagnose. Typical manifestations include skin rashes, arthritis, serositis, and lupus nephritis. Hematological and neuropsychiatric involvement are less frequent. Early diagnosis of SLE is crucial to prevent flares and resultant tissue damage. Treatment response can be variable and difficult to predict.

Despite the improvement in the prognosis of lupus within the last decades, the burden of disease is still determined by both the degree and the severity of the immunologic inflammatory disease and the resultant organ damage, either caused by the disease itself, by comorbidities, and/or by treatments [2,3]. Sustained remission is an important goal.

With the aim of achieving better control of disease activity, new therapeutic alternatives to glucocorticoids and immunosuppressants are being developed. A better understanding of the etiopathogenesis of SLE has led to the introduction of a number of biologic agents that specifically target disease pathways underlying the development and progression of lupus [4,5]. Some of these therapies, such as rituximab and belimumab, are available in clinical practice, while others are being tested in ongoing clinical trials. The use of such biologic agents is recommended in patients with an inadequate response to standard therapies [6].

Rituximab (RTX) is a chimeric mAb that targets CD20, a transmembrane protein on all B cells except pro-B cells and plasma cells, which results in cytotoxicity and B cell depletion [7]. Several case series and retrospective studies have shown improvement in SLE parameters, including lupus nephritis, despite negative results of randomized controlled trials (RCT) [8,9]. RTX efficacy was studied in nonrenal SLE with moderate to severe disease activity and is used off-label in refractory and relapsing SLE based on several observational nonrandomized studies [10,11].

Belimumab is a recombinant, fully human monoclonal antibody (mAb) that blocks the binding of soluble B lymphocyte stimulator to its receptor on B cells, thus, decreasing B cell survival, differentiation, and activation. It was the first biologic to be FDA-approved for SLE and is available as an i.v. infusion or a subcutaneous injection. In several large double-blinded phase III randomized controlled trials RCT, it has been shown to improve musculoskeletal and mucocutaneous manifestations and immunologic parameters in patients with active disease on background standard-of-care therapy. These studies initially excluded severe renal and central nervous system (CNS) forms [12–14]. A recent trial has also demonstrated its beneficial effect on lupus nephritis when added to standard treatment [15]. More recently belimumab has shown efficacy in decreasing SLE exacerbations and reducing glucocorticoid doses, thus, contributing to decreased damage accrual [16,17].

The aim of the present study is to analyze the use of these biologic agents in daily practice in our setting. RELES (Registro Español de Lupus Eritematoso Sistémico) is the first Spanish multicentric inception lupus cohort, a research project of the Group of Autoimmune Diseases within the Spanish Society of Internal Medicine, in which patients with a new diagnosis of SLE have been included since January 2009. Thus, we analyze the indications, baseline predictive factors, efficacy, and side effects of the use of biologic therapy in the RELES cohort.

2. Materials and Methods

A total of 518 patients were enrolled in RELES by the end of 2020. Among them, 425 had completed at least one year of follow up, 371 two years, 268 three years, and 200 four years or more. All patients were attended at Internal Medicine Services of 44 Spanish public hospitals. Patients were enrolled at the time when at least 4 ACR classification criteria were met [18].

Recruitment started in January 2009 and data were prospectively collected and entered in a computerized database. All patients signed an informed consent document at the time of enrolment. The study protocol has been approved by the institutional research ethics boards of the coordinating center (Hospital Universitario Cruces) and all participating centers.

Information on demographic characteristics, clinical manifestations, laboratory results, disease activity measured by the Safety of Estrogens in Lupus Erythematosus National Assessment (SELENA) version of the SLE Disease Activity Index (SLEDAI) [19], and treatments received are registered at the time of enrolment and yearly thereafter. Damage accrual, measured by the Systemic Lupus International Collaborating Clinics (SLICC)/American College of Rheumatology (ACR) Damage Index (SDI) [20], is first recorded after 6 months of enrolment and yearly thereafter.

For the purposes of this study, we considered patients treated with biologics who received at least one dose of rituximab or belimumab. We considered as possible indications of a biological treatment those manifestations registered at the same time or in the previous 2 months of the start of the therapy. We considered biologics-related infections to be those diagnosed within the first year after the administration of rituximab or belimumab.

Statistical Analysis

Descriptive data were generated using percentages, means, and standard deviations (SD). Such data included baseline demographic characteristics, clinical manifestations, and immunological profiles at baseline. Likewise, the indications for biologic use, as defined in the previous section, were summarized.

The comparison of data from patients receiving or not receiving biologic therapy was performed using the Chi-square test, Fisher's exact test, non-paired Student's t-test, or Mann–Whitney test, as appropriate. Those variables with a p value of 0.2 or less in the univariate analysis were subsequently included in a logistic regression model with a backward stepwise selection of variables, in order to identify independent predictive factors at baseline for the use of biologic drugs during the follow up.

The efficacy of biologic therapy was assessed by comparing mean SLEDAI scores just before and 6 months after starting therapy in patients receiving these drugs by paired T-test. Finally, infections after biologic therapy were summarized, and the proportions of treated and untreated patients suffering infections within the same period were compared by a Chi-square test.

All statistical analyses were performed using the IBM SPSS statistics19 software package for Windows.

3. Results

3.1. Baseline Clinical Characteristics at Diagnosis

A total of 518 patients were included in this study. The main clinical characteristics of the cohort and treatments received are shown on Table 1. Overall, 89% of patients were women and 78% were Caucasians. The mean SLEDAI score at diagnosis was 9. Most patients had mucocutaneous (75%) or articular manifestations (78%) followed by hematological disorders (21%), nephritis (19%), and serositis (17%).

Table 1. Baseline clinical characteristics of the Registro Español de Lupus Eritematoso Sistémico (RELES) cohort.

	No Biologics (*n* = 479)	Rituximab (*n* = 26)	Belimumab (*n* = 11)
Age at disease onset, mean (SD)	40 (16)	33 (14)	32 (16)
Female, *n* (%)	426 (89)	23 (88)	11
Caucasian, *n* (%)	372 (78)	19 (73)	10 (91)
Hispanic, *n* (%)	95 (20)	5 (19)	1 (9)
Asian, *n* (%)	7 (1)	2 (8)	
Afro-American (%)	5 (1)		
Cutaneous disease, *n* (%)	360 (75)	19 (73)	10 (91)
Arthritis, *n* (%)	370 (77)	20 (77)	11

Table 1. *Cont.*

	No Biologics (*n* = 479)	Rituximab (*n* = 26)	Belimumab (*n* = 11)
Neurologic disease, *n* (%)	29 (6)	6 (23)	1 (9)
Seizures	7 (1)	0	1 (9)
Psychosis	4 (1)	3 (11)	0
Organic mental syndrome	0	2 (8)	0
Myelitis	4 (1)	1 (4)	0
Serositis, *n* (%)	83 (17)	4 (15)	1 (9)
Pleuritis	67 (14)	3 (11)	0
Pericarditis	50 (10)	4 (15)	1 (9)
Pneumonitis, *n* (%)	15 (3)	2 (8)	0
Glomerulonephritis, *n* (%)	86 (18)	9 (35)	2 (18)
Proliferative glomerulonephritis	51 (11)	5 (19)	1 (9)
Hematological, *n* (%)	86 (18)	15 (58)	5 (45)
Hemolytic anemia	33 (7)	10 (38)	4 (36)
Thrombocytopenia	65 (14)	11 (42)	1 (9)
SLEDAI, mean (SD)	9 (7)	15 (11)	12 (7)

3.2. Main Indications of Biologic Therapies and Concomitant Treatments

In our prospective cohort, 37 (7%) patients received at least one biological treatment. Rituximab was prescribed in 26 patients and belimumab in 11. Six patients received rituximab and belimumab consecutively during the study period. In three patients, treatment was administered for refractory diseases, and the other three received rituximab and belimumab for different organ manifestations.

Rituximab was mainly prescribed for hemolytic anemia and/or thrombocytopenia (11 patients, 42%), followed by lupus nephritis and neuropsychiatric lupus (5 patients each, 19%). Belimumab was mostly used for arthritis in the vast majority of patients (eight patients, 73%). The detailed indications for rituximab and belimumab are shown in Table 2.

Table 2. Indications for rituximab and belimumab.

SLE Manifestations	Rituximab (*n* = 26)	Belimumab (*n* = 11)
Arthritis	2 (8%)	8 (73%)
Hematological	11 (42%)	0
Neuropsychiatric disease	5 (19%)	1 (9%)
Serositis	0	1 (9%)
Proliferative glomerulonephritis	5 (19%)	1 (9%)
Pneumonitis	3 (11%)	0

The mean (SD) time from disease onset to the administration of the biologic treatment was 28 (30) months, 25 (27) months for rituximab, and 38 (33) months for belimumab. Rituximab was administered after a mean of 18, 23, and 39 months after the diagnosis of SLE, respectively, for hematological, neuropsychiatric, and renal involvement, whereas belimumab was administered after a mean of 30 months after the SLE diagnosis for articular symptoms.

All patients received glucocorticoids simultaneously to the biologic treatment, while 92% received hydroxychloroquine and 84% received immunosuppressants (5 azathioprine, 18 mycophenolate, 5 methotrexate, and 3 cyclophosphamide).

3.3. Predictive Factors at Baseline for the Use of Biologic Therapy

In the univariate analysis, the predictive factors at baseline for the eventual use of biologic therapy were younger age (33 vs. 40 years in patients not given biologics, $p = 0.006$), a higher SLEDAI score (14 vs. 9, respectively, $p = 0.001$), and the presence of psychosis, organic mental syndrome (SOCA), hemolytic anemia, or thrombocytopenia (Table 3). In the multivariate model, younger age, psychosis, and hemolytic anemia were independent predictors of the use of biologics (Table 4).

Table 3. Predictive factors at baseline associated with the use of biologic treatment.

	Biologic Treatment ($n = 37$)	No Biologic Treatment ($n = 481$)	p
Age at disease onset, mean (SD)	33 (14)	40 (17)	0.006
Female, n (%)	34 (92)	427 (89)	0.79
Caucasian, n (%)	29 (78)	374 (78)	1
SLEDAI, mean (SD)	14 (10)	9 (7)	0.001
Cutaneous disease, n (%)	28 (76)	362 (75)	1
Arthritis, n (%)	31 (84)	372 (77)	0.42
Neurological disease, n (%)	7 (19)	29 (6)	0.01
Seizures	1 (3)	7 (2)	0.45
Psychosis	3 (8)	4 (1)	0.01
Organic mental syndrome	2 (5)	4 (1)	0.06
Myelitis	1 (3)	4 (1)	0.31
Serositis, n (%)	5 (14)	84 (17)	0.65
Pleuritis	3 (8)	68 (14)	0.45
Pericarditis	5 (13)	51 (11)	0.58
Pneumonitis, n (%)	2 (5)	15 (3)	0.34
Nephritis, n (%)	11 (30)	86 (18)	0.08
Proliferative nephritis	6 (16)	51 (11)	0.27
Hematological, n (%)	20 (54)	87 (18)	<0.001
Hemolytic anemia	14 (38)	34 (7)	<0.001
Thrombocytopenia	12 (32)	65 (14)	0.006

Table 4. Multivariant analysis of predictive factors for the use of biologics at diagnoses.

	Initial Model OR (95% CI)	Final Model OR (95% CI)
Age at disease onsett	1.031 (1.007–1.056)	0.970 (0.945–0.995)
Organic mental syndrome	0.147 (0.026–0.828)	
Psychosis	0.095 (0.020–0.442)	11.07 (1.885–65.07)
Hemolytic anemia	0.125 (0.059–0.265)	7.283 (3.164–16.767)
Thrombocytopenia	0.326 (0.156–0.680)	
Lupus nephritis	1.938 (0.922–4.073)	
SLEDAI	0.939 (0.908–0.971)	

3.4. Efficacy and Safety of Biologic Treatment

Regarding efficacy, we observed a significant reduction in lupus activity according to the mean (SD) SLEDAI scores before and after the administration of biologic treatment, namely 12.9 (8.6) vs. 4.4 (4.7), respectively ($p < 0.001$).

Eleven (28%) patients suffered infections after the administration of biologic treatment: three patients had herpes zoster, seven had bacterial infections (four urinary tract infections, two had pneumonia, and one had pelvic inflammatory disease), while one had a cutaneous leishmaniasis. None of these conditions were lethal. The proportion of patients with infections within the same time span was similar in patients who did not receive biologic treatment (128/481 patients, 27%, $p = 0.85$).

4. Discussion

In our prospective cohort, 7% of patients received biologic agents within the first 5 years of the disease course. Data on the number of patients with SLE requiring treatment with biologic agents are scarce. A French registry showed that 136/2551 patients (5.4%) received at least one dose of rituximab [21]. Even taking into account that our cohort includes patients who received either rituximab or belimumab, our results do not greatly differ from those reported.

Younger age, psychosis, and hemolytic anemia at the time of diagnosis of SLE were the only independent predictive factors of the use of biologics in our cohort. In fact, hematological and neuropsychiatric lupus were also two of the main indications for rituximab, which, although not considered a first-line treatment, is being increasingly used in these scenarios due to the frequent lack of effectiveness of usual therapies [6].

It is noteworthy that although belimumab is the only biologic treatment approved for lupus, rituximab was used more frequently and earlier than belimumab in our cohort. Rituximab is usually prescribed for refractory or relapsing severe lupus manifestations, which also include nephritis and arthritis apart from the already mentioned neuropsychiatric and hematological manifestations [22,23]. It is important to remark that rituximab was given earlier within the course of disease to patients with hematological manifestations than to those with neuropsychiatric lupus or nephritis. This is probably due to the fact that usual first-line therapies are less effective in immune thrombocytopenia and hemolytic anemia [22,24]. The role of rituximab in neuropsychiatric lupus is not well defined [25,26], while it is clearly considered a rescue therapy in lupus nephritis [27,28].

In our cohort, belimumab was mainly used for arthritis. Standard treatments for patients with arthritis and mucocutaneous manifestations include hydroxychloroquine and low-dose prednisone, with immunosuppressants being added in refractory cases or when glucocorticoid maintenance doses cannot be reduced [29]. Recent data could suggest that an earlier use of belimumab in the SLE course could speed up the clinical response, especially in patients with a relapsing–remitting pattern who are taking high prednisone doses [30,31].

It well stablished that modifying the disease course with effective therapies and steroid-sparing regimens may reduce organ damage, improve outcomes and decrease mortality in patients with SLE [16]. However, what should be the role of biologic therapy within the global therapeutic strategy of lupus is not well defined. High early and sustained response rates with "conventional" therapy based on pulses of methyl-prednisolone and reduced doses of oral prednisone have been recently shown [32]. In the RELES cohort, patients receiving biologic therapy had a significantly more active disease at diagnosis and a high concomitant use of other therapies, all suggesting refractory disease. After starting biologics, a significant decrease in activity, as measured by SLEDAI scores, was accomplished. These results support the current EULAR recommendations for the use of belimumab and rituximab, both as a second-line therapy in patients who are refractory or intolerant to non-biologic therapy [6]. It must be remarked upon once more that hydroxychloroquine has convincingly shown long-term effects in reducing damage accrual and improving survival, so its role as a universal therapy for lupus patients cannot be replaced at this time by any other therapy, including biologics [33], despite the promising long-term effects of belimumab [32]. Our data are also reassuring in showing that biologic agents were not associated with an increase in the number of infections, as previously described by other authors [9,21].

We acknowledge some limitations of this study. This study is based on a multicenter Spanish register and, therefore, it does not include a control group comparing the use of biological treatment with the standard of care. The use of biologics was decided by the physicians caring for the patients, without any pre-specified protocol. The main outcome measure was the reduction in the SLEDAI score, without specific data on the evolution of the clinical manifestation leading to the use of biologics. The low number of biologic-treated patients and the diversity of indications made it impossible to offer a detailed statistical analysis on this issue. The long-term effects on damage and glucocorticoid use have not been addressed due to the low numbers of biologic-treated patients with prolonged follow-up.

On the other hand, our real-world data offer a realistic view of the use of rituximab and belimumab in our setting. The high proportion of those biologic-treated patients being on prednisone, hydroxychloroquine, and immunosuppressive drugs point to a second-line indication for patients who are refractory to conventional therapy, thus, following current guidelines [6]. Our study has revealed the main baseline predictors for the use of either rituximab or belimumab, as well as global beneficial effects on lupus activity in patients who are refractory to other therapies.

5. Conclusions

In summary, our study reveals that younger age, neuropsychiatric lupus, and hemolytic anemia at SLE diagnosis predict the use of rituximab or belimumab at some point of their SLE course. The global effects of both drugs are beneficial in these groups of patients, with a significant reduction in SLE activity and a low rate of side effects.

Author Contributions: Conceptualization, O.C. and F.M.; methodology, O.C.; validation, O.C., F.M., G.E. and G.R.-I.; formal analysis, O.C. and F.M.; investigation, resources and data curation, all authors; writing—original draft preparation, O.C., F.M. and G.R.-I.; Review and editing, O.C., F.M., G.E., L.C.-M., A.M.-B., R.G.L., A.C., J.C., B.P., E.F. and G.R.-I.; supervision, O.C., F.M., G.E., L.C.-M., A.C and G.R-I. All authors have read and agreed to the published version of the manuscript.

Funding: Ruiz-Irastorza was supported by the Department of Education of the Basque Government, research grant (Grant number: IT 1512-22).

Institutional Review Board Statement: The study was conducted in accordance with the Declaration of Helsinki and approved by the Ethics Committee of Cruces University Hospital (protocol code CEIC E08/35, 24 June 2008).

Informed Consent Statement: Informed consent was obtained from all subjects involved in the study.

Data Availability Statement: The data used during the current study is available from the corresponding author on reasonable request.

Acknowledgments: We thank all the members of the RELES Registry Coordinating Centre, S&H Medical Science Service, for their quality control data, logistic and administrative support. We thank CERCA Program/Generalitat de Catalunya for institutional support. We also thank the patients included in the current study.

Conflicts of Interest: The authors declare no conflict of interest.

References

1. Bertsias, G.K.; Salmon, J.E.; Boumpas, D.T. Therapeutic opportunities in systemic lupus erythematosus: State of the art and prospects for the new decade. *Ann. Rheum. Dis.* **2010**, *69*, 1603–1611. [CrossRef] [PubMed]
2. Van Vollenhoven, R.F.; Mosca, M.; Bertsias, G.; Isenberg, D.; Kuhn, A.; Lerstrøm, K.; Aringer, M.; Bootsma, H.; Boumpas, D.; Bruce, I.N.; et al. Treat-to-target in systemic lupus erythematosus: Recommendations from an international task force. *Ann. Rheum. Dis.* **2014**, *73*, 958–967. [CrossRef] [PubMed]

3. Medina-Quiñones, C.V.; Ramos-Merino, L.; Ruiz-Sada, P.; Isenberg, D. Analysis of Complete Remission in Systemic Lupus Erythematosus Patients Over a 32-Year Period. *Arthritis Care Res.* **2016**, *68*, 981–987. [CrossRef] [PubMed]
4. Murphy, G.; Isenberg, D.A. New therapies for systemic lupus erythematosus-past imperfect, future tense. *Nat. Rev. Rheumatol.* **2019**, *15*, 403–412, Erratum in *Nat. Rev. Rheumatol.* **2019**, *15*, 509. [CrossRef] [PubMed]
5. Basta, F.; Fasola, F.; Triantafyllias, K.; Schwarting, A. Systemic Lupus Erythematosus (SLE) Therapy: The Old and the New. *Rheumatol. Ther.* **2020**, *7*, 433–446. [CrossRef] [PubMed]
6. Fanouriakis, A.; Kostopoulou, M.; Alunno, A.; Aringer, M.; Bajema, I.; Boletis, J.N.; Cervera, R.; Doria, A.; Gordon, C.; Govoni, M.; et al. 2019 update of the EULAR recommendations for the management of systemic lupus erythematosus. *Ann. Rheum. Dis.* **2019**, *78*, 736–745. [CrossRef] [PubMed]
7. Mok, C.C. Current role of rituximab in systemic lupus erythematosus. *Int. J. Rheum. Dis.* **2015**, *18*, 154–163. [CrossRef]
8. Merrill, J.T.; Neuwelt, C.M.; Wallace, D.J.; Shanahan, J.C.; Latinis, K.M.; Oates, J.C.; Utset, T.O.; Gordon, C.; Isenberg, D.A.; Hsieh, H.J.; et al. Efficacy and safety of rituximab in moderately-to-severely active systemic lupus erythematosus: The randomized, double-blind, phase II/III systemic lupus erythematosus evaluation of rituximab trial. *Arthritis Rheum.* **2010**, *62*, 222–233. [CrossRef]
9. Rovin, B.H.; Furie, R.; Latinis, K.; Looney, R.J.; Fervenza, F.C.; Sanchez-Guerrero, J.; Maciuca, R.; Zhang, D.; Garg, J.P.; Brunetta, P.; et al. Efficacy and safety of rituximab in patients with active proliferative lupus nephritis: The Lupus Nephritis Assessment with Rituximab study. *Arthritis Rheum.* **2012**, *64*, 1215–1226. [CrossRef]
10. Fernández-Nebro, A.; de la Fuente, J.M.; Carreño, L.; Izquierdo, M.G.; Tomero, E.; Rúa-Figueroa, I.; Hernández-Cruz, B.; Narváez, J.; Úcar, E.; Olivé, A.; et al. Multicenter longitudinal study of B-lymphocyte depletion in refractory systemic lupus erythematosus: The LESIMAB study. *Lupus* **2012**, *21*, 1063–1076. [CrossRef]
11. Ramos-Casals, M.; Soto, M.J.; Cuadrado, M.J.; Khamashta, M.A. Rituximab in systemic lupus erythematosus: A systematic review of off-label use in 188 cases. *Lupus* **2009**, *18*, 767–776. [CrossRef]
12. Navarra, S.V.; Guzmán, R.M.; Gallacher, A.E.; Hall, S.; Levy, R.A.; Jimenez, R.E.; Li, E.K.; Thomas, M.; Kim, H.Y.; León, M.G.; et al. Efficacy and safety of belimumab in patients with active systemic lupus erythematosus: A randomised, placebo-controlled, phase 3 trial. *Lancet* **2011**, *377*, 721–731. [CrossRef]
13. Furie, R.; Petri, M.; Zamani, O.; Cervera, R.; Wallace, D.J.; Tegzová, D.; Sanchez-Guerrero, J.; Schwarting, A.; Merrill, J.T.; Chatham, W.W.; et al. A phase III, randomized, placebo-controlled study of belimumab, a monoclonal antibody that inhibits B lymphocyte stimulator, in patients with systemic lupus erythematosus. *Arthritis Rheum.* **2011**, *63*, 3918–3930. [CrossRef]
14. Blair, H.A.; Duggan, S.T. Belimumab: A Review in Systemic Lupus Erythematosus. *Drugs* **2018**, *78*, 355–366. [CrossRef]
15. Furie, R.; Rovin, B.H.; Houssiau, F.; Malvar, A.; Teng, Y.K.O.; Contreras, G.; Amoura, Z.; Yu, X.; Mok, C.-C.; Santiago, M.B.; et al. Two-Year, Randomized, Controlled Trial of Belimumab in Lupus Nephritis. *N. Engl. J. Med.* **2020**, *383*, 1117–1128. [CrossRef]
16. Murimi-Worstell, I.B.; Lin, D.H.; Nab, H.; Kan, H.J.; Onasanya, O.; Tierce, J.C.; Wang, X.; Desta, B.; Alexander, G.C.; Hammond, E.R. Association between organ damage and mortality in systemic lupus erythematosus: A systematic review and meta-analysis. *BMJ* **2020**, *10*, e031850. [CrossRef]
17. Urowitz, M.B.; Ohsfeldt, R.L.; Wielage, R.C.; Kelton, K.A.; Asukai, Y.; Ramachandran, S. Organ damage in patients treated with belimumab versus standard of care: A propensity score-matched comparative analysis. *Ann. Rheum. Dis.* **2019**, *78*, 372–379. [CrossRef]
18. Hochberg, M.C. Updating the American College of Rheumatology revised criteria for the classification of systemic lupus erythematosus. *Arthritis Rheum.* **1997**, *40*, 1725. [CrossRef]
19. Petri, M.; Kim, M.Y.; Kalunian, K.C.; Grossman, J.; Hahn, B.H.; Sammaritano, L.R.; Lockshin, M.; Merrill, J.T.; Belmont, H.M.; Askanase, A.D.; et al. OC-SELENA Trial.Combined Oral Contraceptives in Women with Systemic Lupus Erythematosus. *N. Engl. J. Med.* **2005**, *353*, 2550–2558. [CrossRef]
20. Gladman, D.D.; Goldsmith, C.H.; Urowitz, M.B.; Bacon, P.; Fortin, P.; Ginzler, E.; Gordon, C.; Hanly, J.G.; Isenberg, D.A.; Petri, M.; et al. The Systemic Lupus International Collaborating Clinics/American College of Rheumatology (SLICC/ACR) Damage Index for Systemic Lupus Erythematosus International Comparison. *J. Rheumatol.* **2000**, *27*, 373–376.
21. Terrier, B.; Amoura, Z.; Ravaud, P.; Hachulla, E.; Jouenne, R.; Combe, B.; Bonnet, C.; Cacoub, P.; Cantagrel, A.; De Bandt, M.; et al. Safety and efficacy of rituximab in systemic lupus erythematosus: Results from 136 patients from the French autoimmunity and rituximab registry. *Arthritis Rheum.* **2010**, *62*, 2458–2466. [CrossRef] [PubMed]
22. Serris, A.; Amoura, Z.; Canouï-Poitrine, F.; Terrier, B.; Hachulla, E.; Costedoat-Chalumeau, N.; Papo, T.; Lambotte, O.; Saadoun, D.; Hié, M.; et al. Efficacy and safety of rituximab for systemic lupus erythematosus-associated immune cytopenias: A multicenter retrospective cohort study of 71 adults. *Am. J. Hematol.* **2018**, *93*, 424–429. [CrossRef] [PubMed]
23. Witt, M.; Grunke, M.; Proft, F.; Baeuerle, M.; Aringer, M.; Burmester, G.; Chehab, G.; Fiehn, C.; Fischer-Betz, R.; Fleck, M.; et al. Clinical outcomes and safety of rituximab treatment for patients with systemic lupus erythematosus (SLE)—Results from a nationwide cohort in Germany (GRAID). *Lupus* **2013**, *22*, 1142–1149. [CrossRef]
24. Jung, J.H.; Soh, M.S.; Ahn, Y.H.; Um, Y.J.; Jung, J.Y.; Suh, C.H.; Kim, H.A. Thrombocytopenia in Systemic Lupus Erythematosus: Clinical Manifestations, Treatment, and Prognosis in 230 Patients. *Medicine* **2016**, *95*, e2818. [CrossRef]
25. Dale, R.C.; Brilot, F.; Duffy, L.V.; Twilt, M.; Waldman, A.T.; Narula, S.; Muscal, E.; Deiva, K.; Andersen, E.; Eyre, M.R.; et al. Utility and safety of rituximab in pediatric autoimmune and inflammatory CNS disease. *Neurology* **2014**, *83*, 142–150. [CrossRef] [PubMed]

26. Narváez, J.; Ríos-Rodriguez, V.; de la Fuente, D.; Estrada, P.; López-Vives, L.; Gómez-Vaquero, C.; Nolla, J.M. Rituximab Therapy in Refractory Neuropsychiatric Lupus: Current Clinical Evidence. *Semin. Arthritis Rheum.* **2011**, *41*, 364–372. [CrossRef]
27. Díaz-Lagares, C.; Croca, S.; Sangle, S.; Vital, E.M.; Catapano, F.; Martínez-Berriotxoa, A.; García-Hernández, F.; Callejas-Rubio, J.L.; Rascón, J.; D'Cruz, D.; et al. Autoimmunity Reviews Efficacy of rituximab in 164 patients with biopsy-proven lupus nephritis: Pooled data from European cohorts. *Autoimmun. Rev.* **2012**, *11*, 357–364. [CrossRef]
28. Catapano, F.; Chaudhry, A.N.; Jones, R.B.; Smith, K.G.C.; Jayne, D.W. Long-term efficacy and safety of rituximab in refractory and relapsing systemic lupus erythematosus. *Nephrol. Dial. Transplant.* **2010**, *25*, 3586–3592. [CrossRef]
29. Trentin, F.; Gatto, M.; Zen, M.; Larosa, M.; Maddalena, L.; Nalotto, L.; Saccon, F.; Zanatta, E.; Iaccarino, L.; Doria, A. Effectiveness, Tolerability, and Safety of Belimumab in Patients with Refractory SLE: A Review of Observational Clinical-Practice-Based Studies. *Clin. Rev. Allergy Immunol.* **2018**, *54*, 331–343, Erratum in *Clin. Rev. Allergy Immunol.* **2018**, *55*, 237. [CrossRef]
30. Gatto, M.; Saccon, F.; Zen, M.; Regola, F.; Fredi, M.; Andreoli, L.; Tincani, A.; Urban, M.L.; Emmi, G.; Ceccarelli, F.; et al. Early Disease and Low Baseline Damage as Predictors of Response to Belimumab in Patients with Systemic Lupus Erythematosus in a Real-Life Setting. *Arthritis Rheumatol.* **2020**, *72*, 1314–1324. [CrossRef]
31. Bruce, I.N.; Urowitz, M.; van Vollenhoven, R.; Aranow, C.; Fettiplace, J.; Oldham, M.; Wilson, B.; Molta, C.; Roth, D.; Gordon, D. Long-term organ damage accrual and safety in patients with SLE treated with belimumab plus standard of care. *Lupus* **2016**, *25*, 699–709. [CrossRef]
32. Ruiz-Irastorza, G.; Ruiz-Estevez, B.; Lazaro, E.; Ruiz-Arruza, I.; Duffau, P.; Martin-Cascon, M.; Richez, C.; Ugarte, A.; Blanco, P. Prolonged remission in SLE is possible by using reduced doses of prednisone: An observational study from the Lupus-Cruces and Lupus-Bordeaux inception cohorts. *Autoimmun. Rev.* **2019**, *18*, 102359. [CrossRef]
33. Ruiz-Irastorza, G.; Bertsias, G. Treating systemic lupus erythematosus in the 21st century: New drugs and new perspectives on old drugs. *Rheumatology* **2020**, *59* (Suppl. S5), v69–v81. [CrossRef]

Disclaimer/Publisher's Note: The statements, opinions and data contained in all publications are solely those of the individual author(s) and contributor(s) and not of MDPI and/or the editor(s). MDPI and/or the editor(s) disclaim responsibility for any injury to people or property resulting from any ideas, methods, instructions or products referred to in the content.

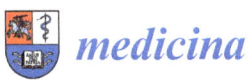

Article

Relationship between Chinese Herbal Medicine Use and Risk of Sjögren's Syndrome in Patients with Rheumatoid Arthritis: A Retrospective, Population-Based, Nested Case-Control Study

Hou-Hsun Liao [1,2,3,†], Hanoch Livneh [4,†], Miao-Chiu Lin [5,†], Ming-Chi Lu [6,7], Ning-Sheng Lai [6,7,*], Hung-Rong Yen [1,8,9,10,11,*] and Tzung-Yi Tsai [3,12,13,*]

1. Graduate Institute of Chinese Medicine, School of Chinese Medicine, College of Chinese Medicine, China Medical University, Taichung 404333, Taiwan; harrisliao@gmail.com
2. Department of Chinese Medicine, Dalin Tzu Chi Hospital, Buddhist Tzu Chi Medical Foundation, Chiayi 62247, Taiwan
3. Department of Nursing, Tzu Chi University of Science and Technology, Hualien 62247, Taiwan
4. Rehabilitation Counseling Program, Portland State University, Portland, OR 97207-0751, USA; livnehh@pdx.edu
5. Department of Nursing, Dalin Tzu Chi Hospital, Buddhist Tzu Chi Medical Foundation, Chiayi 62247, Taiwan; df729376@tzuchi.com.tw
6. School of Medicine, Tzu Chi University, Hualien 97004, Taiwan; dm252940@tzuchi.com.tw
7. Division of Allergy, Immunology and Rheumatology, Dalin Tzu Chi Hospital, Buddhist Tzu Chi Medical Foundation, Chiayi 62247, Taiwan
8. Department of Chinese Medicine, China Medical University Hospital, Taichung 404333, Taiwan
9. Research Center for Traditional Chinese Medicine, Department of Medical Research, China Medical University Hospital, Taichung 404333, Taiwan
10. Chinese Medicine Research Center, China Medical University, Taichung 404333, Taiwan
11. Department of Biotechnology, Asia University, Taichung 41354, Taiwan
12. Department of Environmental and Occupational Health, College of Medicine, National Cheng Kung University, Tainan 70428, Taiwan
13. Department of Medical Research, Dalin Tzu Chi Hospital, Buddhist Tzu Chi Medical Foundation, Chiayi 62247, Taiwan
* Correspondence: q12015@tzuchi.com.tw (N.-S.L.); hungrongyen@gmail.com (H.-R.Y.); dm732024@tzuchi.com.tw (T.-Y.T.); Tel.: +886-5-2648000-8713 (N.-S.L.); +886-4-22053366-3313 (H.-R.Y.); +886-5-2648000-3209 (T.-Y.T.); Fax: +886-5-2648006 (N.-S.L. & T.-Y.T.); +886-4-22037690 (H.-R.Y.)
† These authors contributed equally to this work.

Abstract: *Background and Objectives*: Sjögren's Syndrome (SS) is a common extra-articular feature among subjects with rheumatoid arthritis (RA). While Chinese herbal medicine (CHM) has been used to treat symptoms of RA for many years, few studies have examined its efficacy in guarding against the SS onset. This study aimed to compare risk of SS for RA patients with and without use of CHM. *Materials and Methods*: Data obtained for this nested case-control study were retrieved from Taiwanese nationwide insurance database from 2000–2013. Cases with SS claims were defined and matched to two randomly selected controls without SS from the recruited RA cohorts. Risk of SS in relation to CHM use was estimated by fitting multiple conditional logistic regression. *Results*: Patients aged between 20 and 80 years were included and 916 patients with incident SS were matched to 1832 non-SS controls by age, sex and index year. Among them, 28.1% and 48.4% cases ever received CHM therapy, respectively. After adjusting for baseline characteristics, CHM use was found to be related to a lower risk of SS among them (adjusted odds ratio = 0.40, 95% confidence interval: 0.34–0.47). A dose-dependent, reverse association, was further detected between the cumulative duration of CHM use and SS risk. Those receiving CHM therapy for more than 730 days showed a significantly reduced risk of SS by 83%. *Conclusions*: Findings of this study indicated that the add-on CHM formula, as part of RA care, may be a beneficial treatment for prevention against the incident SS.

Keywords: rheumatoid arthritis; Sjögren's syndrome; Chinese herbal medicines; nested case-control study; risk

Citation: Liao, H.-H.; Livneh, H.; Lin, M.-C.; Lu, M.-C.; Lai, N.-S.; Yen, H.-R.; Tsai, T.-Y. Relationship between Chinese Herbal Medicine Use and Risk of Sjögren's Syndrome in Patients with Rheumatoid Arthritis: A Retrospective, Population-Based, Nested Case-Control Study. *Medicina* **2023**, *59*, 683. https://doi.org/10.3390/medicina59040683

Academic Editor: Daniela Opris-Belinski

Received: 28 February 2023
Revised: 23 March 2023
Accepted: 28 March 2023
Published: 30 March 2023

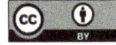

Copyright: © 2023 by the authors. Licensee MDPI, Basel, Switzerland. This article is an open access article distributed under the terms and conditions of the Creative Commons Attribution (CC BY) license (https://creativecommons.org/licenses/by/4.0/).

1. Introduction

Rheumatoid arthritis (RA) is a chronic debilitating inflammatory autoimmune disease that primarily targets joints in the body and other connective tissues. This disorder affects approximately 1% of the population worldwide and is more frequent among women [1]. Just as this chronic disorder has no known cure, estimates indicated that up to 30% of affected patients become permanently work-disabled within the first 2–3 years of symptom onset [2], thus imposing tremendous economic consequences. According to one study conducted in recent year, the economic burden of RA has increased significantly in such a way that the annual economic burden of RA in the United States was $19.3 billion, where the total annual societal cost would rise to nearly 40 billion after adding the intangible and indirect costs [3].

Not only is RA the cause of a profound economic burden, the concomitant systemic inflammation might be responsible for a wide array of comorbid conditions commonly seen in RA, particularly Sjögren's Syndrome [1,4–6]. One meta-analysis of 19 studies reported the pool prevalence of SS among RA patients was as high as 55% [7]. It is also worth noting that the coexistence of RA and SS may pose a higher disease burden than is typical with RA alone. A prior study noted that RA patients with SS may have higher levels of rheumatoid factor or anti-citrullinated peptide antibody than did those with RA alone [8]. Consequently, one recent nationwide survey disclosed that RA subjects with the concomitant SS may have higher risks of comorbidities including cardiovascular disease, malignancies and serious infections [5]. Thus, there is an urgent need for clinical treatments or drugs with safety and efficacy to lessen the disease progression, particularly the incident SS.

Chinese herbal medicine (CHM), long-used in Asian countries to treat RA, has attracted attention for a long time [9]. With the application of omics and bioinformatics to natural herbs research, it had shown that some herb products could exert inhibitory action on inflammatory cytokines that are involved in the pathogenesis of inflammatory diseases [10,11]. Take the Tripterygium wilfordii hook F (TwHF) for example, former studies showed that combination treatment with TwHF and methotrexate (MTX) was more effective than MTX alone in decreasing the secretions of proinflammatory cytokines and tumor necrosis factor-α (TNF-α) [12,13]. Meanwhile, those receiving a combination of TwHF and MTX experienced better control of disease activity when compared to RA patients treated with MTX alone [14]. In light of the aberrant expression of inflammatory mediators that may link RA and SS [15], understanding the relationship between CHM use and sequent SS risk would be of importance in the solution of treatment and clinical management for RA.

As of now, several studies reported that adding CHM to conventional therapy may be beneficial in improving both symptoms burden and lacrimal and salivary dysfunction caused by SS [16]. In contrast, another recent randomized controlled trial identified a null association between CHM use and relief of SS symptoms [17]. Thus, no consensus has been achieved regarding the effect of CHM on the management of SS. Most of the previous studies were based mainly on self-reported questionnaires and chart reviews, and the number of recruited patients was small [16,17]. In accordance with the belief that "an ounce of prevention is worth a pound of cure," early exploration of the impact of CHM on reduction of predisposition to SS, particularly RA subjects, should be stressed. Such documentation would provide an empirically robust ground for health care policymakers to initiate strategies to reduce preventable morbidity among people with SS. To this end, we carried out a nested case-control study using a real-world data to answer this question.

2. Methods

2.1. Data Source and Identification of Study Participants

We applied a retrospective, nested case-control study design using a national health claims from the Longitudinal Health Insurance Database (LHID) in Taiwan. Nowadays, nearly 99% of residents in Taiwan have enrolled in the National Health Insurance Administration Ministry of Health and Welfare's program [18]. LHID is a data subset of the

NHI program and covers the claims of 1 million beneficiaries randomly selected from all beneficiaries under the NHI program. This database contains all NHI enrollment files, claims data, and prescription drug information that provides comprehensive information on all insured subjects.

In the present study, the RA cohort was constructed by identifying all people in the linked claims data set who were 20–80 years of age and had at least three outpatient service claims or one hospital service in which RA was recorded (International Classification of Diseases, 9th Revision, Clinical Modification, ICD-9-CM 714.0) between January 2000 and December 2010. Afterwards, all enrollees were connected to the catastrophic illness registry to ensure diagnostic validity. This is because beneficiaries with major diseases, such as autoimmune disorders, are exempted from the required cost under the NHI program. This approach allowed us to strictly define RA cases and reduce potential misclassification bias. We, therefore, used the date of approval for catastrophic illness registration as the starting point for patients diagnosed with RA. We adhered to the rule that subjects must be excluded if they had any history of SS prior to RA onset. All enrollees were followed up from the date of enrollment to the date of incident SS or the end of follow-up visit, whichever happened first. This article research project was approved by Ethics Committee of the Buddhist Dalin Tzu Chi Hospital (No. B10004021-1) and was conducted with consideration of Helsinki Declaration in all phases of the study. Additionally, the institutional review board waved the need for informed consent for this study since an encrypted database was fully used.

2.2. Identification of Case and Control

The primary outcome measure was first-time diagnosis of SS in which they occurred between 2001 and 2013 (ICD-9-CM code 710.2). The documentation of the SS code was regarded as valid if the enrollee has incurred at least twice in the records of outpatient clinics within 1 year or at least one hospitalization during the study period. We also capitalized on the catastrophic illness registry to ensure the accuracy of enrollees' diagnoses, as conducted in a previous study [19]. We excluded the cases with a diagnosis of SS prior to the onset of RA (n = 144), and removed those patients who were followed for less than one year after cohort entry or those who had missing data (n = 17). The final cohort comprised 10,710 new-onset RA patients. Of them, each SS case was matched, according to age (within 2 years) and sex, using a risk set sampling of 1:2, with two control subjects who were not diagnosed with SS (Figure 1). The outcome date for each case group was assigned as the index date to the control group, for case and control groups with the same probability to occurrence of SS event during the follow-up period.

2.3. Exposure Assessment of CHM Use

To define CHM exposure of subjects, we examined the individual CHM treatment records occurring from the cohort entry date to the index date. Under the NHI program, the medical services used to treat specific diseases that last for 30 days, or more, are considered as one complete course of treatment. In this context, the patients are not required to make copayments for medical services after the first clinic visit throughout the remainder of the treatments. So based on the formerly-established method [20], CHM users were defined as they ever received the relevant CHM treatments being made by the certified Chinese medicine physician for more than 30 days due to RA or its associated symptoms, whereas those visited Western medical doctors only were deemed non-CHM users. For CHM users, we summed up the cumulative days of CHM therapy and categorized them into three levels, low, medium, and high sub-periods, based on the length (in days) of time of receiving CHM therapy, namely, use for 31–365 days, 366–730 days, and 731 days or more. This procedure allowed us to clearly shed light on the dose effect of CHM on the prevention of SS among participants.

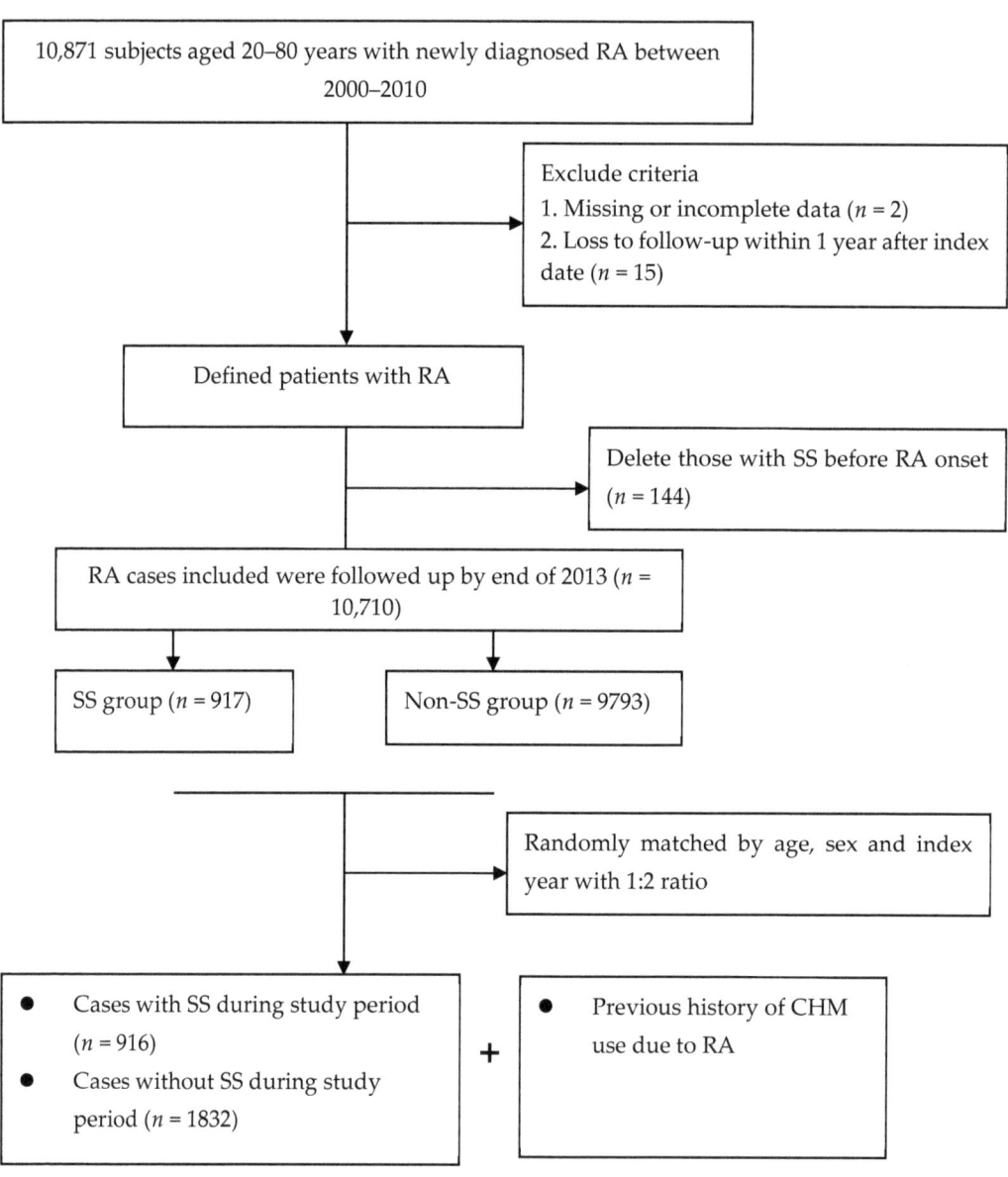

Figure 1. Flowchart of patient screening.

2.4. Measurement of Covariates

Of the covariates considered for the study, it comprised gender, age, income for estimating insurance payment, urbanization of the subject's residential area and former comorbidities. Regarding income, we used the premium category as a proxy and it was transformed to ordinal variables, namely New Taiwan Dollars [NTD] $\leq$ 17,880, 17,881–40,000, and $\geq$ 400,001. Furthermore, we adopted the urbanization rate of insured zone studied by former scholars, and ranging from level 1 (highly urban) to level 7 (highly rural), as the standard to assess personal urbanization [21]. Baseline comorbidities for each subject were assessed on the basis of individual medical records that occurred within one year prior to cohort entry, and all of them were evaluated by the established Charlson–Deyo comorbidity index (CCI) [22]. It contains 17 chronic diseases and scores on a score of 1–6, revealing higher total scores indicated severer burdens of comorbidities. Medication use was separated into two subgroups according to if the enrollee had (vs. not used at all) the disease-modifying anti-rheumatic drugs, or corticosteroids, for more than 180 days after RA onset.

2.5. Statistical Modeling

For baseline characteristics, continuous variables were represented as the mean (standard deviation, SD) and categorical variables reported as frequencies and percentages. The student's *t*-test and Chi-square test were used to evaluate whether there was a significant difference between two groups. Univariate conditional logistic regression analysis was used to estimate the crude odds ratio (OR) and the corresponding confidence interval (CI) of SS events among CHM users. Multivariate conditional logistic regression was then performed in which the results were adjusted for all covariates that were measured in one year preceding the index date, which included age, gender, urbanization level, income and comorbidities. Subgroup analysis stratified by sex and age was also performed. All data processing and statistical analyses were performed using SAS version 9.3 for Windows (SAS Institute Inc., Cary, NC, USA). The statistical significance was determined at two-tailed and $p < 0.05$.

3. Results

A total of 10,710 RA patients who met the selection criteria during 2000–2010 were identified. Among them, 916 and 1832 matched pairs of RA patients with and without SS were recruited. Baseline characteristics are shown in Table 1. The mean age was 53.2 years (SD = 14.4) and the majority were female (86.9%). Additionally, the majority of enrollees had a monthly income of NTD 17,881–43,900 (52.0%) and lived in urbanized areas (57.2%). Collectively, there were no differences in initial demographic data or comorbidities between two groups.

Table 1. Demographic data and selected comorbidities between two groups.

Variables	Total Group	Case N = 916 (%)	Control N = 1832 (%)	p
Age (years)				0.47
≤50	1254 (45.6)	427 (46.6)	827 (45.1)	
>50	1494 (54.4)	489 (53.4)	1005 (54.9)	
Mean (SD)	53.2 (14.4)	53.1 (14.8)	53.3 (13.9)	0.81
Sex				0.99
Female	2388 (86.9)	796 (86.9)	1592 (87.0)	
Male	360 (13.1)	120 (13.1)	240 (13.0)	
Monthly income				0.53
Low	1210 (44.1)	406 (44.3)	804 (43.9)	
Median	1430 (52.0)	469 (51.2)	961 (52.5)	
High	108 (3.9)	41 (4.5)	67 (3.7)	
Residential area				0.66
Urban	1572 (57.2)	516 (56.2)	1057 (57.7)	
Suburban	416 (15.1)	128 (15.9)	270 (14.7)	
Rural	760 (27.7)	272 (27.9)	505 (27.6)	
Medication use				0.67
Yes	2038 (74.2)	684 (74.7)	1354 (73.9)	
No	710 (25.8)	232 (25.3)	478 (26.1)	
CCI	4.73 (7.9)	4.59 (7.8)	4.86 (8.0)	0.40

CCI: Charlson–Deyo Comorbidity Index; SD: standard deviation.

Of the whole study cohort, after using multivariable logistic regression model to explore the association between previous exposure of CHM use and SS risk by the end of 2013 (Table 2), we observed that those who ever received CHM therapy had a lower risk of SS than those who did not use CHM (adjusted OR = 0.40; 95% CI: 0.34–0.47). Notably, this benefit increased with longer exposure to CHM use, from 56% of those using low intensity CHM, to 58% of those using medium intensity CHM, and to 83% for those receiving high intensity CHM, thus suggesting a dose-dependent inverse relationship between CHM use and SS risk. Table 3 presents these results, stratified by age and sex. Multivariable stratified analysis showed that the benefit of CHM therapy in reducing SS appeared to be more predominant in females, with an adjusted OR of 0.38 (95% CI: 0.32–0.46) (Table 3). Furthermore, of the commonly prescribed CHM formulas, uses of several prescriptions may be related to the lower risk of SS, which contained Da Huang, Shu-Jing-Huo-Xue-Tang (SJHXT), Du-Huo-Ji-Sheng-Tang (DHJST), Ge-Gen-Tang (GGT), Ping-Wei-San (PWS), Shao-Yao-Gan-Cao-Tang (SYGCT), and Zhi-Gan-Cao-Tang (ZHCT) (Figure 2).

Table 2. The association between SS onset and use of CHM.

CHM Exposure	Subjects				Crude OR (95% CI)	Adjusted OR * (95% CI)
	Case n = 916		Control n = 1832			
Non-CHM users	659	72%	945	52%	1	1
CHM users	257	28%	887	48%	0.42 (0.35–0.49)	0.40 (0.34–0.47)
Low intensity (31–365 days)	215	23%	720	39%	0.44 (0.30–0.64)	0.44 (0.30–0.65)
Medium intensity (366–730 days)	35	4%	112	6%	0.43 (0.36–0.51)	0.42 (0.35–0.50)
High intensity (731 days or more)	7	1%	55	3%	0.18 (0.09–0.34)	0.17 (0.10–0.32)

OR: odds ratio; CI: confidence interval; CHM: Chinese herbal medicine. * Model adjusted for age, residential area, monthly income, medication use and CCI.

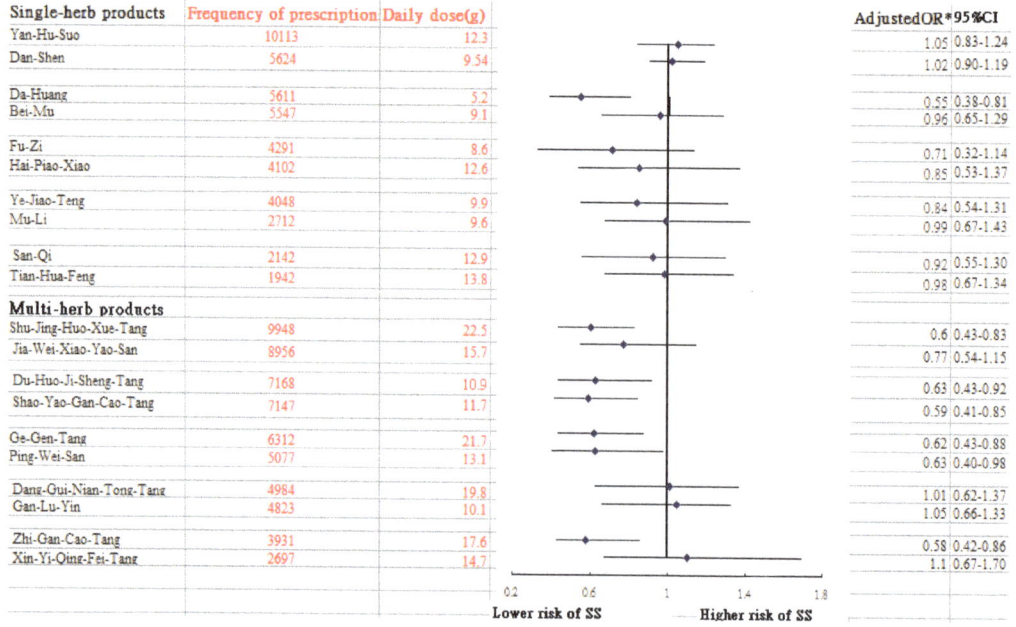

Figure 2. Risk of SS in relation to the 10 most-used single-herb and multi-herb CHM products for RA patients. * Model adjusted for age, residential area, monthly income, medication use and CCI.

Table 3. SS risk for RA patients with and without CHM use stratified by sex and age.

Variables	Subjects, n (%)	Crude OR (95% CI)	Adjusted OR * (95% CI)
Female			
Non-CHM users	566 (71.1)	1	1
CHM users	230 (28.9)	0.39 (0.33–0.47)	0.38 (0.32–0.46)
Male			
Non-CHM users	93 (77.5)	1	1
CHM users	27 (22.5)	0.62 (0.37–1.02)	0.63 (0.37–1.03)
Age ≤ 50			
Non-CHM users	291 (68.1)	1	1
CHM users	136 (31.9)	0.38 (0.30–0.48)	0.37 (0.29–0.47)
Age > 50			
Non-CHM users	368 (75.3)	1	1
CHM users	121 (24.7)	0.44 (0.35–0.56)	0.42 (0.35–0.49)

OR: odds ratio; CI: confidence interval; CHM: Chinese herbal medicine. * Model adjusted for age, residential area, monthly income, medication use and CCI.

4. Discussion

SS is a chronic autoimmune disease characterized by autoantibody production and lymphocytic infiltration, which has been well recognized as one important extra-articular feature of RA to exacerbate the negative clinical prognosis for RA patients. Faced with few specific strategies of prevention of SS in the standard treatment, exploring alternative treatments is of great therapeutic interest. As a whole, in this over 10-year follow-up study, we had provided the first evidence to indicate the integration CHM into the standard treatments was related to the lower risk of having SS. Notably, this benefit could be increased with a long-term exposure to CHM use, from 56% for those using CHM for 31–365 days, to 58% for those using CHM for 366–730 days, and to 83% for those receiving CHM for more than two years. The establishment of dose-response relationship in this observational study may support the causal association between exposure and disease. Despite the lack of comparable literature, the positive effect of CHM on SS prevention among these patients could add to the growing body of literature on the clinical efficacy of complementary therapies among patients diagnosed with rheumatic diseases [23–25]. A variety of natural products from traditional Chinese medicine have been shown to possess effective anti-inflammatory along with antiarthritic activities [26,27], which may explain the beneficial effect of CHM found in our work.

Findings of the present study indicated that female patients benefited more from CHM use than did males. As others have shown, females often display better knowledge, attitudes, and self-care practices [28], and accordingly, they may tend to adhere to the prescribed medical regimen, thus decreasing their chance of developing SS. In addition, sex hormones, especially estrogen, have been shown to exert anti-inflammatory effects. One study showed that high levels of estrogens were beneficial in downregulating the expression of the inflammatory mediators [29], which has been proven to take on the role of development of SS [11].

Of the commonly used single-herb products to treat RA, we noted that the prescription of Da-Huang might lessen the risk of SS. Pharmacological studies have shown that Da-Huang dose-dependently moderates the release of nitric oxide in lipopolysaccharide-stimulated macrophage RAW264.7 cells and remarkably reduces IL-6 and IL-1β secretion via mediation of the PI3K-Akt signaling pathway [30]. This action could account for the positive effect of Da-Huang observed in this study. Of the commonly used multi-herb products, we observed that DHJST use was associated with a decreased chance of SS among RA patients. A previous study reported that DHJST exerts a powerful anti-inflammatory effect [31]. The relevant mechanisms by which DHJST inhibits expression of cytokines, like TNF-α, IL-1β and IL 6, may involve regulation of the toll-like receptor 4 (TLR4)/NF-κB signaling pathway [32]. The TLR4/NF-κB signaling pathway plays a central role in driving inflammation via the differentiation and amplification of T helper17 together with over-expression of inflammatory mediators [33,34], thus promoting susceptibility to SS.

The current study pointed to a lower incidence of SS among RA patients who used SJHXT and SYGCT. Clinically, these CHM products are often prescribed to arthritis patients for the treatment of muscle pain. One earlier study in a rodent model suggested that SJHXT may intensify anti-inflammatory and analgesic effects by modulating the activity of the α-2 adrenoceptor [35]. A review article reported that dysregulation of the α2- adrenoceptor pathway may contribute to the aberrant cytokine gene expression [36]. SYGCT use also correlated with a lower risk of SS. Chang and colleagues reported that this compound markedly inhibited the production of inflammatory mediators in rats with polycystic ovary syndrome by blocking TLR4/NF-κB signal pathway [37]. This pathway promotes proinflammatory activities in immune cells, thereby leading to a variety of other inflammatory and autoimmune disorders [34].

An association between ZGCT and PWS use and a decreased rate of SS development in RA patients was reported as well. Several previous animal experiments have shown that the anti-inflammatory properties of these compounds were also present in compound extracts, including *Radix glycyrrhiza* from ZGCT [38], and *Magnolia officinalis* from PWS [39]. The mechanisms by which these ingredients markedly decrease the secretion of inflammatory cytokines may be due in part to the inhibition of NF-κB and mitogen-associated kinase signaling pathways [38,39]. Ge-Gen-Tang is proposed to exert anti-oxidant and anti-inflammatory activities by suppressing inflammatory signaling. Puerarin, a major ingredient of GGT, has proven to suppress inflammatory mediator release by blocking NF-κB in lipopolysaccharide-induced peripheral blood mononuclear cells [40], decreasing to some extent the risk of SS.

Despite its obvious strengths, several important limitations restrict the significance of our study. First, information regarding family history, lifestyle, body weight, exercise and laboratory parameters were not recorded in the database. Thus, it is possible that one or more confounding variables may be partly responsible for this association. Therefore, caution should be exerted when interpreting the findings, especially regarding daily drug dosage. A randomized controlled trial is warranted in order to examine, more thoroughly, the potential mechanisms underlying the clinical benefits of CHM products in controlling the development of SS. Second, the findings herein are merely based on a nested case-control design within a retrospective cohort study that uses ICD-9-CM diagnostic codes. Thus, bias due to miscoding and misclassification may arise. To minimize this potential error, we selected subjects with either RA or SS only after they were recorded as having at least three ambulatory or inpatient claims reporting consistent diagnoses. It should also be acknowledged that the NHI Bureau of Taiwan has randomly reviewed the charts and audited all medical charges, and given heavy penalties for outlier charges or malpractice to validate the quality of data. Additionally, as the probability of individuals being misclassified is equal for the two groups, a non-differential misclassification would only result in bias toward the null-value. Third, data regarding RA severity were unavailable in the database, and failure to examine this factor might bias any conclusions. To address this concern, we utilized a proxy indicator to confirm RA severity. The indicator was comprised of the prescriptions of biological agents which included adalimumab, etanercept, infliximab, rituximab and tocilizumab. Findings from the reanalysis showed that those who did use CHM still had a lower risk of SS than those who were not receiving CHM treatment (adjusted OR = 0.45; 95% CI = 0.31–0.58), which implied that the severity of RA dose not alter the direction of association between CHM treatment and likelihood of SS. After acknowledging the limitations of the research, this study has several strengths that bolster the value of the findings. The first strength stems from the use of a large population database. Over 90% of the Taiwanese population and healthcare providers are covered by the NHI program, which includes a representative Taiwanese RA sample, leaving little room for non-response or loss to follow-up, especially given the relatively low incidence of RA in the population. The second merit stems from the long observation time used in our study. SS is a chronic disease and the employed longer than 10-year follow-up period allowed us ample opportunity to observe and assess the underlying correlation. Lastly, the nested case-control approach used is a rival alternative to a cohort analysis when studying time-dependent exposure, as in the use of CHM treatments. Hence, our study reflects real-world data that approximate those present in clinical reports using a randomized controlled trial.

5. Conclusions

To summarize our findings, this population-based nested case-control study revealed that the integration of CHM, during routine treatment of RA, lessens the risk of developing SS by approximately 60%. We believe that these findings may help to plan interventions to make complementary therapies more responsive to the needs of individuals living with RA. Future research efforts should adopt prospective randomized trials to overcome the disadvantages of this study, thus providing more robust insights in clinical practice.

Author Contributions: Conceptualization, H.-H.L., H.L., M.-C.L. (Miao-Chiu Lin) and T.-Y.T.; methodology, H.-H.L., H.L., N.-S.L. and T.-Y.T.; software, H.-H.L., M.-C.L. (Ming-Chi Lu), H.-R.Y. and T.-Y.T.; validation, H.-H.L., H.-R.Y., N.-S.L. and T.-Y.T.; formal analysis, H.L., M.-C.L. (Miao-Chiu Lin) and T.-Y.T.; investigation, H.-H.L., M.-C.L. (Miao-Chiu Lin) and T.-Y.T.; resources, M.-C.L. (Ming-Chi Lu), H.-R.Y., and N.-S.L.; data curation, M.-C.L. (Ming-Chi Lu), H.-R.Y. and T.-Y.T.; writing—original draft preparation, H.-H.L., H.L., M.-C.L. (Miao-Chiu Lin), N.-S.L., H.-R.Y. and T.-Y.T.; writing—review and editing, H.-H.L., H.L., M.-C.L. (Miao-Chiu Lin), N.-S.L., H.-R.Y., M.-C.L. (Ming-Chi Lu) and T.-Y.T.; visualization, M.-C.L. (Ming-Chi Lu), H.-R.Y. and T.-Y.T.; supervision, N.-S.L., H.-R.Y. and T.-Y.T.; project administration, N.-S.L., H.-R.Y. and M.-C.L. (Ming-Chi Lu). All authors have read and agreed to the published version of the manuscript.

Funding: This work did not receive any specific grant from funding agencies in the public, commercial, or not-for-profit sectors.

Institutional Review Board Statement: This article research project was approved by Ethics Committee of the Buddhist Dalin Tzu Chi Hospital (No. B10004021-1) and was conducted with consideration of Helsinki Declaration in all phases of the study. Additionally, the institutional review board waved the need for informed consent for this study since an encrypted database was fully used.

Informed Consent Statement: Not applicable.

Data Availability Statement: The datasets analyzed in this article are not publicly available. Data are available from the National Health Insurance Research Database (NHIRD) published by Taiwan National Health Insurance (NHI) Bureau. Due to legal restrictions imposed by the government of Taiwan in relation to the "Personal Information Protection Act", data cannot be made publicly available. Requests to access the datasets should be directed to the NHIRD and the corresponding authors.

Acknowledgments: This study obtained data from the National Health Insurance Research Database provided by the Bureau of National Health Insurance, managed by the Department of Health and Welfare, Taiwan. The main mission of the authority is to ensure that universal participation and equal-opportunity of medical care are being fulfilled. The interpretation and conclusions contained herein do not represent those of the Bureau of National Health Insurance, Department of Health, or of the National Health Research Institutes.

Conflicts of Interest: The authors declare no conflict of interest.

References

1. Almutairi, K.; Nossent, J.; Preen, D.; Keen, H.; Inderjeeth, C. The global prevalence of rheumatoid arthritis: A meta-analysis based on a systematic review. *Rheumatol. Int.* **2021**, *41*, 863–877. [CrossRef]
2. Sokka, T. Work disability in early rheumatoid arthritis. *Clin. Exp. Rheumatol.* **2003**, *21*, S71–S74.
3. Chen, C.I.; Wang, L.; Wei, W.; Yuce, H.; Phillips, K. Burden of rheumatoid arthritis among US medicare population: Co-morbidities, health-care resource utilization and costs. *Rheumatol. Adv. Pract.* **2018**, *2*, I1–I9. [CrossRef] [PubMed]
4. Santosh, K.; Dhir, V.; Singh, S.; Sood, A.; Gupta, A.; Sharma, A.; Sharma, S. Prevalence of secondary Sjögren's syndrome in Indian patients with rheumatoid arthritis: A single-center study. *Int. J. Rheum. Dis.* **2017**, *20*, 870–874. [CrossRef] [PubMed]

5. Harrold, L.R.; Shan, Y.; Rebello, S.; Kramer, N.; Connolly, S.E.; Alemao, E.; Kelly, S.; Kremer, J.M.; Rosenstein, E.D. Prevalence of Sjögren's syndrome associated with rheumatoid arthritis in the USA: An observational study from the Corrona registry. *Clin. Rheumatol.* **2020**, *39*, 1899–1905. [CrossRef] [PubMed]
6. Andonopoulos, A.P.; Drosos, A.A.; Skopouli, F.N.; Moutsopoulos, H.M. Sjögren's syndrome in rheumatoid arthritis and progressive systemic sclerosis. A comparative study. *Clin. Exp. Rheumatol.* **1989**, *7*, 203–205.
7. Alani, H.; Henty, J.R.; Thompson, N.L.; Jury, E.; Ciurtin, C. Systematic review and meta-analysis of the epidemiology of polyautoimmunity in Sjögren's syndrome (secondary Sjögren's syndrome) focusing on autoimmune rheumatic diseases. *Scand. J. Rheumatol.* **2018**, *47*, 141–154. [CrossRef]
8. Brown, L.E.; Frits, M.L.; Iannaccone, C.K.; Weinblatt, M.E.; Shadick, N.A.; Liao, K.P. Clinical characteristics of RA patients with secondary SS and association with joint damage. *Rheumatology* **2015**, *54*, 816–820. [CrossRef]
9. Lee, W.Y.; Chen, H.Y.; Chen, K.C.; Chen, Y.C. Treatment of rheumatoid arthritis with traditional Chinese medicine. *BioMed. Res. Int.* **2014**, *2014*, 11. [CrossRef]
10. Zhang, L.W.; Zhou, P.R.; Wei, P.; Cong, X.; Wu, L.L.; Hua, H. Expression of interleukin-17 in primary Sjögren's syndrome and the correlation with disease severity: A systematic review and meta-analysis. *Scand. J. Immunol.* **2018**, *87*, e12649. [CrossRef]
11. Benchabane, S.; Boudjelida, A.; Toumi, R.; Belguendouz, H.; Youinou, P.; Touil-Boukoffa, C. A case for IL-6, IL-17A, and nitric oxide in the pathophysiology of Sjögren's syndrome. *Int. J. Immunopathol. Pharmacol.* **2016**, *29*, 386–397. [CrossRef] [PubMed]
12. Wang, S.; Li, R.; He, S.; He, L.; Zhao, H.; Deng, X.; Chen, Z. Tripterygium wilfordii glycosides upregulate the new anti-inflammatory cytokine IL-37 through ERK1/2 and p38 mapk signal pathways. *Evid. Based Complement. Alternat. Med.* **2017**, *2017*, 9148523. [CrossRef] [PubMed]
13. Tang, Y.; Liu, Q.; Feng, Y.; Zhang, Y.; Xu, Z.; Wen, C.; Zhang, Y. Tripterygium ingredients for pathogenicity cells in rheumatoid arthritis. *Front. Pharmacol.* **2020**, *11*, 583171. [CrossRef]
14. Zhou, Y.Z.; Zhao, L.D.; Chen, H.; Zhang, Y.; Wang, D.F.; Huang, L.F.; Lv, Q.W.; Liu, B.; Li, Z.; Wei, W.; et al. Comparison of the impact of Tripterygium wilfordii Hook F and Methotrexate treatment on radiological progression in active rheumatoid arthritis: 2-year follow up of a randomized, non-blinded, controlled study. *Arthritis Res. Ther.* **2018**, *20*, 70. [CrossRef]
15. Patel, R.; Shahane, A. The epidemiology of Sjögren's syndrome. *Clin. Epidemiol.* **2014**, *6*, 247–255. [PubMed]
16. Luo, H.; Li, X.; Liu, J.; Andrew, F.; George, L. Chinese Herbal medicine in treating primary sjogren's syndrome: A systematic review of randomized trials. *Evid. Based Complement. Alternat. Med.* **2012**, *2012*, 640658. [CrossRef] [PubMed]
17. Chen, H.H.; Lai, J.N.; Yu, M.C.; Chen, C.Y.; Hsieh, Y.T.; Hsu, Y.F.; Wei, J.C. Traditional Chinese medicine in patients with primary sjogren's syndrome: A randomized, double-blind, placebo-controlled clinical trial. *Front. Med.* **2021**, *8*, 744194. [CrossRef]
18. National Health Insurance Database. LHID 2000. Available online: https://nhird.nhri.org.tw/en/Data_Subsets.html (accessed on 7 January 2022).
19. Chung, Y.J.; Wei, C.K.; Livneh, H.; Lai, N.S.; Lu, M.C.; Liao, H.H.; Tsai, T.Y. Relationship between the use of Chinese herbal medicines and Sjögren syndrome risk among women with menopause: A retrospective cohort study. *Menopause* **2020**, *28*, 58–64. [CrossRef]
20. Li, H.H.; Livneh, H.; Chen, W.J.; Fan, W.L.; Lu, M.C.; Guo, H.R.; Tsai, T.Y. Effect of Chinese herbal medicines on hearing loss risk in rheumatoid arthritis patients: Retrospective claims analysis. *Front. Med.* **2021**, *8*, 683211. [CrossRef]
21. Liu, C.Y.; Hung, Y.T.; Chuang, Y.L.; Chen, Y.J.; Weng, W.S.; Liu, J.S.; Liang, K.Y. Incorporating development stratification of Taiwan townships into sampling design of large scale health interview survey. *J. Health Manag.* **2006**, *4*, 1–22.
22. Deyo, R.A.; Cherkin, D.C.; Ciol, M.A. Adapting a clinical comorbidity index for use with ICD-9-CM administrative databases. *J. Clin. Epidemiol.* **1992**, *45*, 613–619. [CrossRef] [PubMed]
23. Pan, H.D.; Xiao, Y.; Wang, W.Y.; Ren, R.T.; Leung, E.L.; Liu, L. Traditional Chinese medicine as a treatment for rheumatoid arthritis: From empirical practice to evidence-based therapy. *Engineering* **2019**, *5*, 895–906. [CrossRef]
24. Tognolo, L.; Coraci, D.; Fioravanti, A.; Tenti, S.; Scanu, A.; Magro, G.; Maccarone, M.C.; Masiero, S. Clinical impact of balneotherapy and therapeutic exercise in rheumatic diseases: A lexical analysis and scoping review. *Appl. Sci.* **2022**, *12*, 7379. [CrossRef]
25. Maccarone, M.C.; Magro, G.; Solimene, U.; Scanu, A.; Masiero, S. From in vitro research to real life studies: An extensive narrative review of the effects of balneotherapy on human immune response. *Sport Sci. Health.* **2021**, *17*, 817–835. [CrossRef] [PubMed]
26. Pan, M.H.; Chiou, Y.S.; Tsai, M.L.; Ho, C.T. Anti-inflammatory activity of traditional Chinese medicinal herbs. *J. Tradit. Complement. Med.* **2011**, *1*, 8–24. [CrossRef] [PubMed]
27. Luo, J.; Ming, B.; Zhang, C.; Deng, X.; Li, P.; Wei, Z.; Xia, Y.; Jiang, K.; Ye, H.; Ma, W.; et al. IL-2 Inhibition of Th17 generation rather than induction of treg cells is impaired in primary sjögren's syndrome patients. *Front. Immunol.* **2018**, *9*, 1755. [CrossRef]
28. Shih, C.C.; Liao, C.C.; Su, Y.C.; Tsai, C.C.; Lin, J.G. Gender differences in traditional Chinese medicine use among adults in Taiwan. *PLoS ONE* **2012**, *7*, e32540. [CrossRef]
29. Shivers, K.Y.; Amador, N.; Abrams, L.; Hunter, D.; Jenab, S.; Quiñones-Jenab, V. Estrogen alters baseline and inflammatory-induced cytokine levels independent from hypothalamic-pituitary-adrenal axis activity. *Cytokine* **2015**, *72*, 121–129. [CrossRef]
30. Hu, B.; Zhang, H.; Meng, X.; Wang, F.; Wang, P. Aloe-emodin from rhubarb (*Rheum rhabarbarum*) inhibits lipopolysaccharide-induced inflammatory responses in RAW264.7 macrophages. *J. Ethnopharmacol.* **2014**, *153*, 846–853. [CrossRef]
31. Wenjin, C.; Jianwei, W. Protective effect of gentianine, a compound from Du Huo Ji Sheng Tang, against freund's complete adjuvant-induced arthritis in rats. *Inflammation* **2017**, *40*, 1401–1408. [CrossRef]

32. Wang, N.; Liu, Y.; Jia, C.; Gao, C.; Zheng, T.; Wu, M.; Zhang, Q.; Zhao, X.; Li, Z.; Chen, J.; et al. Machine learning enables discovery of Gentianine targeting TLR4/NF-κB pathway to repair ischemic stroke injury. *Pharmacol. Res.* **2021**, *173*, 105913. [CrossRef] [PubMed]
33. Kiripolsky, J.; Kramer, J.M. Current and emerging evidence for toll-like receptor activation in sjögren's syndrome. *J. Immunol. Res.* **2018**, *2018*, 1246818. [CrossRef] [PubMed]
34. Sisto, M.; Ribatti, D.; Lisi, S. Understanding the complexity of sjögren's syndrome: Remarkable progress in elucidating NF-κB mechanisms. *J. Clin. Med.* **2020**, *9*, 2821. [CrossRef] [PubMed]
35. Shu, H.; Arita, H.; Hayashida, M.; Zhang, L.; An, K.; Huang, W.; Hanaoka, K. Anti-hypersensitivity effects of Shu-jing-huo-xue-tang, a Chinese herbal medicine, in CCI-neuropathic rats. *J. Ethnopharmacol.* **2010**, *131*, 464–470. [CrossRef]
36. Scanzano, A.; Cosentino, M. Adrenergic regulation of innate immunity: A review. *Front. Pharmacol.* **2015**, *6*, 171. [CrossRef]
37. Chang, Z.P.; Deng, G.F.; Shao, Y.Y.; Xu, D.; Zhao, Y.N.; Sun, Y.F.; Zhang, S.Q.; Hou, R.G.; Liu, J.J. Shaoyao-gancao decoction ameliorates the inflammation state in polycystic ovary syndrome rats via remodeling gut microbiota and suppressing the TLR4/NF-κB pathway. *Front. Pharmacol.* **2021**, *12*, 670054. [CrossRef] [PubMed]
38. Yang, X.L.; Liu, D.; Bian, K.; Zhang, D.D. Study on in vitro anti-inflammatory activity of total flavonoids from glycyrrhizae radix et rhizoma and its ingredients. *Zhongguo Zhong Yao Za Zhi* **2013**, *38*, 99–104.
39. Zhang, Z.; Cao, H.; Shen, P.; Liu, J.; Cao, Y.; Zhang, N. Ping weisan alleviates chronic colitis in mice by regulating intestinal microbiota composition. *J. Ethnopharmacol.* **2020**, *255*, 112715. [CrossRef]
40. Zhang, S.; Wang, J.; Zhao, H.; Luo, Y. Effects of three flavonoids from an ancient traditional Chinese medicine radix puerariae on geriatric diseases. *Brain Circ.* **2018**, *4*, 174–184.

Disclaimer/Publisher's Note: The statements, opinions and data contained in all publications are solely those of the individual author(s) and contributor(s) and not of MDPI and/or the editor(s). MDPI and/or the editor(s) disclaim responsibility for any injury to people or property resulting from any ideas, methods, instructions or products referred to in the content.

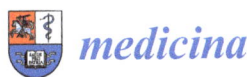

Article

Association of Clinical Manifestations of Systemic Lupus Erythematosus and Complementary Therapy Use in Taiwanese Female Patients: A Cross-Sectional Study

Ming-Chi Lu [1,2], Chia-Wen Hsu [3], Hui-Chin Lo [3], Hsiu-Hua Chang [3] and Malcolm Koo [4,5,*]

1. Division of Allergy, Immunology and Rheumatology, Dalin Tzu Chi Hospital, Buddhist Tzu Chi Medical Foundation, Dalin, Chiayi 622401, Taiwan; e360187@yahoo.com.tw
2. School of Medicine, Tzu Chi University, Hualien City 97004, Taiwan
3. Department of Medical Research, Dalin Tzu Chi Hospital, Buddhist Tzu Chi Medical Foundation, Dalin, Chiayi 622401, Taiwan; chiawen0114@yahoo.com.tw (C.-W.H.); df289469@tzuchi.com.tw (H.-C.L.); df274760@tzuchi.com.tw (H.-H.C.)
4. Graduate Institute of Long-Term Care, Tzu Chi University of Science and Technology, Hualien City 970302, Taiwan
5. Dalla Lana School of Public Health, University of Toronto, Toronto, ON M5T 3M7, Canada
* Correspondence: m.koo@utoronto.ca

Abstract: *Background and Objectives*: Systemic lupus erythematosus (SLE) is a chronic systemic autoimmune disease that affects predominantly women in the childbearing years. Patients may seek complementary therapies to manage their health and to reduce symptoms. However, to our knowledge, no studies have explored the association between clinical manifestations of SLE and complementary therapies. Therefore, this study aimed to investigate the association of complementary therapies with common clinical manifestations in Taiwanese female patients with SLE. *Materials and Methods*: A cross-sectional study was conducted at a regional teaching hospital in southern Taiwan. Outpatients from the rheumatology clinic who met the inclusion criteria were consecutively recruited. Demographic data, clinical manifestations of SLE, and types of complementary therapy use were determined using paper-based questionnaire. Multiple logistic regression analyses were conducted to investigate the use of complementary therapies associated with clinical manifestations of SLE. *Results*: Of the 317 female patients with SLE, 60.9% were 40 years or older. The five SLE clinical manifestations with the highest prevalence were Raynaud's phenomenon (61.2%), photosensitivity (50.2%), Sjögren's syndrome (28.4%), arthralgia and arthritis (22.1%), and renal involvement (14.5%). Multiple logistic regression analyses revealed that Raynaud's phenomenon was significantly associated with fitness walking or strolling (adjusted odds ratio [aOR] 1.77; $p = 0.027$) and fish oil supplements (aOR 3.55, $p < 0.001$). Photosensitivity was significantly and inversely associated with the use of probiotics (aOR 0.49; $p = 0.019$). Renal involvement was significantly associated with the use of probiotics (aOR 2.43; $p = 0.026$) and visit to the Chinese medicine department in a hospital (aOR 3.14, $p = 0.026$). *Conclusions*: We found that different clinical manifestations of SLE were associated with the use of different complementary therapies. Health care providers should have up-to-date knowledge of common complementary therapies and be ready to provide evidence-based advice to patients with SLE.

Keywords: systemic lupus erythematosus; complementary medicine; clinical manifestations; probiotics; Raynaud's phenomenon

Citation: Lu, M.-C.; Hsu, C.-W.; Lo, H.-C.; Chang, H.-H.; Koo, M. Association of Clinical Manifestations of Systemic Lupus Erythematosus and Complementary Therapy Use in Taiwanese Female Patients: A Cross-Sectional Study. *Medicina* 2022, 58, 944. https://doi.org/10.3390/medicina58070944

Academic Editor: Shoenfeld Yehuda

Received: 7 June 2022
Accepted: 13 July 2022
Published: 17 July 2022

Publisher's Note: MDPI stays neutral with regard to jurisdictional claims in published maps and institutional affiliations.

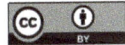

Copyright: © 2022 by the authors. Licensee MDPI, Basel, Switzerland. This article is an open access article distributed under the terms and conditions of the Creative Commons Attribution (CC BY) license (https://creativecommons.org/licenses/by/4.0/).

1. Introduction

Systemic lupus erythematosus (SLE) is a complex, chronic, systemic autoimmune disease that mainly affects women of childbearing age. The worldwide prevalence of SLE varied considerably from 2 to 7 per 10,000 people [1]. In Taiwan, the reported incidence of SLE in 2011 was 8.1 per 10,000 people with 14.3 and 1.6 per 10,000 women and men, respectively [2]. Many organs or systems can be involved, leading to multiple clinical manifestations in patients with SLE. In addition, poor body image, severe fatigue, and psychological morbidity could negatively affect health-related quality of life, resulting in a high prevalence of disability among patients with SLE [3,4].

Despite the substantial progress in the medical treatment of SLE, patients continue to live with a range of clinical symptoms, such as fatigue, joint pain, and skin rash [5]. In addition to conventional pharmacological therapies, patients may seek various complementary therapies to manage their chronic symptoms. While there is not yet a universal accepted operational definition of complementary therapies [6], it was estimated that more than half of patients with SLE had used complementary therapies to manage their health and to reduce symptoms [7]. A nationwide survey in the United Kingdom of 2527 people with SLE revealed that 32% of them sought complementary therapies, with acupuncture, massage, and vitamin supplements being the most commonly used [8]. Moreover, our previous study showed that over 85% of Taiwanese patients with SLE used complementary therapies on a regular basis. The top five popular types of complementary therapies used were fitness walking or strolling, Buddhist prayer or attending temples, vitamins, calcium supplements, and fish oil [9]. Nevertheless, while there is some evidence that certain complementary therapies could be beneficial for certain clinical conditions, studies on their efficacy and long-term safety are still limited [10].

Motivation to use complementary therapies in patients with SLE is complex. A study conducted in a tertiary-care rheumatology center in Singapore revealed that there were two types of users—those who intended to use complementary therapies to treat SLE and those who used them for general health maintenance [11]. Furthermore, a systematic review of randomized controlled trials of non-pharmacologic therapies, predominantly psychological interventions, in patients with SLE revealed that these therapies were significantly associated with an improvement in fatigue, anxiety and depression, and pain in some studies [12]. However, to our knowledge, there were no studies on the association between common clinical manifestations of SLE and the use of various complementary therapies. Therefore, the aim to this study was to investigate the association of prevalent SLE clinical manifestations and complementary therapy use in Taiwanese female patients with SLE.

2. Materials and Methods

2.1. Study Design and Population

This cross-sectional study was a sub-study of our previous investigation of factors associated with the use of complementary therapies among Taiwanese patients with SLE [9]. In the present study, we focused on the use of complementary therapy in female patients with different clinical manifestations of SLE. Only female patients were analyzed because the clinical manifestations of SLE are different between the sexes [13].

Outpatients attending the rheumatology clinic in a regional teaching hospital in southern Taiwan were consecutively recruited into the study between April and August 2019. A paper-based questionnaire was used to obtain information from the patients. Two rheumatology clinic research nurses were available to assist with the completion of the questionnaire, if necessary.

The sample size was estimated using G*Power software (version 3.1.9.4) [14]. For a multiple regression analysis with 20 predictors, α of 0.05, power of 90%, and Cohen's f^2 effect size of 0.09, 307 participants would be needed. The f^2 was set at halfway between a small effect size (0.02) and a medium (0.15) effect size [15].

The study was conducted according to the guidelines of the Declaration of Helsinki, and all patients signed an informed consent. The study protocol was approved by the institutional review board of Dalin Tzu Chi Hospital, Buddhist Tzu Chi Medical Foundation (No. B10801017).

2.2. Inclusion and Exclusion Criteria

The inclusion criteria for this study were female patients aged ≥ 20 years, those who met clinician-confirmed diagnosis of SLE according to the 1997 American College of Rheumatology revised criteria [16] or the 2012 Systemic Lupus International Collaborating Clinics Classification Criteria [17]. Patients who had previously been diagnosed with other important systemic autoimmune diseases, including rheumatoid arthritis, systemic sclerosis, spondyloarthritis, dermatomyositis, polymyositis, or juvenile idiopathic arthritis were excluded from the study.

2.3. Clinical Manifestations of Systemic Lupus Erythematosus

The clinical manifestations of SLE were defined in advance and evaluated at the time of enrollment by attending physicians and research nurses. Common clinical manifestations were selected based on the definition of the SLE Disease Activity Index 2000 (SLEDAI-2K) [18] and their frequency of occurrence [19,20]. In addition, we chose those symptoms that are more likely to have a direct impact on patients' quality of life. A total of 10 clinical manifestations were investigated in this study, including Raynaud's phenomenon, photosensitivity, Sjögren's syndrome, arthralgia or arthritis, renal involvement, malar rash, oral ulcer, alopecia, skin vasculitis, and discoid lesion. Manifestations such as leukopenia, thrombocytopenia, low complement, and elevated dsDNA level were omitted from this study because patients with SLE are less likely to seek complementary therapies that do not directly affect their quality of life. Clinical manifestations were considered present only when patients were experiencing them at the time of the survey.

2.4. Measurement of Demographic Variables

The following demographic information was determined from the questionnaire: age, body mass index, educational level, marital status, employment status, self-perceived health status, age at the diagnosis of SLE, smoking habit, alcohol use in the past year, regular vigorous exercise in the past year, and daily duration of sleep. In this study, overweight ($24 \leq$ body mass index < 27 kg/m^2) and obesity (body mass index ≥ 27 kg/m^2) were defined according to the Ministry of Health and Welfare, Taiwan [21]. Regarding the question about exercise, the respondents were asked whether they had engaged in exercise that lasted at least 20 minutes that made them breathe faster and sweat in the past year. The response categories were never, once a month or fewer, several times a month, several times a week, and daily. The last two categories were combined and defined as regular vigorous exercise.

2.5. Use of Complementary Therapy

Complementary therapies were presented as seven broad categories in the questionnaire, as described in our previous study [9] (Table 1). A Likert-type scale with four response choices was used. These four response categories were collapsed into two responses by treating the "always use" category as "use" while the remaining three categories (sometimes use, had tried previously, and never use) as "not use".

Table 1. Categories of complementary therapies.

Complementary Therapy Category	Description
1. Body-based and energy therapy	massage therapy or Tui Na (Chinese massage), chiropractic or osteopathic manipulation, Gua Sha therapy or cupping, acupuncture or moxibustion, and far-infrared therapy
2. Mind-body therapy	qigong or Tai Chi, meditation, relaxation therapy, and aromatherapy

Table 1. Cont.

Complementary Therapy Category	Description
3. Folk remedies and religious practices	divination and nameology, exorcise, Buddhist chanting, and praying
4. Exercise therapy	dancing, fitness workout, jogging, fitness walking or strolling, swimming, and cycling
5. Chinese medicine	visit to the Chinese medicine department in a hospital, visit to Chinese medicine clinics, Chinese medicinal herbs shop, and herbal remedies
6. Nutrient supplements	vitamins, fish oil supplements, ginkgo, calcium supplements, glucosamine, turmeric, and probiotics
7. Diet therapy	raw food diet, organic diet, Mediterranean diet, low-carbohydrate diet, and ketogenic diet

2.6. Data Analysis

The basic characteristics of the study participants were summarized as frequencies with percentages. The 10 most popular types of complementary therapies were identified based on their frequency of use by patients in this study. The five SLE clinical manifestations with the highest prevalence were treated as outcome variables and analyzed using multiple logistic regression analysis. The independent variables were the 10 types of complementary therapies with the highest prevalence and all demographic variables listed in Table 1. A backward variable selection method based on likelihood ratios was used to obtain the final regression model. All statistical analyses were performed using IBM SPSS Statistics for Windows, version 27.0.1.0 (IBM Corp., Armonk, NY, USA). $p < 0.05$ was considered statistically significant.

3. Results

The basic characteristics of the 317 patients with SLE are summarized in Table 2. Most of them (60.9%) were 40 years or older. About 74% of the patients reported that their health status was average, poor, or very poor. The prevalence of the 10 clinical manifestations of SLE in our patients is shown in Figure 1. The five clinical manifestations with the highest prevalence were Raynaud's phenomenon (61.2%), photosensitivity (50.2%), Sjögren's syndrome (28.4%), arthralgia and arthritis (22.1%), and renal involvement (14.5%). Furthermore, the 10 most popular types of complementary therapies used by patients in this study were the following: fitness walking or strolling (37.5%), Buddhist chanting (37.2%), vitamins (31.9%), calcium supplements (24.6%), fish oil supplements (19.6%), probiotics (17.7%), massage therapy or Tui Na (11.7%), fitness workout (11.0%), visit to Chinese medicine clinics (8.8%), and visit to the Chinese medicine department in a hospital (7.9%).

Table 2. Basic characteristics of female patients with systemic lupus erythematosus ($n = 317$).

Variable	n (%)
Age interval, years	
20–39	124 (39.1)
≥40	193 (60.9)
Body mass index	
Normal	167 (52.7)
Underweight	45 (14.2)
Overweight or obese	105 (33.1)

Table 2. *Cont.*

Variable	n (%)
Educational level	
High school or below	158 (49.8)
College or above	159 (50.2)
Marital status	
Single	106 (33.4)
Being married, widowed, or divorced	211 (66.6)
Employment status	
Employed	200 (63.1)
Unemployed	117 (36.9)
Self-perceived health status	
Very good and good	83 (26.2)
Average, poor and very poor	234 (73.8)
Age at SLE diagnosis, years	
20–29	172 (54.3)
≥30	145 (45.7)
Smoking habit	
No	296 (93.4)
Daily or occasionally	21 (6.6)
Alcohol use in the past year	
No	248 (78.2)
Daily or occasionally	69 (21.8)
Regular vigorous exercise in the past year	
No	169 (53.3)
Yes	148 (46.7)
Duration of sleep/day, hours	
≥8	59 (18.6)
≤7	258 (81.4)

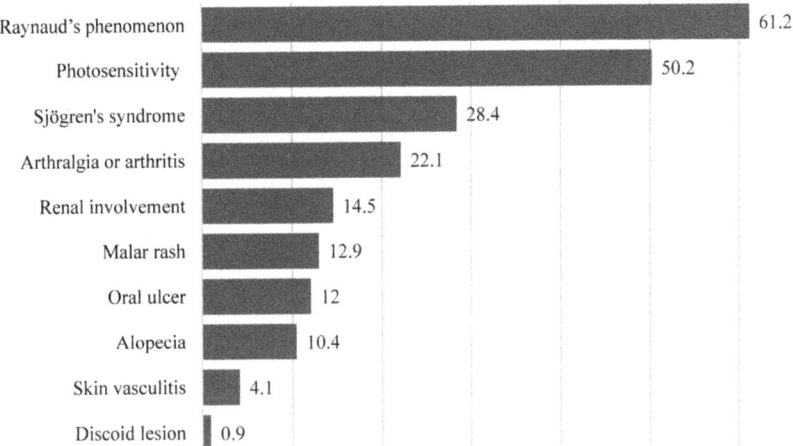

Figure 1. Prevalence of different clinical symptoms in Taiwanese female patients with systemic lupus erythematosus. Numbers shown are percentages.

The results of multiple logistic regression analyses of the clinical manifestations of SLE are shown in Table 2. Of the five SLE clinical manifestations with the highest prevalence, two of them (Sjögren's syndrome, arthralgia or arthritis) were not significantly associated with the use of any of the 10 complementary therapies. Therefore, only the results of the remaining three clinical manifestations of SLE are shown in Table 3. First, Raynaud's phenomenon was significantly associated with fitness walking or strolling (adjusted odds ratio [aOR] 1.77; $p = 0.027$) and fish oil supplements (aOR 3.55; $p < 0.001$), adjusted for age at diagnosis of SLE. Second, photosensitivity was significantly associated with probiotics (aOR 0.49; $p = 0.019$). Third, renal involvement was significantly associated with probiotics (aOR 2.43; $p = 0.026$) and visit to the Chinese medicine department in a hospital (aOR 3.14; $p = 0.026$), adjusted for body mass index, educational level, and marital status.

Table 3. Multiple logistic regression analyses of factors associated with clinical manifestations with significant use of complementary therapies in Taiwanese female patients with systemic lupus erythematosus ($n = 319$).

Variable	Raynaud's Phenomenon		Photosensitivity		Renal Involvement	
	Adjusted odds ratio (95% CI)	p	Adjusted odds ratio (95% CI)	p	Adjusted odds ratio (95% CI)	p
Body mass index						
Normal					1	
Underweight					2.67 (1.13–6.28)	0.025
Overweight or obese					1.61 (0.73–3.54)	0.237
Educational level						
High school or below					1	
College or above					2.64 (1.00–6.92)	0.049
Marital status						
Being married, widowed, or divorced					1	
Single					3.32 (1.70–6.46)	<0.001
Age at SLE diagnosis, years						
≥30	1					
20–29	1.76 (1.09–2.84)	0.022				
Fitness walking or strolling	1.77 (1.07–2.92)	0.027				
Fish oil supplements	3.55 (1.75–7.19)	<0.001				
Probiotics			0.49 (0.27–0.89)	0.019	2.43 (1.11–5.30)	0.026
Visit Chinese medicine department in a hospital					3.14 (1.15–8.58)	0.026

CI: confidence interval. In the multiple regression logistic model, the following variables were evaluated: age interval, body mass index, educational level, marital status, employment status, self-perceived health status, age at diagnosis of SLE, smoking habit, alcohol use in the past year, regular exercise in the past year, duration of sleep per day, and 10 types of complementary therapies (fitness walking or strolling, Buddhist chanting, vitamins, calcium supplements, fish oil supplements, probiotics, massage therapy or Tui Na, fitness workout, visit to Chinese medicine clinics, and visit to the Chinese medicine department in a hospital).

4. Discussion

In this cross-sectional study of Taiwanese women with SLE, we reported the association between the use of complementary therapies and common clinical manifestations of SLE. Patients with SLE are often present with various systemic manifestations, and many of them are not SLE-specific, such as fatigue and fever. In our study, two of the five clinical manifestations with the highest prevalence, namely Sjögren's syndrome and arthralgia or arthritis, were not associated with the use of any of the complementary therapies.

In our female patients, the most common clinical manifestation of SLE with significant use of complementary therapies was Raynaud's phenomenon, which affected 61.2% of them. The Raynaud phenomenon is a nonspecific skin manifestations of SLE, resulting from a vasospasm typically triggered by cold conditions or emotional stress. The present study showed that the presence of Raynaud's phenomenon was associated with fitness walking or strolling and fish oil supplements. Although there is no specific research that evaluates the efficacy of exercise in the treatment of Raynaud's phenomenon, a meta-analysis of 11 trials with a total of 355 participants revealed that exercise could significantly improve microvascular and macrovascular function in patients with autoimmune diseases [22]. In the present study, we observed a significant increased use of fitness walking or strolling in our patients, as low-impact may improve blood circulation and may thereby improve Raynaud's phenomenon. We also noted that the use of fish oil supplements was significantly associated with the presence of Raynaud's phenomenon. A prospective double-blind, randomized, control study using 32 patients with Raynaud's phenomenon showed that taking fish oil could improve tolerance to cold exposure and delay the onset of vasospasm in patients with primary, but not secondary, Raynaud's phenomenon [23]. However, the beneficial effect of fish oil in patients with secondary Raynaud's phenomenon has not been validated in further studies. In addition, a number of food items, such as garlic, ginkgo biloba, L-carnitine, inositol nicotinate, and evening primrose oil had been reported to increase skin blood flow or hand skin temperature. Overall, evidence from rigorous studies is still lacking to support any food ingredients in alleviating Raynaud's phenomenon [24]. Nevertheless, given the general beneficial health effects of fish oil on cardiovascular disease [25], and possibly on several autoimmune diseases, such as multiple sclerosis [26], rheumatoid arthritis [27], and psoriasis [28], future intervention studies on the association between fish oil and SLE should also include the evaluation of Raynaud's phenomenon as an outcome [29].

The second most prevalent clinical manifestation of SLE with significant use of complementary therapies was photosensitivity. Photosensitivity is a highly complex condition and is a common clinical manifestation of SLE. Exposure to ultraviolet radiation can lead to increased skin disease flares and systemic symptoms, such as joint pain and fatigue [30]. In this study, the use of probiotics was significantly and inversely associated with the presence of photosensitivity. Previous research suggested that probiotics could potentially be used in the prevention and management of allergic diseases [31], allergic inflammation, skin hypersensitivity, and UV-induced skin damage [32]. As photosensitivity is often referred to sun allergy by the general population, it is surprised to observe an increased use of complementary therapies that are thought to be able to alleviate allergy reaction. However, the opposite association was observed in our study—patients with photosensitivity were associated with decreased use of probiotics. The reduction could possibly be related to the concern of stimulating the immune response by probiotics [33,34]. Animal studies have shown that probiotics could modify various immune parameters, such as the innate immune response of macrophages and dendritic cells [35], and the cell wall structure of probiotic *Lactobacillus casei* could potently induce IL-12 production [36]. In contrast, animal studies suggested that intake of *Lactobacillus casei* Shirota could alleviate SLE symptoms and their cardiovascular and renal complications [37]. More research is required to establish the safety and efficacy of probiotics for the prevention and treatment of photosensitivity in patients with SLE.

The third most prevalent clinical manifestation of SLE with significant use of complementary therapies was renal involvement. The kidney is the most commonly affected visceral organ in SLE, and renal failure and sepsis are two of the main causes of mortality in patients with SLE [38]. In the present study, the use of probiotics and visits to the Chinese medicine department in a hospital were significantly associated with renal involvement. A meta-analysis of 13 randomized controlled trials showed that the intake of probiotics, prebiotics, and synbiotics could reduce the formation of uremic toxin, p-cresol, and their serum levels [39]. Another meta-analysis of 13 clinical trials revealed that prebiotic, probiotic, and synbiotic supplementation could significantly decrease urea and blood urea nitrogen, but uric acid was increased. No significant changes in the glomerular filtration rate were observed [40]. However, no studies have specifically examined the effect of probiotics on renal function in patients with SLE. Furthermore, as safety reporting in studies assessing probiotics, prebiotics, and synbiotics is still inadequate [41], the potential risk in using probiotics in immunocompromised patients must be carefully evaluated.

In the present study, renal involvement was significantly associated with a more frequent visit to the Chinese medicine department in a hospital. A meta-analysis of six randomized controlled trials with 470 patients showed that the combination application of traditional Chinese and Western Medicine could improve the clinical efficacy of treatment of lupus nephritis with lower 24-hour urine protein, serum creatinine, and decrease adverse drug reactions [42]. Based on the secondary analysis of 16,645 newly diagnosed SLE patients identified from the Taiwan National Health Insurance Research Database, the combined use of conventional medicine and traditional Chinese medicine was found to significantly decrease the risk of lupus nephritis among Taiwanese patients with SLE [43]. Additional studies are warranted to explore the type of Chinese medicine prescriptions that were commonly used in SLE patients with renal involvement and their efficacy when combined with Western medicine.

There were some limitations in this study. First, due to the cross-sectional design of the present study, causal inferences between the SLE manifestations and their associated factors could not be established. Second, the findings of the study might not be generalizable to other countries with different health care systems and cultural dimensions.

5. Conclusions

In conclusion, the prevalence of SLE clinical manifestations and the use of complementary therapies were identified in female Taiwanese patients with SLE. It is important that health care providers have up-to-date knowledge of common complementary therapies and be ready to provide evidence-based advice to patients with SLE. Furthermore, given the increasing use of fish oil supplements for Raynaud's phenomenon and probiotics for renal involvement, their safety and efficacy should be investigated in future studies.

Author Contributions: Conceptualization, M.-C.L.; formal analysis, M.K. and C.-W.H.; investigation, H.-C.L. and H.-H.C.; writing—original draft preparation, M.-C.L.; writing—review and editing, M.K. and M.-C.L. All authors have read and agreed to the published version of the manuscript.

Funding: This research was funded by grants from Dalin Tzu Chi Hospital, Buddhist Tzu Chi Medical Foundation [No: DTCRD109-I-21, DTCRD109-I-23], and Buddhist Tzu Chi Medical Foundation [No. TCMF-A 108-05].

Institutional Review Board Statement: The study was conducted in accordance with the Declaration of Helsinki, and the study protocol was approved by the institutional review board of Dalin Tzu Chi Hospital, Buddhist Tzu Chi Medical Foundation (No. B10801017, date of approval 29 March 2019).

Informed Consent Statement: Informed consent was obtained from all subjects involved in the study.

Data Availability Statement: The data that support the findings of this study are available on request from the corresponding author.

Conflicts of Interest: The authors declare no conflict of interest.

References

1. Pons-Estel, G.J.; Alarcon, G.S.; Scofield, L.; Reinlib, L.; Cooper, G.S. Understanding the epidemiology and progression of systemic lupus erythematosus. *Semin. Arthritis Rheum.* **2010**, *39*, 257–268. [CrossRef] [PubMed]
2. Leong, P.Y.; Huang, J.Y.; Chiou, J.Y.; Bai, Y.C.; Wei, J.C. The prevalence and incidence of systemic lupus erythematosus in Taiwan: A nationwide population-based study. *Sci. Rep.* **2021**, *11*, 5631. [CrossRef] [PubMed]
3. Pereira, M.G.; Duarte, S.; Ferraz, A.; Santos, M.; Fontes, L. Quality of life in patients with systemic lupus erythematosus: The mediator role of psychological morbidity and disease activity. *Psychol. Health Med.* **2020**, *25*, 1247–1257. [CrossRef]
4. Schmeding, A.; Schneider, M. Fatigue, health-related quality of life and other patient-reported outcomes in systemic lupus erythematosus. *Best Pract. Res. Clin. Rheumatol.* **2013**, *27*, 363–375. [CrossRef]
5. Cornet, A.; Andersen, J.; Myllys, K.; Edwards, A.; Arnaud, L. Living with systemic lupus erythematosus in 2020: A European patient survey. *Lupus Sci. Med.* **2021**, *8*, e000469. [CrossRef] [PubMed]
6. Wieland, L.S.; Manheimer, E.; Berman, B.M. Development and classification of an operational definition of complementary and alternative medicine for the Cochrane collaboration. *Altern. Ther. Health Med.* **2011**, *17*, 50–59. [PubMed]

7. Greco, C.M.; Nakajima, C.; Manzi, S. Updated review of complementary and alternative medicine treatments for systemic lupus erythematosus. *Curr. Rheumatol. Rep.* **2013**, *15*, 378. [CrossRef]
8. Morgan, C.; Bland, A.R.; Maker, C.; Dunnage, J.; Bruce, I.N. Individuals living with lupus: Findings from the LUPUS UK Members Survey 2014. *Lupus* **2018**, *27*, 681–687. [CrossRef]
9. Lu, M.C.; Lo, H.C.; Chang, H.H.; Hsu, C.W.; Koo, M. Factors associated with the use of complementary therapies in Taiwanese patients with systemic lupus erythematosus: A cross-sectional study. *BMC Complement. Med. Ther.* **2021**, *21*, 247. [CrossRef]
10. Patavino, T.; Brady, D.M. Natural medicine and nutritional therapy as an alternative treatment in systemic lupus erythematosus. *Altern. Med. Rev.* **2001**, *6*, 460–471.
11. Leong, K.P.; Pong, L.Y.; Chan, S.P. Why lupus patients use alternative medicine. *Lupus* **2003**, *12*, 659–664. [CrossRef] [PubMed]
12. Fangtham, M.; Kasturi, S.; Bannuru, R.R.; Nash, J.L.; Wang, C. Non-pharmacologic therapies for systemic lupus erythematosus. *Lupus* **2019**, *28*, 703–712. [CrossRef] [PubMed]
13. Yacoub Wasef, S.Z. Gender differences in systemic lupus erythematosus. *Gend. Med.* **2004**, *1*, 12–17. [CrossRef]
14. Faul, F.; Erdfelder, E.; Buchner, A.; Lang, A.G. Statistical power analyses using G*Power 3.1: Tests for correlation and regression analyses. *Behav. Res. Methods* **2009**, *41*, 1149–1160. [CrossRef] [PubMed]
15. Cohen, J. *Statistical Power Analysis for the Behavioral Sciences*; Lawrence Erlbaum Associates: Hillsdale, NJ, USA, 1988.
16. Hochberg, M.C. Updating the American College of Rheumatology revised criteria for the classification of systemic lupus erythematosus. *Arthritis Rheum.* **1997**, *40*, 1725. [CrossRef]
17. Petri, M.; Orbai, A.M.; Alarcón, G.S.; Gordon, C.; Merrill, J.T.; Fortin, P.R.; Bruce, I.N.; Isenberg, D.; Wallace, D.J.; Nived, O.; et al. Derivation and validation of the Systemic Lupus International Collaborating Clinics classification criteria for systemic lupus erythematosus. *Arthritis Rheum.* **2012**, *64*, 2677–2686. [CrossRef]
18. Gladman, D.D.; Ibañez, D.; Urowitz, M.B. Systemic lupus erythematosus disease activity index 2000. *J. Rheumatol.* **2002**, *29*, 288–291.
19. Bertsias, G.K.; Pamfil, C.; Fanouriakis, A.; Boumpas, D.T. Diagnostic criteria for systemic lupus erythematosus: Has the time come? *Nat. Rev. Rheumatol.* **2013**, *9*, 687–694. [CrossRef]
20. Nossent, J.; Kiss, E.; Rozman, B.; Pokorny, G.; Vlachoyiannopoulos, P.; Olesinska, M.; Marchesoni, A.; Mosca, M.; Påi, S.; Manger, K.; et al. Disease activity and damage accrual during the early disease course in a multinational inception cohort of patients with systemic lupus erythematosus. *Lupus* **2010**, *19*, 949–956. [CrossRef]
21. Health Promotion Administration. Ministry of Health and Welfare. Taiwan Taiwan's Obesity Prevention and Management Strategy. Available online: https://www.hpa.gov.tw/File/Attach/10299/File_11744.pdf (accessed on 6 June 2022). (In Chinese)
22. Peçanha, T.; Bannell, D.J.; Sieczkowska, S.M.; Goodson, N.; Roschel, H.; Sprung, V.S.; Low, D.A. Effects of physical activity on vascular function in autoimmune rheumatic diseases: A systematic review and meta-analysis. *Rheumatology* **2021**, *60*, 3107–3120. [CrossRef]
23. DiGiacomo, R.A.; Kremer, J.M.; Shah, D.M. Fish-oil dietary supplementation in patients with Raynaud's phenomenon: A double-blind, controlled, prospective study. *Am. J. Med.* **1989**, *86*, 158–164. [CrossRef]
24. Wright, C.I.; Kroner, C.I.; Draijer, R. Raynaud's phenomenon and the possible use of foods. *Food Sci.* **2005**, *70*, R67–R75. [CrossRef]
25. Ghasemi Fard, S.; Wang, F.; Sinclair, A.J.; Elliott, G.; Turchini, G.M. How does high DHA fish oil affect health? A systematic review of evidence. *Crit. Rev. Food Sci. Nutr.* **2019**, *59*, 1684–1727. [CrossRef] [PubMed]
26. AlAmmar, W.A.; Albeesh, F.H.; Ibrahim, L.M.; Algindan, Y.Y.; Yamani, L.Z.; Khattab, R.Y. Effect of omega-3 fatty acids and fish oil supplementation on multiple sclerosis: A systematic review. *Nutr. Neurosci.* **2021**, *24*, 569–579. [CrossRef]
27. Gioxari, A.; Kaliora, A.C.; Marantidou, F.; Panagiotakos, D.P. Intake of ω-3 polyunsaturated fatty acids in patients with rheumatoid arthritis: A systematic review and meta-analysis. *Nutrition* **2018**, *45*, 114–124.e4. [CrossRef]
28. Chen, X.; Hong, S.; Sun, X.; Xu, W.; Li, H.; Ma, T.; Zheng, Q.; Zhao, H.; Zhou, Y.; Qiang, Y.; et al. Efficacy of fish oil and its components in the management of psoriasis: A systematic review of 18 randomized controlled trials. *Nutr. Rev.* **2020**, *78*, 827–840. [CrossRef]
29. de Medeiros, M.C.S.; Medeiros, J.C.A.; de Medeiros, H.J.; Leitão, J.C.G.D.C.; Knackfuss, M.I. Dietary intervention and health in patients with systemic lupus erythematosus: A systematic review of the evidence. *Crit. Rev. Food Sci. Nutr.* **2019**, *59*, 2666–2673. [CrossRef]
30. Kim, A.; Chong, B.F. Photosensitivity in cutaneous lupus erythematosus. *Photodermatol. Photoimmunol. Photomed.* **2013**, *29*, 4–11. [CrossRef]
31. Kalliomäki, M.; Antoine, J.M.; Herz, U.; Rijkers, G.T.; Wells, J.M.; Mercenier, A. Guidance for substantiating the evidence for beneficial effects of probiotics: Prevention and management of allergic diseases by probiotics. *J. Nutr.* **2010**, *140*, 713S–721S. [CrossRef]
32. Roudsari, M.R.; Karimi, R.; Sohrabvandi, S.; Mortazavian, A.M. Health effects of probiotics on the skin. *Crit. Rev. Food Sci. Nutr.* **2015**, *55*, 1219–1240. [CrossRef]
33. Senok, A.C.; Ismaeel, A.Y.; Botta, G.A. Probiotics: Facts and myths. *Clin. Microbiol. Infect.* **2005**, *11*, 958–966. [CrossRef] [PubMed]
34. Doron, S.; Snydman, D.R. Risk and safety of probiotics. *Clin. Infect. Dis.* **2015**, *60* (Suppl. 2), S129–S134. [CrossRef] [PubMed]
35. Galdeano, C.M.; Perdigón, G. The probiotic bacterium *Lactobacillus casei* induces activation of the gut mucosal immune system through innate immunity. *Clin. Vaccine Immunol.* **2006**, *13*, 219–226. [CrossRef] [PubMed]

36. Shida, K.; Nanno, M.; Nagata, S. Flexible cytokine production by macrophages and T cells in response to probiotic bacteria: A possible mechanism by which probiotics exert multifunctional immune regulatory activities. *Gut Microbes* **2011**, *2*, 109–114. [CrossRef]
37. Guo, X.; Yang, X.; Li, Q.; Shen, X.; Zhong, H.; Yang, Y. The microbiota in systemic lupus erythematosus: An update on the potential function of probiotics. *Front. Pharmacol.* **2021**, *12*, 759095. [CrossRef]
38. Cojocaru, M.; Cojocaru, I.M.; Silosi, I.; Vrabie, C.D. Manifestations of systemic lupus erythematosus. *Maedica* **2011**, *6*, 330–336.
39. Zheng, H.J.; Guo, J.; Wang, Q.; Wang, L.; Wang, Y.; Zhang, F.; Huang, W.J.; Zhang, W.; Liu, W.J.; Wang, Y. Probiotics, prebiotics, and synbiotics for the improvement of metabolic profiles in patients with chronic kidney disease: A systematic review and meta-analysis of randomized controlled trials. *Crit. Rev. Food Sci. Nutr.* **2021**, *61*, 577–598. [CrossRef]
40. Firouzi, S.; Haghighatdoost, F. The effects of prebiotic, probiotic, and synbiotic supplementation on blood parameters of renal function: A systematic review and meta-analysis of clinical trials. *Nutrition* **2018**, *51–52*, 104–113. [CrossRef]
41. Bafeta, A.; Koh, M.; Riveros, C.; Ravaud, P. Harms reporting in randomized controlled trials of interventions aimed at modifying microbiota: A systematic review. *Ann. Intern. Med.* **2018**, *169*, 240–247. [CrossRef]
42. Heng, M.; Tu, J.; Hao, Y.; Zhao, Y.; Tian, J.; Bu, H.; Wang, H. Effects of Integrated traditional Chinese and western medicine for the treatment of lupus nephritis: A meta-analysis of randomized trials. *Evid. Based Complement. Altern. Med.* **2016**, *2016*, 1502107. [CrossRef] [PubMed]
43. Chang, C.M.; Wu, P.C.; Chiang, J.H.; Wei, Y.H.; Chen, F.P.; Chen, T.J.; Pan, T.L.; Yen, H.R.; Chang, H.H. Integrative therapy decreases the risk of lupus nephritis in patients with systemic lupus erythematosus: A population-based retrospective cohort study. *J. Ethnopharmacol.* **2017**, *196*, 201–212. [CrossRef] [PubMed]

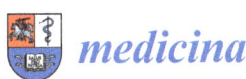

Article

Efficacy of Siwan Traditional Therapy on Erythrocyte Sedimentation Rate, Lipid Profile, and Atherogenic Index as Cardiac Risk Factors Related to Rheumatoid Arthritis

Noha F. Mahmoud [1,*], Nashwa M. Allam [2], Islam I. Omara [3] and Howida A. Fouda [4,*]

[1] Rehabilitation Sciences Department, Health and Rehabilitation Sciences College, Princess Nourah bint Abdulrahman University, P.O. Box 84428, Riyadh 11671, Saudi Arabia
[2] Orthopedics and Orthopedic Surgery Department, Physical Therapy Faculty, Ahram Canadian University, Giza P.O. Box 12451, Egypt
[3] Department of Animal Production, Faculty of Agriculture, Cairo University, Giza P.O. Box 12613, Egypt
[4] Physical Therapy for Internal Diseases Department, Physical Therapy Faculty, October 6 University, Giza P.O. Box 12585, Egypt
* Correspondence: nfmahmoud@pnu.edu.sa (N.F.M.); howida.fouda@gmail.com (H.A.F.)

Abstract: *Background and Objectives*: The most frequent cause of mortality in rheumatoid arthritis (RA) patients is cardiovascular disease (CVD). Inflammation, dyslipidemia, and decreased physical activity are some of the main risk factors for CVD. Siwan sand therapy is a type of traditional therapy used in Egypt to treat RA. The approach of this therapy depends on the experience of the healers. The aim of the current study was to compare the effects of three sessions of Siwan traditional therapy to five sessions on common CVD risk factors and physical function in rheumatoid arthritis patients. *Materials and Methods*: Thirty patients (9 male and 21 female) were assigned into two groups of equal size: group (A) received three sessions of Siwan traditional therapy in the form of a sand bath. Group (B) received the same form of therapy for five days. Erythrocyte sedimentation rate (ESR), lipid profile, atherogenic index of plasma (AIP), and a health assessment questionnaire (HAQ) were measured before and after treatment. *Results*: There was a significant increase above normal within group (A) for ESR ($p = 0.001$), triglycerides (TG; $p = 0.015$), total cholesterol (Tot-Chol; $p = 0.0001$), and low-density lipoprotein (LDL; $p = 0.0001$). However, there were no considerable differences in high-density lipoprotein (HDL; $p = 0.106$), very low-density lipoprotein (VLDL; $p = 0.213$), AIP ($p = 0.648$), and HAQ ($p = 0.875$). For the second group, there were significant changes within group B only in Tot-Chol ($p = 0.0001$), HDL ($p = 0.0001$), VLDL ($p = 0.0001$), AIP ($p = 0.008$), and HAQ ($p = 0.014$). There was a significant difference between both groups regarding HDL ($p = 0.027$), LDL ($p = 0.005$), AIP ($p = 0.029$), ESR ($p = 0.016$), and HAQ ($p = 0.036$). *Conclusions*: For RA patients, five days of Siwan traditional therapy caused significant changes regarding inflammation, Tot-Chol, LDL, HDL, AIP, and functional activity when compared to three days of Siwan hot sand therapy.

Keywords: Siwa; Siwan traditional therapy; psammotherapy; cardiac risk factors; lipid profile; atherogenic index; physical function; rheumatoid arthritis

Citation: Mahmoud, N.F.; Allam, N.M.; Omara, I.I.; Fouda, H.A. Efficacy of Siwan Traditional Therapy on Erythrocyte Sedimentation Rate, Lipid Profile, and Atherogenic Index as Cardiac Risk Factors Related to Rheumatoid Arthritis. *Medicina* **2023**, *59*, 54. https://doi.org/10.3390/medicina59010054

Academic Editors: Ming-Chi Lu and Malcolm Koo

Received: 3 November 2022
Revised: 15 December 2022
Accepted: 22 December 2022
Published: 27 December 2022

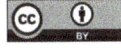

Copyright: © 2022 by the authors. Licensee MDPI, Basel, Switzerland. This article is an open access article distributed under the terms and conditions of the Creative Commons Attribution (CC BY) license (https://creativecommons.org/licenses/by/4.0/).

1. Introduction

Rheumatoid arthritis (RA) is a systemic, chronic, progressive autoimmune disease that primarily affects the linings of the joints (synovial membranes) [1,2]. The most affected populations with RA are women, smokers, and people with RA family history [3]. In developed countries, RA affects 0.5–1% of the adult population [1], with 40 new cases for every 100,000 people each year [4]. Considering that low-to-middle-income countries account for the vast majority of the world's population, the number of affected people is significant and is expected to grow in the coming years [5].

Pathogenic pathways underpin the etiology of inflammatory rheumatic diseases, which are initiated by a systemic decrease in immunological tolerance and a subsequent disruption in the immune system. Multiple disorders outside of the joints are linked to systemic inflammation [6], such as vasculitis and uveitis, rheumatoid nodules, pericarditis, osteoporosis, rheumatoid lung [7], cardiovascular events, anemia, atherosclerosis, and type 2 diabetes mellitus [6].

Patients diagnosed with RA are 30–60% more likely to develop cardiovascular disease (CVD) than the general population [8]. In individuals with rheumatoid arthritis, the incidence of myocardial infarction and stroke was nearly doubled. Patients with rheumatoid arthritis exhibited a 30% increase in CVD mortality [9]. Approximately 30% of asymptomatic RA patients in a study group in upper Egypt had atherosclerosis compared to only 5% of normal control. Between the disease activity index and atherosclerosis, there was a strong statistically significant correlation [10]. CVD is a major mortality causing factor in RA patients [9]. The relationship between RA and CVD might be thought of as a "natural experiment" that, if properly analyzed, could shed light on the underlying processes by which inflammation speeds up the development of atherosclerosis, as well as heart disease [11]. Hence, the inflammation in RA is not confined to the joints but also present in the vessel wall. Previously believed to be a passive illness caused by lipid buildup, atherosclerosis is now widely understood to be a dynamic inflammatory process that starts with endothelial activation, leukocyte recruitment, and lipid oxidation and ends with plaque instability and thrombosis [12].

When compared to the general population, patients with RA have a 1.5–2.0-fold greater risk of developing coronary artery disease (CAD) [9], which is comparable to the risk posed by diabetes mellitus [13]. This elevated CAD risk is evident even before the clinical diagnosis of RA: before diagnosis, persons with RA were more than three times more likely to have had a previous MI than participants without RA. A European League Against Rheumatism expert group has advised that CV risk ratings in certain RA patients be multiplied by 1.5 to reflect their elevated risk of heart disease [14]. In individuals with RA, diastolic dysfunction may be linked to systemic inflammation, increasing the risk of heart failure [15].

In the general population, an unfavorable lipid profile, often called dyslipidemia, is a major risk factor for cardiovascular disease (CVD) [15,16]. Researchers found that the risk of cardiovascular disease steadily rose in correlation with blood cholesterol levels [17]. Convincing data suggests that people with rheumatoid arthritis (RA) have an increased risk of cardiovascular disease [9]. On the other hand, systemic inflammation appears to play a significant role in the lipid profile alterations seen in RA, making the relationship between lipids and cardiovascular risk in this disease more complicated than in the general population. Total cholesterol (Tot-Chol), low-density lipoprotein (LDL), and high-density lipoprotein (HDL) values are all lower in individuals with active, untreated RA, according to mounting data [18]. However, rising blood lipid levels may occur simultaneously with decreasing inflammation [19]. Uncertainty surrounds the effects of these modifications on cardiovascular risk, as well as the relative contributions of dyslipidemia and systemic autoimmune inflammation to this risk in RA [20].

Inflammatory indicators such as CRP, erythrocyte sedimentation rate, rheumatoid factor, anti-citrullinated protein antibodies, and more active or severe RA are all linked to an increased risk of cardiac disease in RA patients [21]. Even in people without rheumatic illnesses, rheumatoid factor and anti-nuclear antibodies are linked to heart disease and overall mortality [22]. Reduced muscle mass as well as an abnormal body mass index, which could be the result of uncontrolled inflammation, increase the likelihood that people with RA will engage in less physical activity [23]. HAQ, which measures functional activity, is a predictor of CVD and death [24]. The HAQ disability index (HAQ-DI) is a self-reported measurement of physical function. When evaluating the level of physical impairment caused by RA, the HAQ Disability Index (HAQ-DI) is the disability assessment component of the HAQ [25].

RA is a costly chronic systemic disease; therefore, it is important to explore different effective, cheap, and safe methods of therapy. Traditional sand therapy is one of the well-known traditional therapies in eastern countries, and Siwan sand therapy in Egypt is one such therapy. Siwan therapy is related to the word "Siwa", which is an oasis in the western desert of Egypt. Siwan families have special skills in traditional healing. They pass their knowledge from generation to generation [26]. Siwan sand therapy was found to be more effective in improving functional activity and decreasing pain in RA patients than traditional physical therapy [27]. Generally, sand therapy can increase internal body temperature, decrease peripheral vascular resistance, increase tissue metabolism and venous return, and improve cardiac output, which in turn, increases the excretion of waste [28]. Despite the previously mentioned effects of sand therapy, it is not a popular intervention. Siwa Oasis has several traditional healing centers where sand therapy is applied. The centers receive patients from different governates in the country, most of them from rural areas or indigenous tribes on the borders of Egypt. Despite its great heritage value, there have not been enough studies conducted to validate its ideal approach and discover its underlying mechanism.

Per the authors' knowledge, the current study is the first conducted to investigate the effect of Siwan sand therapy on some cardiac risk factors such as inflammation, lipid profile, atherogenic index, and physical function. Although cardiac events are the main cause of death in RA patients, the mechanism of their death is not well understood. Evidence suggests that people with RA are less likely to obtain either primary or secondary heart preventative medicine due to a lack of awareness among health providers and patients [15]. The current study aims to discover more about the effect of a cheap and safe treatment, sand therapy, on RA patients' cardiac risk factors, considering that RA patients die mostly from CVD [9]. The study helps design the best practice protocol for such rare natural therapies.

2. Materials and Methods

2.1. Study Design

This study is a prospective single-blind pretest–posttest clinical trial. It was approved by the Ethics Committee of Cairo University's Faculty of Physical Therapy, Egypt (P.T. REC/012/00947). The research adhered to the Declaration of Helsinki's standards for the treatment of research participants. Research was conducted from March 2021 to August 2022. Siwan traditional therapy starts from June until the beginning of September annually.

2.2. Participants

Thirty RA patients, 9 males and 21 females, participated in this study according to the 2010 American College of Rheumatology/European League Against Rheumatism classification criteria for RA [29]. Patients were recruited from seven traditional healing centers in Siwa, Marsa Matrouh Governorate. They were interviewed and evaluated individually to assess their eligibility to be included in the study. Positive RA patients on a stable anti-rheumatic drug regimen; age range of 40 to 60 years; and BMI of 25 to 40 were the inclusion criteria. Patients who were known to have one of the following criteria were excluded from the study: uncontrolled diabetes, uncontrolled hypertension, renal disorders, unstable angina, heart failure, pregnancy, and bleeding disorders. Patients were assigned into two groups according to the number of treatment sessions.

2.3. Randomization

Patients were randomly assigned into two equal groups according to the number of treatment sessions. The authors did not interfere in selecting the number of sessions because it depended on the patient's budget, tolerance, and preference after discussion with the traditional healers. However, a random list was generated within each group in an Excel sheet according to the patient order. Despite that, the principal healer knew the number of sessions for each group. The healer assistants who applied the process for the patients were blinded and did not know about the patients' grouping till the end of the treatment day. All subjects gave their informed written permission before the initial assessment.

2.4. Intervention

Group (A) (*n* = 15) received Siwan sand therapy for three days, and Group (B) received Siwan sand therapy for five days. Sessions were conducted every day between 1 p.m. and 4 p.m. when the temperature of the sand was between 45 and 60 °C. It began with orientation the day before the sand baths began. Patients were advised not to take a shower or use body lotion or cream before the bath and not to use a fan or air conditioning during the sand bathing period and for three days after treatment. The patients were instructed to cover their bodies well to prevent air drafts and drink a significant amount of hot or warm fluids before and after every session to prevent dehydration. In the early morning of the next day, healers traveled to El Dakrour Mountain to dig holes in the sand. The hot radiation of the sun increases the sand temperature until noon. The patients were asked to lay supine in the hole. Then, healers covered their bodies with sand, except for the neck and head regions, which were kept under a small umbrella. The sand bath continued for 15–30 min as tolerated by the patient, then they were well wrapped and transferred to a dry tent close to the hole. The patients were seated inside the tent for 10–15 min and were given herbal warm drinks such as anise and lemon juice. Sweating and a number of physiological changes take place for two hours from the beginning of the session. After the sweating stopped, patients were able to change clothes into dry and heavy ones and were allowed to go to the hotel for rest. After three and five sessions of sand bathing, groups (A) and (B) received a whole-body massage with olive oil. Patients rested until the morning and were then allowed to travel back home.

2.5. Outcome Measures

2.5.1. Lipid Profile

Composed of Tot-Chol, TG, HDL, LDL, and VLDL were assessed according to standard laboratory protocol [30]. Interpretations of the lipid profile:

- Tot-Chol: normal, up to 200 mg/dL; borderline, 200–239 mg/dL; high, more than 240 mg/dL.
- TG: normal female, 35–135 mg/dL; normal male, 40–160 mg/dL.
- HDL: 45–65 mg/dL is considered normal.
- LDL: normal, less than 100–130 mg/dL; borderline high, 130–159 mg/dL; high, 160–189 mg/dL.
- VLDL: normal, 25–50 mg/dL.

2.5.2. Atherogenic Index of Plasma (AIP)

Measured by (AIP = log10 TG/HDL) [31,32].

- Lower values are associated with a lower risk of cardiovascular disease.
- Values between 0.11 and 0.21 are associated with intermediate risks.
- High risks are associated with values greater than 0.21.

2.5.3. Inflammatory Marker

As a common and cheap hematology test, the erythrocyte sedimentation rate (ESR) was used to indicate and monitor the increased inflammatory activity, according to the International Council for Standardization in Hematology (ICSH) [33]. The ESR fast detector machine was used for the test. Its normal value is up to 7 mm/s.

2.5.4. Physical Function

The HAQ disability index examines a patient's functional capacity and includes questions on fine upper-extremity movements, locomotor activities of the lower limb, and tasks that include both the upper and lower extremities. Twenty questions are broken down into eight different categories of functioning, each of which represents a full set of functional tasks. These categories include clothing, getting up, eating, walking, hygiene, reaching, and gripping, as well as daily activities. Each question begins with the phrase

"Are you able to...?" before moving on to the specific activity. On a scale from 0 (no disability) to 3 (severe impairment) (completely disabled), the patient's answers are written down. At least two distinct component questions are included in each of the categories [34]. The HAQ-Arabic version was employed in the present investigation [35].

- 0 to 1, 0 indicates mild to moderate difficulty
- 1 to 2 indicates moderate to severe difficulty
- 2 to 3 indicates severe to very severe difficulty.

2.6. Sample Size Effect

The appropriate sample size for this study is 30 patients (15 patients in each group). The G*Power software version 3.1.9 (G*Power program version 3.1, Heinrich-Heine-University, Düsseldorf, Germany) was used to calculate the two-tailed test sample size. The sample size calculation was dependent on t-tests (means: difference between two independent means for two groups), type I error (alpha = 0.05), power (1-βeta = 90%), and the effect size d = 0.95.

3. Results

3.1. Statistical Analysis

In the current study, data were normally distributed after using the Shapiro–Wilk test ($p > 0.05$) and Levene's test for testing the homogeneity of variance ($p > 0.05$). SPSS Package, version 25 for Windows, was used to conduct the statistical analysis (SPSS, Inc., Chicago, IL, USA). Statistical measures for continuous data are the mean and standard deviation, whereas those for discrete data are numbered categories (percentage). For numerical data, a paired t-test was utilized to compare the two groups pre- and post-treatment, and an unpaired t-test was utilized to compare the two groups pre- and post-treatment. For categorical data, the Chi-square test was utilized for within-group, between-group, and subgroup comparisons. When the level of probability is less than or equal to 0.05 ($p \leq 0.05$), the data is considered significant.

3.2. Results

An overall number of 30 rheumatoid patients from both genders (9 males and 21 females) were involved in this study and randomized into two groups (15 patients per group). The statistical analysis for demographic data (Table 1) revealed that there were no significant differences ($p > 0.05$) in age ($p = 0.617$), BMI ($p = 0.834$), disease duration ($p = 0.407$), gender ($p = 0.690$), diabetes ($p = 0.624$), hypertension ($p = 0.409$), heart problems ($p = 0.143$), poor lipids ($p = 0.232$), medication ($p = 0.464$), academic level ($p = 0.295$), and history of previous Siwan Traditional Therapy ($p = 0.705$) between the two experimental groups.

The distribution of lipid profiles, AIP, and ESR in (Table 2) revealed that there were significant differences between before and after treatment for triglycerides ($p = 0.015$), Tot-Chol ($p = 0.0001$), LDL ($p = 0.0001$), and 1st hour ESR ($p = 0.001$) in group (A) pairwise comparison tests. However, there were no significant differences in HDL ($p = 0.106$), VLDL ($p = 0.213$), and AIP ($p = 0.648$) within the 3-day group. In group (B) (Table 2), pairwise comparison testing showed that there were significant differences between pre- and post-treatment for Tot-Chol ($p = 0.0001$), HDL ($p = 0.0001$), VLDL ($p = 0.0001$), and AIP ($p = 0.008$) but no significant differences in TG ($p = 0.406$), LDL ($p = 0.580$), and 1st hour ESR ($p = 0.878$) within the 5-day group. Group (B) recorded fewer changes in all laboratory investigations (TG, Tot-Chol, HDL, LDL, VLDL, and 1st hour ESR) (5.63, 29.76, 3.98, 3.10, 3.88, and 1.04, respectively) compared to group (A) (31.37, 35.25, 6.76, 31.01, 5.79, and 28.17, respectively). At pre-treatment (Table 2), pairwise comparison tests (group effect) revealed no significant differences in all studied laboratory investigations. After treatment (Table 2), HDL ($p = 0.027$), LDL ($p = 0.005$), AIP ($p = 0.029$), and 1st ESR ($p = 0.016$) were affected significantly ($p < 0.05$) between both groups. However, there were no substantial differences among the 3-day group and the 5-day group in Siwan traditional therapy, TG ($p = 0.340$), ($p = 0.559$), VLDL ($p = 0.503$). A further subgroup analysis is seen in Table 3.

Table 1. Rheumatoid patient's general characteristics in 3-day group and 5-day group.

Items	Groups		p-Value
	Group A (n = 15) 3-Day Group	Group B (n = 15) 5-Day Group	
Age (year)	48.89 ± 8.38	49.80 ± 9.34	0.617
BMI (kg/m^2)	30.83 ± 6.42	32.37 ± 5.77	0.834
Disease duration (year)	10.40 ± 2.71	11.11 ± 3.29	0.407
Gender (Males:Females)	5 (33.3%):10 (66.7%)	4 (26.7%):11 (73.3%)	0.690
Diabetes (Yes:No)	2 (13.3%):13 (86.7%)	3 (20.0%):12 (80.0%)	0.624
Hypertension (Yes:No)	3 (20.0%):12 (80.0%)	5 (33.3%):10 (66.7%)	0.409
Heart problem (Yes:No)	0 (0%):15 (100%)	2 (13.3%):13 (86.7%)	0.143
Poor lipids (Yes:No)	6 (40.0%):9 (60.0%)	3 (20.0%):12 (80.0%)	0.232
Medication (Medicated:Non-medicated)	7 (%):8 (53.3%)	9 (60.0%):6 (40.0%)	0.464
Academic level (Educated:Non-educated)	13 (86.7%):2 (13.3%)	10 (66.7%):5 (33.3%)	0.195
Have you ever been through STT before (Yes:No)	6 (40%):9 (60%)	5 (33.3%):10 (66.7%)	0.705

Unpaired t-test is used to compare numerical data expressed as mean ± standard deviation. Chi-square test is used to compare categorical data expressed as numbers (percentage). p-value: probability value; NS: non-significant; STT: Siwan Traditional Therapy.

Table 2. Inter- and intra-groups comparison for laboratory investigations.

Items		Groups (Mean ± SD)		Change (MD)	p-Value
		Group (A) 3-Days (n = 15)	Group (B) 5-Days (n = 15)		
TG	Before-treatment	160.00 ± 23.89	161.30 ± 61.99	1.30	0.968
	After-treatment	128.63 ± 92.08	155.67 ± 66.58	27.04	0.340
	Change (MD)	31.37	5.63		
	Change %	19.60%	3.49%		
	p-value	0.015 *	0.406		
Tot-Chol	Before-treatment	161.62 ± 48.29	160.90 ± 35.63	0.72	0.959
	After-treatment	196.87 ± 35.98	190.67 ± 24.80	6.20	0.559
	Change (MD)	35.25	29.76		
	Change %	21.81%	18.60%		
	p-value	0.0001 *	0.0001 *		
HDL	Before-treatment	48.87 ± 18.06	46.10 ± 9.79	2.77	0.560
	After-treatment	55.63 ± 22.77	42.11 ± 9.01	13.52	0.027 *
	Change (MD)	6.76	3.98		
	Change %	13.83%	8.63%		
	p-value	0.106	0.002 *		
LDL	Before-treatment	146.43 ± 23.52	142.54 ± 42.22	3.89	0.744
	After-treatment	115.42 ± 24.15	139.44 ± 21.98	24.02	0.005 *
	Change (MD)	31.01	3.10		
	Change %	21.17%	2.17%		
	p-value	0.0001 *	0.580		
VLDL	Before-treatment	30.45 ± 29.88	32.16 ± 12.40	1.71	0.817
	After-treatment	24.66 ± 19.51	28.28 ± 10.90	3.62	0.503
	Change (MD)	5.79	3.88		
	Change %	19.01%	12.06%		
	p-value	0.213	0.0001 *		
AIP Before treatment	Low risk (<0.11)	2 (13.3%)	0 (0.0%)		
	Moderate risk (0.11–0.21)	2 (13.3%)	6 (40.0%)		0.122
	High risk (>0.21)	11 (73.3%)	9 (60.0%)		
AIP after treatment	Low risk (<0.11)	2 (13.3%)	5 (33.3%)		
	Moderate risk (0.11–0.21)	4 (26.7%)	8 (53.4%)		0.029 *
	High risk (>0.21)	9 (60.00%)	2 (13.3%)		
	p-value	0.648	0.008 *		
ESR (1st hour)	Before-treatment	41.53 ± 13.98	44.33 ± 28.86	2.80	0.715
	After-treatment	69.70 ± 3 2.44	43.29 ± 26.50	25.41	0.016 *
	Change (MD)	28.17	1.04		
	Change %	67.83%	2.35%		
	p-value	0.001 *	0.878		

Data are expressed as mean ± standard deviation (SD) for TG, Tot-Chol, HDL, LDL, VLDL, and ESR. Data are expressed as number percentage for atherogenic index. MD: mean difference, p-value: probability value, * Significant ($p < 0.05$).

Table 3. Subgroup comparison of lipid profiles.

Lipid Profiles	Categories	Group A (3-Days) (n = 15)		p-Value	Group B (5-Days) (n = 15)		p-Value
		Before-Treatment	After-Treatment		Before-Treatment	After-Treatment	
TG	Low	0%	0%	-	0%	0%	-
	Normal	83%	75%	0.835	42%	58%	0.439
	High	17%	25%	0.705	58%	42%	0.439
Tot-Chol	Low	100%	75%	0.433	92%	67%	0.414
	Normal	0%	0%	-	0%	0%	-
	Borderline	0%	17%	-	0%	33%	-
	High	0%	8%	-	8%	0%	-
HDL	Low	44%	55.3%	0.796	66.6%	46.66%	0.046 *
	Normal	33.33%	11.36%	0.257	33.3%	53.33%	0.041 *
	High	22.6%	33.33%	0.480	0%	0%	-
LDL	Low	33.33%	11.36%	0.257	11.11%	0%	-
	Normal	55.31%	55.31%	1.000	44.44%	53.33%	0.796
	Borderline	0%	11.11%	-	33.33%	40.00%	0.763
	High	11.36%	22.22%	0.655	11.11%	6.67%	0.564
VLDL	Low	42%	38%	0.989	25%	17%	0.705
	Normal	42%	54%	0.593	67%	83%	0.670
	High	17%	8%	0.317	8%	0%	-
AIP	Low risk	13.30%	13.30%	1.000	0.00%	33.30%	-
	Moderate risk	13.30%	26.70%	0.414	40.00%	53.40%	0.593
	High risk	73.30%	60.00%	0.655	60.00%	13.30%	0.035 *

Data are expressed as number percentage p-value: probability value * Significant ($p < 0.05$).

Table 3 shows the comparison of lipid profiles and AIP in subgroups; there was a significant ($p = 0.041$) increase in normal HDL values after Siwan Traditional Therapy and a non-significant increase in normal TG ($p = 0.439$), LDL ($p = 0.796$), and VLDL ($p = 0.670$) values in group (B). In group A, there was a non-significant increase in normal values of VLDL ($p = 0.593$) and a non-significant decrease in normal values of TG ($p = 0.835$) and HDL ($p = 0.257$), but there was no change in normal values of LDL ($p = 1.000$). Moreover, no change was noted in total cholesterol profiles in both groups. In group B, there was a significant decrease in high AIP risk ($p = 0.035$) and a non-significant increase in moderate risk ($p = 0.593$) while increasing the percentage of low risk. However, in group A, there was a non-significant decrease in high risk ($p = 0.655$), a non-significant increase in moderate risk ($p = 0.414$), and no change in low risk ($p = 1.000$). In general, there were significant improvements in HDL and AIP and non-significant improvements in TG, LDL, and VLDL due to the treatment of rheumatoid patients with 5-day traditional sand therapy (Group B) compared with 3-day traditional sand therapy (Group A).

The distributions of HAQ (Table 4) did not differ significantly between before and after treatment within the 3-day group ($p = 0.875$), but there were substantial differences in HAQ within the 5-day group ($p = 0.014$). There were no significant differences in HAQ before treatment ($p = 0.656$), but there were substantial differences in HAQ at post-treatment ($p = 0.036$) between Groups (A) and (B).

Table 4. Inter- and intra-groups comparison for HAQ.

Variables		Categories	Groups		p-Value
			Group (A) 3-Days Group (n = 15)	Group (B) 5-Days Group (n = 15)	
HAQ	Before-treatment	Mild—moderate difficulty (0–1) Moderate—severe disability (1–2) Severe—very severe disability (2–3)	5 (33.3%) 8 (53.3%) 2 (13.3%)	4 (26.70%) 7 (46.7%) 4 (26.7%)	0.656
	After-treatment	Mild—moderate difficulty (0–1) Moderate—severe disability (1–2) Severe—very severe disability (2–3)	5 (33.3%) 7 (46.7%) 3 (20.0%)	12 (80.0%) 2 (13.3%) 1 (6.7%)	0.036 *
	p-value		0.875	0.014 *	

Data are expressed as number (percentage). p-value: probability value * Significant ($p < 0.05$).

4. Discussion

Sand therapy has been used for centuries to improve function and reduce pain in patients [36]. Siwa is a place that embraces that practice. However, modern science has not investigated its benefits and hazards extensively. Therefore, the current study evaluated the efficacy of Siwan traditional sand therapy on some cardiac risk factors. It is a trial to uncover few physiological changes that happen to RA patients because of that approach, which is directed mainly toward pain and function rather than its mechanism or other effects. In a trial to standardize this method, the study also compares the effects of 3 days versus 5 days of treatment, as traditional healers usually, from their experience, recommend an odd number of sessions: three, five, or seven.

The main risk factors for CVD in the overall population include dyslipidemia, hypertension, obesity, lack of physical activity, poor nutrition, and smoking [37]. Disease activity scores and inflammation are important risk factors for CVD in RA patients as there is a significant association between them [38]. Therefore, controlling inflammation is important to reduce CV events [39]. Inflammation was assessed using the ESR test. An elevated ESR is an important detector of coronary artery disease [40].

The results of the current study revealed that in the 3-day group, there was a significant increase when comparing before and after treatment for ESR (p = 0.001), while there was an insignificant decrease in the second group (p > 0.05), showing that ESR (a measure of inflammation) went up in the 3-day group and went down in the 5-day group. The increase in inflammatory biomarkers (ESR) in the 3-day group may be due to the immediate effect of generalized hyperthermia. The patient is exposed to a high temperature (from 45 to 60 °C) for 15 to 30 min, which might have stimulated thermo-nociceptors called Transient Receptor Potential Vanilloid 1 (TRPV1), which in turn, can increase inflammation by the production of interleukin-6, interleukin-8, and prostaglandin, thereby reducing inflammation [41]. Thermal therapy might reduce inflammation and repair cartilage damage by preventing the binding of serum tumor necrosis factor-a (TNF) to activated cells that produce pro-inflammatory cytokines [42].

The Siwan sand mineral constituents may explain the beneficial effect of the current study when augmented by the effect of hot sand. The hot sand bath increases skin permeability, which might aid the transport of the sand's mineral constituents to the skin's deeper layers, allowing them to do their work [43]. Siwan sand was analyzed in a previous study in 2018, and it was found to be rich in carbon, silicon, Ca, and Mg, plus other microelements [27]. The elements Ca (in ionic form) and Zn (in covalent form) can enter the dermis and be absorbed by skin cells. Ca^{2+} plays an important role in maintaining healthy muscle and nervous system function, as well as regular cardiovascular function. Calcium treatment in conjunction with vitamin D treatment is also known to improve calcium absorption. As a result, sand treatment is beneficial to human health and may have a role in reducing musculoskeletal disease and enhancing functional impairment. Sand walking is a great way to exercise and obtain vitamin D from the sun [44], which in turn, might have affected the results of HAQ.

Low magnesium (Mg) levels are linked to increased inflammation [45]. For example, magnesium salts in Dead Sea water have a beneficial effect on inflammatory diseases [46]. Moreover, in 1966, the German chemist Bedouno Sanouni analyzed the sands near Siwa. Radon levels were reportedly greater than in neighboring areas. Geological research revealed silica carbonates, iron, and magnesium in quite high concentrations. Radon therapy is recommended for rheumatoid arthritis and has been used in rheumatoid arthritis treatment since the beginning of the 20th century [47]. Radon is taken up by transcutaneous resorption, which may be facilitated by carbon dioxide or heat [48], and then it is distributed all over the body by the blood. Radon stimulates the release of anti-inflammatory cytokines. These cytokines act as antagonists against the pro-inflammatory cytokines [49].

Results of the lipid profile of the current study showed that in Group (A), there was no significant increase in the normal value before and after treatment for VLDL, while there was no significant increase in the abnormal values of TG, Tot-Chol, HDL, and LDL. In Group (B), there was a significant increase in normal values of HDL pre- and post-treatment but no significant increase in normal values of VLDL pre- and post-treatment.

The plasma lipid profile is a major risk factor and predictor of CVD [50]. A strong association was found between low values of HDL, high levels of LDL, and cardiovascular events [51]. Chronic inflammation in RA leads to quantitative as well as qualitative changes in TG, LDL, and HDL [52]. It leads to a condition of "reverse epidemiology". Patients in remission from their RA no longer have the "lipid paradox" of high CV risk among those with low LDL cholesterol [53]. Therefore, the increased inflammation in the 3-day group in the current study might explain the increased number of patients with abnormal values of TG, Tot-Chol, HDL, and LDL. Group (B) results are aligned with a study conducted on healthy young males who received 10 hot sauna sessions. LDL and cholesterol fraction levels dropped throughout the sauna sessions. However, after sauna sessions, some people noticed a small (but not statistically significant) increase in HDL and a temporary decrease in TG [54]. The present study contradicted a study that showed a statistically significant rise in blood Tot-Chol with small as well as statistically insignificant shifts in LDL and HDL fractions in a group of middle-aged patients subjected to a set of 20-min bathing sessions in natural hot springs with temperatures of 42 °C two times a week for three months [55]. The difference between this result and the current study result may be due to differences in both temperature and/or treatment approach.

One factor that may explain the tendency of the lipid profile toward normal values in the 5-day group is the presence of magnesium, which is very important for human health. Under the form of Mg^{+2}, magnesium produces well-known effects based on animal experimentation "in vivo", reducing cardiovascular pathologies since it has an important role in the metabolism of fats or lipids [44]. Although both groups took the same sessions at different doses, the results were different. It might be recommended that patients suffering from dyslipidemia need higher doses of thermal and magnesium therapy. The impact of lipid fluctuation due to the variable grade of chronic inflammation on CV risk is less well understood throughout the disease process [56]. The fluctuations in increased inflammation in the 3-day group and a decrease in the 5-day group might have affected the lipid profile results and made them even more difficult to explain, especially with the known lipid paradox in RA patients. Therefore, the AIP may be a better choice for assessing the relative impact of lipids on CV risk in those patients than the specific cholesterol fraction tests [44,56].

The atherogenic index of plasma (AIP) is a powerful predictor of atherosclerosis, as well as coronary heart disease. It reflects the genuine link between protective and atherogenic lipoproteins and is related to the particle size of pre- and anti-atherosclerotic lipoproteins. It may be determined using the log (TG/HDL-C) equation [51]. The results showed that there was a non-significant change in Group A and a significant change in the second group. A significant difference was also found between groups. The non-significant decrease in AIP in Group (A) might be related to the increased inflammation in that group, which affected the results of TG and HDL, while the significant improvement in AIP in Group (B) might be related to the decreased inflammation and its effect on TG and HDL. ESR is positively correlated with AIP in RA patients and is a predictor of AIP. Rheumatoid arthritis is linked to an altered lipid profile, particularly in individuals with elevated inflammatory markers, as well as autoimmune antibodies [57].

Fatigue, anemia, and muscle wasting accompany chronic inflammation with other specific disease symptoms, leading to deconditioned muscles. Comorbidities exacerbate inflammation, which in turn, negatively affects physical activity and cardiovascular performance. This is the "vicious cycle" of chronic inflammation underlying inflammatory rheumatic disorders [58]. Physical inactivity is one of the risk factors for cardiac events in RA patients, and these results can be explained by the fact that inflammation was lower in group B than in group A. The results might also be attributed to the physiological effects of sand therapy, as hot sand baths can significantly increase body temperature, which in turn, improves muscle tonicity and decreases pain [34]. It also reduces peripheral arterial resistance and increases blood flow [59], which in turn, increases tissue metabolism and oxygenation [60]. These results are in agreement with a previous study where seven sessions of Siwan sand therapy improved functional disability in RA patients [27]. However, it came into conflict with the short-term measures of another previous study [61], which found that seven sessions of Siwan sand therapy on RA patients decreased functional activity. Both studies were conducted in Siwa, but the measurement was performed after different treatment durations and/or treatment protocols from the current study.

Increasing physical activity could lead to better disease control, as recommended by recent international guidelines, and thus, improve the CV profile. Physical function measured by HAQ could be an indicator of physical activity, as HAQ is significantly associated with physical activity [34]. Physical function measured by HAQ in the first group improved but not significantly. It has, however, significantly improved in group B, as well as between the two groups.

These results can be explained by the fact that inflammation was lower in group B compared to group A. The results might also be attributed to the physiological effects of sand therapy, as hot sand baths can significantly increase body temperature, which in turn, improves muscle tonicity and decreases pain [34]. It also reduces peripheral arterial resistance and increases blood flow [59], which in turn, increases tissue metabolism and oxygenation [60]. These results are in agreement with a previous study where seven sessions of Siwan sand therapy improved functional disability in RA patients [27]. However, it came in conflict with the short-term measures of another previous study [61], which found that seven sessions of Siwan sand therapy on RA patients decreased functional activity. Both studies were conducted in Siwa, but the measurement was performed after different treatment durations and/or treatment protocols different from the current study.

Hippocrates, known as the "Father of Natural Medicine," thought that because man is part of the Cosmos, nature may heal him. He viewed health as the perfect condition of equilibrium among natural forces, and he felt that physicians should consider the curative power of vital energy. He suggested sunbathing, water, and detoxifying to attain this purpose [44]. It is worth mentioning that there is something else beyond the effect of hot sands that might have boosted the results of this study, which is the harmony between natural forces that is found in Siwa. Maybe it is the special location, below sea level by up to 18 m, the very dry and hot weather, the ecological architecture, the mineral springs, and the salt lakes that work together to encourage body self-healing [36] in a way that is known as climatotherapy rather than sand therapy.

5. Conclusions, Limitations, and Recommendation

The study found that 5-days Siwan hot sand therapy caused significant changes regarding inflammation, Tot-Chol, LDL, HDL, AIP, and functional activity when compared to 3-days of Siwan hot sand therapy. Five sessions of Siwan sand therapy might be able to reduce cardiovascular risk factors more than three sessions of therapy. More investigations are needed to explore the underlying mechanisms of such measured effects. The clinical implementation of the current results still needs further research and comparison between RA patients, a normal subject group, and a RA placebo group. Further studies are needed to evaluate the chronic effects of longer sand therapy sessions and to establish a standardized sand bath therapy protocol for the various clinical conditions and different approaches to setting an effective treatment session.

The authors considered that the measured biological variables could be changed because of the climate of the place (climatotherapy) rather than only sand therapy. That is why the control group should be in Siwa. However, the current study is limited to the two experimental groups without a control group, which was not convenient for the patients (due to the long distance and the fatigability of the disease, as well as for the research budget). It was also considered unethical to transport patients over long distances without providing treatment. Further randomized control trials with a larger sample size are recommended for future research. The research is limited to 30 patients. However, this type of intervention is only available 70 days a year and for a limited number of patients.

It is also important to highlight that this study aimed to investigate the effect of Siwan sand therapy, which is a non-invasive, known, and widely used approach by RA patients. It did not aim to assess its effectiveness. Rheumatoid patients usually target symptomatic relief rather than the risk factors. The current study measured inflammation, lipid profile, atherogenic index, and physical function as a trial to give a deep look inside the physiological changes due to this kind of therapy. More research is needed to extensively explore the underlying effects of such interventions. Cardiac risk factors were selected as the leading cause of death among RA patients.

Author Contributions: Conceptualization, N.F.M., N.M.A., H.A.F. and I.I.O.; formal analysis, I.I.O.; funding acquisition, N.F.M.; project supervision and administration, N.F.M.; investigation, N.M.A., H.A.F. and N.M.A.; methodology, H.A.F., N.M.A. and N.F.M.; methodology resources, H.A.F., N.M.A., I.I.O. and H.A.F.; writing—original draft, H.A.F.; writing—review and editing, N.F.M., H.A.F. and N.M.A. All authors have read and agreed to the published version of the manuscript.

Funding: This work was funded by Princess Nourah bint Abdulrahman University Researchers Supporting Project Number PNURSP2022R206, Princess Nourah bint Abdulrahman University, Riyadh, Saudi Arabia.

Institutional Review Board Statement: The study was carried out in accordance with the Helsinki Declaration guidelines and was approved by the Ethics Committee of Cairo University's Faculty of Physical Therapy, Egypt (P.T.REC/012/00947).

Informed Consent Statement: Informed consent was obtained from all subjects involved in the study.

Data Availability Statement: We declare that the data considered for this research are original and were collected by the authors for gaining insights.

Acknowledgments: The authors express their gratitude to Princess Nourah bint Abdulrahman University Researchers Supporting Project Number PNURSP2022R206, Princess Nourah bint Abdulrahman University, Riyadh, Saudi Arabia.

Conflicts of Interest: The authors stated no possible conflict of interest regarding this article's study, authorship, and/or publication.

References

1. Choy, E. Understanding the Dynamics: Pathways Involved in the Pathogenesis of Rheumatoid Arthritis. *Rheumatology* **2012**, *51* (Suppl. S5), v3–v11. [CrossRef]
2. Bonafede, M.; Johnson, B.H.; Tang, D.H.; Harrison, D.J.; Stolshek, B.S. Compliance and Cost of Biologic Therapies for Rheumatoid Arthritis. *Am. J. Pharm. Benefits* **2017**, *9*, 84–90.
3. Wasserman, A.M. Diagnosis and Management of Rheumatoid Arthritis. *Am. Fam. Physician* **2011**, *84*, 1245–1252. [PubMed]
4. Peschken, C.A.; Esdaile, J.M. Rheumatic Diseases in North America's Indigenous Peoples. *Semin. Arthritis Rheum.* **1999**, *28*, 368–391. [CrossRef] [PubMed]
5. Rudan, I.; Sidhu, S.; Papana, A.; Meng, S.J.; Xin-Wei, Y.; Wang, W.; Campbell-Page, R.M.; Demaio, A.R.; Nair, H.; Sridhar, D.; et al. Prevalence of Rheumatoid Arthritis in Low- and Middle-Income Countries: A Systematic Review and Analysis. *J. Glob. Health* **2015**, *5*, 010409. [CrossRef]

6. Weiss, G.; Schett, G. Anaemia in Inflammatory Rheumatic Diseases. *Nat. Rev. Rheumatol.* **2013**, *9*, 205–215. [CrossRef]
7. Hochberg, M.C.; Johnston, S.S.; John, A.K. The Incidence and Prevalence of Extra-Articular and Systemic Manifestations in a Cohort of Newly-Diagnosed Patients with Rheumatoid Arthritis between 1999 and 2006. *Curr. Med. Res. Opin.* **2008**, *24*, 469–480. [CrossRef]
8. Sárvári, A.K.; Doan-Xuan, Q.-M.; Bacsó, Z.; Csomós, I.; Balajthy, Z.; Fésüs, L. Interaction of Differentiated Human Adipocytes with Macrophages Leads to Trogocytosis and Selective IL-6 Secretion. *Cell Death Dis.* **2015**, *6*, e1613. [CrossRef]
9. Solomon, D.H.; Goodson, N.J.; Katz, J.N.; Weinblatt, M.E.; Avorn, J.; Setoguchi, S.; Canning, C.; Schneeweiss, S. Patterns of Cardiovascular Risk in Rheumatoid Arthritis. *Ann. Rheum. Dis.* **2006**, *65*, 1608–1612. [CrossRef]
10. Elshereef, R.R.; Darwish, A.; Ali, A.; Abdel-Kadar, M.; Hamdy, L. Asymptomatic Atherosclerosis in Egyptian Rheumatoid Arthritis Patients and Its Relation to Disease Activity. *Int. J. Rheumatol.* **2015**, *2015*, 381931. [CrossRef]
11. Hürlimann, D.; Enseleit, F.; Ruschitzka, F. Rheumatoid Arthritis, Inflammation, and Atherosclerosis. *Herz* **2004**, *29*, 760–768. [CrossRef]
12. Libby, P. Role of Inflammation in Atherosclerosis Associated with Rheumatoid Arthritis. *Am. J. Med.* **2008**, *121*, S21–S31. [CrossRef] [PubMed]
13. Peters, M.J.L.; van Halm, V.P.; Voskuyl, A.E.; Smulders, Y.M.; Boers, M.; Lems, W.F.; Visser, M.; Stehouwer, C.D.A.; Dekker, J.M.; Nijpels, G.; et al. Does Rheumatoid Arthritis Equal Diabetes Mellitus as an Independent Risk Factor for Cardiovascular Disease? A Prospective Study. *Arthritis Care Res.* **2009**, *61*, 1571–1579. [CrossRef] [PubMed]
14. Peters, M.J.L.; Symmons, D.P.M.; McCarey, D.; Dijkmans, B.A.C.; Nicola, P.; Kvien, T.K.; McInnes, I.B.; Haentzschel, H.; Gonzalez-Gay, M.A.; Provan, S.; et al. EULAR Evidence-Based Recommendations for Cardiovascular Risk Management in Patients with Rheumatoid Arthritis and Other Forms of Inflammatory Arthritis. *Ann. Rheum. Dis.* **2010**, *69*, 325–331. [CrossRef]
15. Crowson, C.S.; Liao, K.P.; Davis III, J.M.; Solomon, D.H.; Matteson, E.L.; Knutson, K.L.; Hlatky, M.A.; Gabriel, S.E. Rheumatoid Arthritis and Cardiovascular Disease. *Am. Heart J.* **2013**, *166*, 622–628. [CrossRef] [PubMed]
16. Third Report of the National Cholesterol Education Program (NCEP) Expert Panel on Detection, Evaluation, and Treatment of High Blood Cholesterol in Adults (Adult Treatment Panel III) Final Report. *Circulation* **2002**, *106*, 3144–3421. [CrossRef]
17. Stamler, J.; Daviglus, M.L.; Garside, D.B.; Dyer, A.R.; Greenland, P.; Neaton, J.D. Relationship of Baseline Serum Cholesterol Levels in 3 Large Cohorts of Younger Men to Long-Term Coronary, Cardiovascular, and All-Cause Mortality and to Longevity. *JAMA* **2000**, *284*, 311–318. [CrossRef]
18. Choy, E.; Sattar, N. Interpreting Lipid Levels in the Context of High-Grade Inflammatory States with a Focus on Rheumatoid Arthritis: A Challenge to Conventional Cardiovascular Risk Actions. *Ann. Rheum. Dis.* **2009**, *68*, 460–469. [CrossRef] [PubMed]
19. Steiner, G.; Urowitz, M.B. Lipid Profiles in Patients with Rheumatoid Arthritis: Mechanisms and the Impact of Treatment. *Semin. Arthritis Rheum.* **2009**, *38*, 372–381. [CrossRef]
20. Myasoedova, E.; Crowson, C.S.; Kremers, H.M.; Roger, V.L.; Fitz-Gibbon, P.D.; Therneau, T.M.; Gabriel, S.E. Lipid Paradox in Rheumatoid Arthritis: The Impact of Serum Lipid Measures and Systemic Inflammation on the Risk of Cardiovascular Disease. *Ann. Rheum. Dis.* **2011**, *70*, 482–487. [CrossRef] [PubMed]
21. Maradit-Kremers, H.; Nicola, P.J.; Crowson, C.S.; Ballman, K.v.; Gabriel, S.E. Cardiovascular Death in Rheumatoid Arthritis: A Population-Based Study. *Arthritis Rheum.* **2005**, *52*, 722–732. [CrossRef]
22. Liang, K.P.; Kremers, H.M.; Crowson, C.S.; Snyder, M.R.; Therneau, T.M.; Roger, V.L.; Gabriel, S.E. Autoantibodies, and the Risk of Cardiovascular Events. *J. Rheumatol.* **2009**, *36*, 2462–2469. [CrossRef]
23. Kremers, H.M.; Nicola, P.J.; Crowson, C.S.; Ballman, K.V.; Gabriel, S.E. Prognostic Importance of Low Body Mass Index in Relation to Cardiovascular Mortality in Rheumatoid Arthritis. *Arthritis Rheum.* **2004**, *50*, 3450–3457. [CrossRef]
24. Turesson, C.; Matteson, E.L. Cardiovascular Risk Factors, Fitness and Physical Activity in Rheumatic Diseases. *Curr. Opin. Rheumatol.* **2007**, *19*, 190–196. [CrossRef]
25. Bruce, B.; Fries, J.F. The Stanford Health Assessment Questionnaire: A Review of Its History, Issues, Progress, and Documentation. *J. Rheumatol.* **2003**, *30*, 167–178.
26. Malim, F. Oasis Siwa: From the Inside: Traditions, Customs, and Magic. Al Katan: Egypt, 2001. Available online: https://www.amazon.com/Oasis-Inside-Traditions-Customs-Magic/dp/B000W8I0R0 (accessed on 2 November 2022).
27. Allam, N.M.; Koura, G.M.R.; Alrawaili, S.M.; Hamada, H.A.; Khater, H.A.; Balbaa, A.A. The Effect of Siwan Therapy in Management of Patients with Rheumatoid Arthritis: A Single Blind Randomized Controlled Trial. *Biomed. Res.* **2018**, *29*, 1400–1406. [CrossRef]
28. Dilixat, Y.; Aytulun, S.; Ibadet, R.; Arkin, S.; Mayiram, S.; Sekine, M.; Kagamimori, S. Effects of Sand Bathing on Some Physiological Parameters with Special Reference to Its Use in the Treatment of Rheumatoid Arthritis. *J. Jpn. Assoc. Phys. Med. Balneol. Climatol.* **2002**, *65*, 107–113.
29. Aletaha, D.; Neogi, T.; Silman, A.J.; Funovits, J.; Felson, D.T.; Bingham III, C.O.; Birnbaum, N.S.; Burmester, G.R.; Bykerk, V.P.; Cohen, M.D. 2010 Rheumatoid Arthritis Classification Criteria: An American College of Rheumatology/European League Against Rheumatism Collaborative Initiative. *Arthritis Rheum.* **2010**, *62*, 2569–2581. [CrossRef] [PubMed]
30. Lemieux, I.; Lamarche, B.; Couillard, C.; Pascot, A.; Cantin, B.; Bergeron, J.; Dagenais, G.R.; Després, J.-P. Total Cholesterol/HDL Cholesterol Ratio vs LDL Cholesterol/HDL Cholesterol Ratio as Indices of Ischemic Heart Disease Risk in Men: The Quebec Cardiovascular Study. *Arch. Intern. Med.* **2001**, *161*, 2685–2692. [CrossRef] [PubMed]

31. Onat, A.; Can, G.; Kaya, H.; Hergenç, G. "Atherogenic Index of Plasma" (Log10 Triglyceride/High-Density Lipoprotein–Cholesterol) Predicts High Blood Pressure, Diabetes, and Vascular Events. *J. Clin. Lipidol.* **2010**, *4*, 89–98. [CrossRef] [PubMed]
32. Dobiášová, M.; Frohlich, J.; Šedová, M.; Cheung, M.C.; Brown, B.G. Cholesterol Esterification and Atherogenic Index of Plasma Correlate with Lipoprotein Size and Findings on Coronary Angiography. *J. Lipid Res.* **2011**, *52*, 566–571. [CrossRef] [PubMed]
33. International Council for Standardization in Haematology (Expert Panel on Blood Rheology). ICSH Recommendations for Measurement of Erythrocyte Sedimentation Rate. *J. Clin. Pathol.* **1993**, *46*, 198–203. [CrossRef] [PubMed]
34. Piva, S.R.; Almeida, G.J.M.; Wasko, M.C.M. Association of Physical Function and Physical Activity in Women with Rheumatoid Arthritis. *Arthritis Care Res.* **2010**, *62*, 1144–1151. [CrossRef]
35. Ferraz, M.B.; Quaresma, M.R.; Aquino, L.R.; Atra, E.; Tugwell, P.; Goldsmith, C. Reliability of Pain Scales in the Assessment of Literate and Illiterate Patients with Rheumatoid Arthritis. *J. Rheumatol.* **1990**, *17*, 1022–1024. [PubMed]
36. Van Tubergen, A.; van der Linden, S. A Brief History of Spa Therapy. *Ann. Rheum. Dis.* **2002**, *61*, 273. [CrossRef]
37. Deaton, C.; Froelicher, E.S.; Wu, L.H.; Ho, C.; Shishani, K.; Jaarsma, T. The Global Burden of Cardiovascular Disease. *Eur. J. Cardiovasc. Nurs.* **2011**, *10* (Suppl. S2), S5–S13. [CrossRef]
38. Gabriel, S.E.; Crowson, C.S. Risk Factors for Cardiovascular Disease in Rheumatoid Arthritis. *Curr. Opin. Rheumatol.* **2012**, *24*, 171–176. [CrossRef]
39. Smolen, J.S.; Landewé, R.; Breedveld, F.C.; Dougados, M.; Emery, P.; Gaujoux-Viala, C.; Gorter, S.; Knevel, R.; Nam, J.; Schoels, M. EULAR Recommendations for the Management of Rheumatoid Arthritis with Synthetic and Biological Disease-Modifying Antirheumatic Drugs. *Ann. Rheum. Dis.* **2010**, *69*, 964–975. [CrossRef]
40. Yayan, J. Erythrocyte Sedimentation Rate as a Marker for Coronary Heart Disease. *Vasc. Health Risk Manag.* **2012**, *8*, 219. [CrossRef]
41. Terenzi, R.; Romano, E.; Manetti, M.; Peruzzi, F.; Nacci, F.; Matucci-Cerinic, M.; Guiducci, S. Neuropeptides Activate TRPV1 in Rheumatoid Arthritis Fibroblast-like Synoviocytes and Foster IL-6 and IL-8 Production. *Ann. Rheum. Dis.* **2013**, *72*, 1107–1109. [CrossRef]
42. Bellometti, S.; Galzigna, L.; Richelmi, P.; Gregotti, C.; Bertè, F. Both Serum Receptors of Tumor Necrosis Factor Are Influenced by Mud Pack Treatment in Osteoarthrotic Patients. *Int. J. Tissue React.* **2002**, *24*, 57–64.
43. Williams, A.C.; Barry, B.W. Penetration Enhancers. *Adv. Drug Deliv. Ststems Rev.* **2004**, *56*, 603–618. [CrossRef] [PubMed]
44. Gomes, C.D.S.F. Naturotherapies Based on Minerals. *Geomaterials* **2013**, *3*, 1–14. [CrossRef]
45. Ridker, P.M. Inflammatory Biomarkers and Risks of Myocardial Infarction, Stroke, Diabetes, and Total Mortality: Implications for Longevity. *Nutr. Rev.* **2007**, *65* (Suppl. S3), S253–S259. [CrossRef] [PubMed]
46. Proksch, E.; Nissen, H.; Bremgartner, M.; Urquhart, C. Bathing in a Magnesium-rich Dead Sea Salt Solution Improves Skin Barrier Function, Enhances Skin Hydration, and Reduces Inflammation in Atopic Dry Skin. *Int. J. Dermatol.* **2005**, *44*, 151–157. [CrossRef] [PubMed]
47. van Tubergen, A.; Landewé, R.; van der Heijde, D.; Hidding, A.; Wolter, N.; Asscher, M.; Falkenbach, A.; Genth, E.; Thè, H.G.; van der Linden, S. Combined Spa–Exercise Therapy Is Effective in Patients with Ankylosing Spondylitis: A Randomized Controlled Trial. *Arthritis Care Res. Off. J. Am. Coll. Rheumatol.* **2001**, *45*, 430–438. [CrossRef]
48. Franke, A.; Reiner, L.; Pratzel, H.G.; Franke, T.; Resch, K.L. Long-Term Efficacy of Radon Spa Therapy in Rheumatoid Arthrirtis—A Randomized, Sham-Controlled Study and Follow-Up. *Rheumatology* **2000**, *39*, 894–902. [CrossRef]
49. Franke, A.; Reiner, L.; Resch, K.-L. Long-Term Benefit of Radon Spa Therapy in the Rehabilitation of Rheumatoid Arthritis: A Randomised, Double-Blinded Trial. *Rheumatol. Int.* **2007**, *27*, 703–713. [CrossRef]
50. Katараki, P.; Pharm, I.J.; Sci, B.; Vishnu Madhuri, K.; Sreekanth Varma, V. Study of Serum Lipid Profile in Individuals Residing in and Around Nalgonda. *Int. J. Pharm. Biol. Sci.* **2012**, *2*, 110–116. [CrossRef]
51. Nwagha, U.I.; Ikekpeazu, E.J.; Ejezie, F.E.; Neboh, E.E.; Maduka, I. Atherogenic Index of Plasma as Useful Predictor of Cardiovascular Risk among Postmenopausal Women in Enugu, Nigeria. *Afr. Health Sci.* **2010**, *10*, 248–252.
52. Rodríguez-Carrio, J.; Alperi-López, M.; López, P.; López-Mejías, R.; Alonso-Castro, S.; Abal, F.; Ballina-García, F.J.; González-Gay, M.Á.; Suárez, A. High Triglycerides and Low High-Density Lipoprotein Cholesterol Lipid Profile in Rheumatoid Arthritis: A Potential Link among Inflammation, Oxidative Status, and Dysfunctional High-Density Lipoprotein. *J. Clin. Lipidol.* **2017**, *11*, 1043–1054. [CrossRef]
53. Choy, E.; Ganeshalingam, K.; Semb, A.G.; Szekanecz, Z.; Nurmohamed, M. Cardiovascular Risk in Rheumatoid Arthritis: Recent Advances in the Understanding of the Pivotal Role of Inflammation, Risk Predictors and the Impact of Treatment. *Rheumatology* **2014**, *53*, 2143–2154. [CrossRef] [PubMed]
54. Gryka, D.; Pilch, W.; Szarek, M.; Szygula, Z.; Tota, Ł. The Effect of Sauna Bathing on Lipid Profile in Young, Physically Active, Male Subjects. *Int. J. Occup. Med. Environ. Health* **2014**, *27*, 608–618. [CrossRef] [PubMed]
55. Sakurai, R.; Fujiwara, Y.; Saito, K.; Fukaya, T.; Kim, M.; Yasunaga, M.; Kim, H.; Ogawa, K.; Tanaka, C.; Tsunoda, N. Effects of a Comprehensive Intervention Program, Including Hot Bathing, on Overweight Adults: A Randomized Controlled Trial. *Geriatr. Gerontol. Int.* **2013**, *13*, 638–645. [CrossRef] [PubMed]
56. Popa, C.; van Tits, L.J.H.; Barrera, P.; Lemmers, H.L.M.; van den Hoogen, F.H.J.; van Riel, P.; Radstake, T.; Netea, M.G.; Roest, M.; Stalenhoef, A.F.H. Anti-Inflammatory Therapy with Tumour Necrosis Factor Alpha Inhibitors Improves High-Density Lipoprotein Cholesterol Antioxidative Capacity in Rheumatoid Arthritis Patients. *Ann. Rheum Dis.* **2009**, *68*, 868–872. [CrossRef] [PubMed]
57. Xue, C.; Liu, W.L.; Sun, Y.H.; Ding, R.J.; Hu, D.Y. Association between Systemic Inflammation and Autoimmunity Parameters and Plasma Lipid in Patients with Rheumatoid Arthritis. *Zhonghua Xin Xue Guan Bing Za Zhi* **2011**, *39*, 941–945.
58. Petersen, A.M.W.; Pedersen, B.K. The Anti-Inflammatory Effect of Exercise. *J. Appl. Physiol.* **2005**, *98*, 1154–1162. [CrossRef]

59. Nadler, S.F.; Weingand, K.; Kruse, R.J. The Physiologic Basis and Clinical Applications of Cryotherapy and Thermotherapy for the Pain Practitioner. *Pain Physician* **2004**, *7*, 395–400. [CrossRef]
60. Hutter, J.J.; Mestril, R.; Tam, E.K.W.; Sievers, R.E.; Dillmann, W.H.; Wolfe, C.L. Overexpression of Heat Shock Protein 72 in Transgenic Mice Decreases Infarct Size in Vivo. *Circulation* **1996**, *94*, 1408–1411. [CrossRef]
61. Saleh, M.S.; Mahrous, R.M.; El Keblawy, M.M. Effect of Siwa Sand Baths versus Sulphurous Water Bath on Inflammatory Biomarkers, Pain, and Physical Function in Patients with Rheumatoid Arthritis: A Randomized, Single-Blind Controlled Trial. *Fizjoterapia Pol.* **2022**, *22*, 18–24.

Disclaimer/Publisher's Note: The statements, opinions and data contained in all publications are solely those of the individual author(s) and contributor(s) and not of MDPI and/or the editor(s). MDPI and/or the editor(s) disclaim responsibility for any injury to people or property resulting from any ideas, methods, instructions or products referred to in the content.

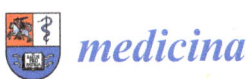

Review

Role of Inflammatory Cytokines in Rheumatoid Arthritis and Development of Atherosclerosis: A Review

Dražen Bedeković [1,2,*], Ivica Bošnjak [1], Sandra Šarić [1,2], Damir Kirner [1,2] and Srđan Novak [3,4]

1. Department of Cardiovascular Diseases Internal Medicine Clinic, University Hospital Osijek, J. Huttlera 4, 31000 Osijek, Croatia; dribosnjak79@gmail.com (I.B.); smakarovic36@gmail.com (S.Š.); damir.kirner@gmail.com (D.K.)
2. Faculty of Medicine Osijek, Department of Internal Medicine, Josip Juraj Strossmayer University, J. Huttlera 4, 31000 Osijek, Croatia
3. Department of Rheumatology and Clinical Immunology, University Hospital Rijeka, Braće Branchetta 20/1, 51000 Rijeka, Croatia; srdan.novak@gmali.com
4. Faculty of Medicine Rijeka, Department of Internal Medicine, University of Rijeka, Braće Branchetta 20/1, 51000 Rijeka, Croatia
* Correspondence: drbedekovic@yahoo.com; Tel.: +385-31-511-714

Abstract: Uncontrolled chronic inflammation results in cardiovascular disease and early death. In this review, we studied the impact of rheumatoid arthritis on the cardiovascular system, including the early and accelerated development of atherosclerosis and its clinical manifestations, focusing on the inflammatory mechanisms leading to arterial wall damage, rapid atherosclerotic plaque formation, and thrombosis. Furthermore, the effect of medications used to treat rheumatoid arthritis on the cardiovascular system was studied. The effect of chronic inflammation and medication on traditional cardiovascular risk factors is not the main subject of this review. We observed that uncontrolled chronic inflammation and some medications directly impact all the stages of atherosclerosis. In conclusion, reducing inflammation and maintaining long-term remission in rheumatoid arthritis may prevent early atherosclerosis. We believe that this review will encourage a better interdisciplinary approach to the management of these patients and further research in this field.

Keywords: rheumatoid arthritis; chronic inflammation mechanisms; cardiovascular risk; cardiovascular mortality; medications used in rheumatoid arthritis

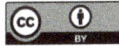

1. Introduction

Rheumatoid arthritis (RA) is a chronic inflammatory systemic disease that primarily affects the synovial membrane, cartilage, and bones of small- and medium-sized joints, leading to chronic damage and pannus formation; however, blood vessels and various internal organs are also often affected [1–5]. The prevalence of RA in the general population is approximately 1%, and women are predominantly affected. RA results in significant disability, socioeconomic consequences, and a short lifespan of 5 to 18 years, mainly attributable to increased cardiovascular (CV) morbidity and mortality [1,6,7]. The causes of RA remain unknown, but being of female sex and a family history of RA are known risk factors. Known triggers for RA include exposure to bacterial or viral infections, especially bacteria that cause periodontal disease or the Epstein–Barr virus; trauma, bone, or joint fractures; cigarette smoking; and obesity. Typically, the symptoms of RA develop slowly over several weeks or months and can range from mild to severe. They include articular symptoms, such as pain and swelling; morning stiffness or stiffness after prolonged rest lasting >30 min; symmetrical involvement and loss of function; general symptoms such as fatigue, fever, and weight loss; and extra-articular symptoms such as rheumatoid nodules, cardiopulmonary disease, eye disease, Sjogren's syndrome, rheumatoid vasculitis, neurological manifestations, and Felty's syndrome [1–16].

Atherosclerosis and its complications are the most common CV manifestations of RA and are the leading cause of death in patients with RA. Moreover, two major mechanisms of chronic inflammation have a substantial impact on CV risk causing direct damage to the CV system, especially the arteries, and an indirect effect through traditional CV risk factors. These factors synergistically increase CV risk, morbidity, and premature mortality. The traditional risk factors include arterial hypertension, cigarette smoking, dyslipidemia, low levels of physical activity, and diabetes/insulin resistance [17]. Compared with healthy individuals, patients with RA experience adverse effects on the development of CV disease (CVD) due to traditional CV risk factors, including arterial hypertension that increases the risk by 53–73% (in most but not all studies); cigarette smoking increases risk by 25–50%; dyslipidemia increases risk by 73% (difficulty in assessment due to "lipid paradox"); low physical activity is neutral to the increased risk; diabetes/insulin resistance is double; and obesity increases risk by 16% (in most but not all studies) [18–37]. However, the effects of chronic inflammation in RA and of medications used for its treatment on traditional CV risk factors are not the subjects of this article. The focus of this review was to gather all relevant data and knowledge, analyze and discuss the role and mechanisms of chronic inflammation, as well as the effect of medications used for treating RA, on the CV system. We believe that this review will contribute to an improved understanding and encourage further research to prevent early atherosclerosis development and its consequences in patients with RA.

2. Materials and Methods

2.1. Objective

To systematically gather and analyze all relevant data regarding the direct effects of chronic inflammation associated with RA, as well as the effect of RA medications on the cardiovascular system.

2.2. Data Sources

A systematic search and review of the available relevant literature was conducted in the medical databases Web of Science, Scopus, PubMed, and Cochrane Library.

2.3. Keywords Used in Article Selection

Rheumatoid arthritis, chronic inflammation mechanisms, cardiovascular risk, cardiovascular mortality, coagulation mechanisms, medications in rheumatoid arthritis, non-steroidal anti-inflammatory drugs (NSAIDs), glucocorticoids/corticosteroids, methotrexate, hydroxychloroquine, leflunomide, cyclosporine, azathioprine, biologic medications, infliximab, etanercept, adalimumab, tocilizumab, abatacept, rituximab, certolizumab, tofacitinib, golimumab, sarilumab, anakinra, canakinumab, baricitinib, and statins.

2.4. Article Selection: Inclusion and Exclusion Criteria

Inclusion criteria: Data from meta-analyses, large randomized controlled trials, prospective clinical trials, relevant reviews, as well as data from the European Society of Cardiology and European Alliance of Associations for Rheumatology guidelines, were considered to be the most relevant. Smaller studies were included only if no other data were available or if we considered them crucial. Only two case reports, one expert opinion, and one meta-analysis (critics) were included on specific topics. All the known study limitations are listed in Table S1. The selected and analyzed articles consisted of important data on the following topics: mechanisms of chronic inflammation in RA and its effect on the CV system, cardiovascular disease development in RA, and the effect of medications used to treat RA on the CV system.

Exclusion criteria: Case reports, pilot projects, studies, meta-analyses, and reviews with questionable methodology or reliability; underpowered studies; studies with no full-text available; studies with a population aged <18 years; and studies not directly related to the investigation topics were generally excluded.

We selected abstracts of published studies according to the inclusion criteria; if suitable, we analyzed the full text. All important data were extrapolated and copied into pre-prepared tables and were analyzed by at least one cardiologist and rheumatologist. Special attention was paid to the statistical data in articles, which were reviewed by at least one of two employed statisticians. The statistician assessed the size and representativeness of the sample and the use of statistical methods and their adequacy. The final analysis was performed by all the authors. The precise selection process is described in Section 3.1 and in the Supplementary Materials.

2.5. Limitations

We accepted all articles written in English or German. Studies involving populations under 18 years of age were excluded from the review. Some studies did not declare the number of participants in a meta-analysis or review but were accepted because of the importance of the topic, or because only a few articles were available on certain topics. Some limitations of the included studies were identified.

2.6. Study Design

Review.

2.7. Review Period

Studies from 1986 to 2022.

3. Results

3.1. Article Selection Process

More than 500,000 published articles were initially crudely screened in databases using the pre-selected keywords. We initially selected 375 abstracts by narrowing the search parameters and carefully combining the main keywords with others (e.g., rheumatoid arthritis and biologic medications) and concurrently included or excluded article types according to the inclusion and exclusion criteria. From 375 abstracts, including 61 meta-analyses, we identified 145 articles that were suitable for this review according to the inclusion and exclusion criteria (Figure 1). We excluded 3 articles that were not in English or German, along with 24 that lacked full-text accessibility, 1 that constituted a letter to the editor, 2 based on the recommendation of a statistician, 2 involving pediatric study population, 2 studies describing obsolete diagnostic procedures, and 194 that were not closely related to our topic or were repetitive. We divided the articles into four categories. The first two categories provided general information about RA and CVD and traditional risk factors, and they served as an introduction, whereas the last two categories were analyzed for the effects of chronic inflammation mechanisms in RA (52 articles) and the effects of medications used in RA (62 articles) on the CV system.

3.2. Analysis Results

We analyzed 52 articles for the effect of RA and 62 for the effect of medications on the CV system. Article characteristics are presented in Table S1.

3.2.1. Chronic Inflammation

RA arises from the interplay between genetic susceptibility and environmental triggers. The most important genetic risk is the presence of the DRB1*04:01 gene, a shared epitope that induces the binding of post-translationally modified (citrullinated) proteins, and the PTPN22 gene, which increases citrullination [38]. The major environmental risk factors include tobacco smoking, being of female sex, being of advanced age, and certain foods [38–40]. Autoimmune processes include the recognition of synovial tissue self-antigens, such as type II collagen, proteoglycans, and cartilage protein gp39 [41–43]. First, the joint intimal lining expands, causing synoviocyte activation and proliferation; they then begin to secrete pro-inflammatory cytokines, such as tumor necrosis factor

(TNF), interleukin-1 (IL-1), interleukin-6 (IL-6), metalloproteinases, prostaglandins, and leukotrienes. Synovial invasion into the adjacent articular structures damages the cartilage and bone, manifesting as joint swelling. Second, synovial layer proliferation contributes to the activation of neutrophils and T- and B-lymphocytes, which infiltrate the joints and secrete cytokines and proteinases that further damage the extracellular matrix. Effector CD4+ T cells play a crucial role in disease progression and are characterized by an imbalance between Th1/Th17 and regulatory T cells [44,45]. Atherosclerosis and synovial inflammation in RA share a common pathway, and sustained synovial secretion of inflammatory mediators elicits chronic low-grade activation and dysfunction of the vascular endothelium, thereby expediting the development of atherosclerosis in RA [46].

With initial crude search of medical databased by keywords we found >500,000 articles related to our topic.

By narrowing search parameters using careful selected keywords combination and including/excluding article types we selected 375 articles for further analyses by authors and statisticians.

By reading abstracts (and full text if needed) we excluded articles: if full text was not available, case reports, pilot projects, studies and reviews with questionable methodology or reliability, underpowered studies, studies with population under 18 years, and studies not directly related to investigation topic.

We accepted in review two case reports and one expert opinion do to relevance of analyzed topic.

We also excluded 3 articles due to language, they were not written in English or German.

Total of 145 full text articles were submitted to analyses.

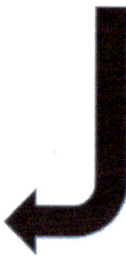

Figure 1. Article selection process for review—schematics.

Citrullinated synovial proteins induce the production of RA-specific autoantibodies (anti-CCP) [47,48], which can increase the risk of ischemic heart disease (6.5% vs. 2.6%, odds ratio [OR]: 2.58, 95% confidence interval [CI]: 1.17–5.65) [49]. Anti-CCP antibodies are associated with early subclinical atherosclerosis and promote atherosclerotic plaque formation by targeting citrullinated sarcomeric proteins, fibrinogen, and vimentin [50–52]. Several studies addressing anti-CCP positivity reported that it is associated with higher total mortality and an increase in fatal CV outcomes but not with heart failure or recurrent ischemia [52–55]; however, large studies did not confirm this finding [56,57]. Other antibodies are also possibly associated with CVD risk, such as antibodies against carbamylated proteins (anti-CarP) and malondialdehyde–acetaldehyde adducts [53]. The combination of genetic and environmental triggers also leads to constant activation and clonal expansion of specific CD4 + CD28 null T cell subsets, and especially the loss of CD28, a co-stimulatory molecule required for normal T cell activation, which correlates with seropositivity and extra-articular RA manifestations [58]. The possible direct cytotoxic effects of these cells on endothelial cells, along with their induced dysfunction, can cause early atherosclerosis and its complications [59–61]. This strongly stimulates the activity and recruitment of macrophages and T cells to the plaque, contributing to reactive oxygen species production, inhibiting collagen production, stimulating matrix metalloproteinases, and inducing tissue factor expression that is an independent predictor of future acute coronary events in patients with RA (OR: 3.01, 95% CI: 1.1–8.25, p = 0.023) [62,63]. The activated endothelium promotes the binding of neutrophils, monocytes, and platelets, which is further potentiated with neutrophils, IL-8, and monocyte CCL2 chemokines. Adherent neutrophils and monocytes promote further activation of the vascular endothelium with PAR-1. Neutrophils exposed to activated platelets form intravascular neutrophil extracellular traps, which by the expression of endothelium-activating proteases, histones, and tissue factors, promotes the creation of intravascular pro-inflammatory and prothrombotic milieus [14].

C-reactive protein (CRP) and fibrinogen are less likely to be causally associated with atherogenesis according to newer studies; however, pro-inflammatory cytokines, interleukin-6 (IL-6), interleukin-18 (IL-18), and tumor necrosis factor-α (TNF-α) could be directly etiologically associated with atherogenesis through the regulation of inflammatory cascades [64,65]. One prospective study, and a meta-analysis of 29 studies investigating six pro-inflammatory cytokines (IL-6, IL-18, matrix metalloproteinase-9 [MMP-9], soluble CD40 ligand [sCD40L], and TNF-α) in coronary heart disease, concluded that higher baseline levels of IL-6, IL-18, and TNF-α were associated with a 10–25% higher risk of non-fatal myocardial infarction and CV death [66].

Chronic inflammation also has pro-coagulant and pro-oxidant effects mediated using several mechanisms, including increased expression of adhesion molecules for tissue factors, reduced synthesis of nitrogen oxide and thrombomodulin, and induction of nicotinamide adenine dinucleotide phosphate (NADPH) oxidases, causing further endothelium dysfunction [67,68]. Significantly increased levels of tissue factors, fibrinogen, von Willebrand factor, factor (F) VIII, activated FXIIa, and markers of thrombin synthesis have been observed in patients with RA with high inflammatory activity [67,69]. Activated platelets are a crucial element in the development of acute CV syndromes, as well as in atherosclerotic plaque formation, and elevated platelet counts could serve to assess RA activity [70,71]. Collectively, these mechanisms shift the hemostatic balance towards a prothrombotic state in RA [52]. CV risk estimation in the general population is based on different risk scores that underestimate CV risk in patients with RA. This phenomenon is believed to be primarily driven by chronic inflammation, and it has been observed in various studies, such as the HOOM and CARRÉ studies, thereby affecting risk assessment models such as the Framingham score or SCORE system [72].

IL-6 and TNF-α are independently associated with a higher coronary calcium score and increased CV risk [52,73,74]. Cytokine influence begins very early in RA, mostly affecting the carotid and coronary arteries, and it is associated with a significant proportion of acute CV events [46]. High-grade inflammation is associated with increased CV morbidity and mortality, with the CRP level and erythrocyte sedimentation rate (ESR) being independent markers [57,75–77]. The use of CRP, or highly sensitive CRP, as a predictor of CV risk in modified CV risk calculators has not been adopted in standard cardiology practice [78].

Endothelial dysfunction and signs of atherosclerosis present very early in RA and is the result of complex interactions among modifiable CV risk factors, genetic predisposition, chronic inflammation, pro-oxidative stress, prothrombotic status, and metabolic abnormalities (insulin resistance and dyslipidemia) [78–81]. According to Gonzalez-Gay et al., endothelial dysfunction is worsened by long-standing RA of >20 years compared with RA of <7 years; however, the success of inflammation control has not been investigated [81]. Recently, critical limb ischemia was reported in a 27-year-old man with psoriasis who presented without any CV risk factors [82]. Endothelial dysfunction in RA can be assessed measuring circulating soluble adhesive molecules, such as E-selectin, P-selectin, intracellular adhesion molecule-1 (ICAM-1), vascular cell type 1 adhesion molecule (VCAM-1), and flow-mediated arterial dilatation, all of which are suggested for use in CV risk assessment; these methodologies are supported by a meta-analysis involving 20 studies including 852 patients with RA [83].

Duplex atherosclerosis screening is a widely used method for the detection of atherosclerotic plaques that are predictive of CV disease [83]. Assessing CV burden in RA by measuring carotid intima–media thickness is no longer recommended [17,27]; however, detection of carotid plaque formation has a predictive value, with a pronounced effect in early RA and among male patients with a higher inflammatory burden [17,84]. Flow-mediated dilatation, augmentation index, pulse wave velocity, coronary artery calcification score (CAC), SPECT/CT, PET/CT, and PET/MRI are also used to assess atherosclerotic burden; however, non-imaging methods have many limitations and confounding factors [36]. CAC, a measure of coronary artery calcification and subclinical atherosclerosis, is closely related to the degree of atherosclerotic plaque burden and is a strong predictor of CV events [36,85]. Coronary artery calcification was independently associated with older age and hypertension, whereas abdominal aorta calcification was independently associated with older age and erosive arthritis [85].

3.2.2. Influence of Medications

NSAIDs

Non-steroidal anti-inflammatory drugs (NSAIDs) and cyclooxygenase-2 inhibitors (COX2 inhibitors) have good anti-inflammatory and analgesic effects, but they increase the risk of acute CV diseases, particularly stroke and myocardial infarction; this occurs particularly with diclofenac and rofecoxib [32,86–92]. Other adverse effects, such as an increased risk of atrial fibrillation and heart failure, can induce or aggravate arterial hypertension, acute or chronic kidney damage, and gastrointestinal complications, especially in older patients with multiple comorbidities [90–94]. Inhibition of different isoenzymes of cyclooxygenase (COX) and a decrease in prostaglandins at inflammatory sites increase thromboxane A2 (COX-1) and decrease prostaglandin I2 (COX-2) production, which may lead to vasoconstriction, platelet activation, hypertension, accelerated atherosclerosis, renal sodium retention with peripheral edema and heart failure, and increased CV morbidity and mortality [88,92,94–96]. The Vioxx Gastrointestinal Outcomes Research (VIGOR) and the Adenomatous Polyp Prevention on Vioxx (APPROVe) trials led to rofecoxib withdrawal due to the high risk of thrombotic events. This was supported by a meta-analysis involving 28 RA studies that reported an 18% increased risk of all CV events (RR, 1.18; 95% CI 1.01 to 1.38; $p = 0.04$) and strokes with a greater effect with COX-2 inhibitors (RR, 1.36; 95% CI 1.10 to 1.67; $p = 0.004$) than that with nonselective NSAIDs (RR, 1.08; 95% CI 0.94 to 1.24; $p = 0.28$) [88,89,91]. An analysis of 19 studies including patients with RA and osteoarthritis revealed a significantly increased risk of CV events with diclofenac and rofecoxib and a non-significant increased risk with celecoxib [97]. NSAIDs should be prescribed at the lowest effective doses and for the shortest possible duration [72,91,93]. Gastric prophylaxis is also recommended, especially if NSAIDs are combined with glucocorticoids, in older adults and in patients with a moderate to high risk of peptic ulcer disease [93]. The use of acetylsalicylic acid for the primary prevention of CV disease in patients with RA is not recommended [17,78].

Glucocorticoids

Glucocorticoids have potent anti-inflammatory and immunosuppressive effects and are widely used in RA treatment. The addition of low-dose glucocorticoids (below 7.5 mg/daily prednisone) to disease-modifying antirheumatics (DMARDs) in early RA slows the radiological progression of bone destruction [92,98]. Long-term use of glucocorticoids at high and low doses significantly increases CV risk, with an unfavorable impact on lipid metabolism, obesity, insulin production, insulin resistance, and blood pressure [22,36,99]. Numerous studies have found an increased incidence of all-cause and CV mortality, hypertension, hyperglycemia, diabetes, osteoporosis, and myocardial infarction with dose- and time-dependent glucocorticoid usage [22,88,92,100]. According to current guidelines, glucocorticoids should be used at the lowest possible dose, continuation should be regularly reassessed, and remission withdrawal should be considered [101,102].

Classical DMARDs

DMARDs, especially methotrexate (MTX), sulfasalazine, and hydroxychloroquine, have beneficial effects on CV risk [36,83,100,103–105]. MTX is an antifolate immunosuppressive drug that inhibits neutrophil chemotaxis and synthesis of pro-inflammatory cytokines, as well as exerts antiatherogenic and cardioprotective effects [102,105]. MTX was associated with a 21% lower overall risk of CV events (95% CI 0.73–0.87, $p < 0.001$) and an 18% lower risk of myocardial infarction (95% CI: 0.71–0.96, $p = 0.01$) [103]. A study on CAC, using computed tomography, reported a lower coronary calcification burden with MTX use in patients with RA [85]. Another meta-analysis including 28 studies reported an overall 21% CV risk reduction with MTX (RR, 0.72; 95% CI 0.57 to 0.91; $p = 0.007$) as well as an 18% risk reduction in myocardial infarction—a trend towards a decreasing risk of heart failure, whereas it revealed no effect on strokes and major adverse cardiac events [88]. An older meta-analysis including 18 studies also reported a similar reduced risk of CV events in patients with RA treated with MTX [106,107]. Several studies have reported that MTX increases total cholesterol, LDL, HDL, and triglyceride levels in RA, with a possible explanation suggesting that it reflects the normalization of lipid levels due to the suppression of inflammation, without increasing CV risk [74]. Hydroxychloroquine exerts antirheumatic effects by targeting autoantigen processing in macrophages, suppressing T-lymphocytes, and neutralizing the prothrombotic effects of antiphospholipid antibodies [91,104]. Hydroxychloroquine improves lipid and glycemic indices and reduces the risk of thromboembolic events and CV risk [72,91,104,108,109]. Several reports have asserted the consideration of hydroxychloroquine cardiotoxicity (restrictive cardiomyopathy and conduction disorders). However, in those cases, patients had prolonged use of large cumulative doses; notably, the use of hydroxychloroquine is considered safe at therapeutic doses with periodic ECG monitoring [104]. Combination therapy with MTX, sulfasalazine, and hydroxychloroquine also decreases CV risk by improving the reduction in inflammation, increase in HDL, and decrease in LDL and by enhancing the ratio of total cholesterol to HDL. Notably, this combination therapy has shown superiority over MTX monotherapy or a combination of MTX and etanercept; however, the study only included patients with early RA with high disease activity who were naïve to DMARDs [110]. Azathioprine, cyclosporine, and leflunomide increase the risk of CV events by 80% that of MTX monotherapy [111,112]. Leflunomide has potent anti-inflammatory and immunomodulatory effects; however, it increases the risk of hypertension, which has been reported in 2.1–10.6% of cases in different studies [91,113]. Cyclosporine is used for the treatment of severe early RA and has many adverse effects; careful monitoring is advised when using cyclosporine [91,113]. Azathioprine is a purine analog with rare adverse effects, which include angina, renal and subclavian vein thrombosis, hypotension, and cardiogenic shock [91,113].

Biologic Agents

Biologics target inflammatory cytokines (TNF-α and IL-6) and cytokine receptors, interrupting the vicious cycle of inflammation, and are recommended even in early RA with low-severity inflammatory arthritis [91,112]. By suppressing inflammation and maintaining low disease activity, they significantly reduce the risk of CV and incidence of myocardial infarction, heart failure, and cerebrovascular events in patients with RA [91,113–117]. Anti-TNF agents neutralize soluble- and/or membrane-bound TNF and act as monoclonal antibodies or soluble receptors [91]. In addition to the anti-inflammatory effect of anti-TNF-α therapy, and the consequential improvement in joint function, they may indirectly lead to increased levels of physical activity, which will subsequently decrease the incidence of other CV risk factors, such as diabetes mellitus and hypertension [114]. Karpouzas et al. reported slower non-calcified coronary plaque progression with longer usage of biologics, independent of inflammation, prednisone dose, and statin use [118].

A recently published meta-analysis, including 26 longitudinal studies addressing the question of anti-TNF therapy's effect on body mass index (BMI), found a small increase in body weight and BMI—on average 0.90 kg, 2.34 kg, and 2.27 kg for infliximab, etanercept, and adalimumab, respectively, at 4 and 104 weeks of follow-up [119]. The ATTACH study reported that anti-TNF therapy increased mortality or worsened heart failure in patients with moderate to severe chronic heart failure, especially those with an ischemic etiology, but the RENAISSANCE and RECOVER clinical trials did not confirm this for etanercept [120]. A possible reduction in insulin resistance with anti-TNF therapy was reported in a meta-analysis of 12 studies [121]. A meta-analysis of studies considering the impact of biologics (tocilizumab, abatacept, rituximab, and TNF inhibitors) on CV risk and safety reported fewer CV events with rituximab [122]. A large meta-analysis, which included 43 biological registers and 27 publications, addressed the issue of biologics' safety and effect on mortality. It reported that overall mortality and CV events were significantly reduced in patients treated with anti-TNFs with relative risk (RR) = 0.60 [95% CI 0.38–0.94] and RR = 0.62 [95% CI 0.44–0.88], respectively, with no effect on the risk of neoplasm but a significant increase in infections during anti-TNF treatment (RR = 1.48 [1.18–1.85]) compared to those who were treated with classical DMARDs [123]. Another meta-analysis including 28 studies of patients with RA reported that anti-TNF treatment was significantly associated with an overall CV risk reduction of approximately 30% [88]. Cheung et al. analyzed the effect of anti-TNF therapy on subclinical atherosclerosis, and six studies measured at least one parameter before and after treatment (24th and 52nd weeks), which included intima–media thickness, pulse wave velocity, and an augmentation index; they observed that anti-TNF therapy had no effect on all three parameters at the 24th week and on intima–media thickness at the 52nd week [124]. An older meta-analysis including 32 studies by Daien et al. demonstrated increased total cholesterol and HDL levels and unchanged LDL levels with long-term anti-TNF therapy, with uncertain effects on CV risk [125]; however, the total cholesterol/HDL ratio was not significantly altered with anti-TNF therapy [74]. A meta-analysis by Zhao et al. reported an increased incidence of hypertension associated with some anti-TNF therapies (OR = 1.8896, 95% CI: 1.35–2.65), as well as an increased incidence of hypertension with longer therapy durations, associated with certolizumab but not with etanercept, tofacitinib, infliximab, and golimumab [126]. Results from a new Korean observational study revealed no increase in the incidence of hypertension with biologics than that with classical DMARDs, in general [127]. A neutral effect of anti-TNF agents on HA incidence was reported by Desai et al. from a large cohort study [128].

The effect of non-anti-TNF agents—abatacept, tocilizumab, sarilumab, anakinra, and rituximab—on CV risk has also been evaluated; abatacept was found to have a 20% greater CV risk reduction than that of anti-TNF agents; tocilizumab had the same effect on CV risk as MTX monotherapy; anakinra showed improved vascular and left ventricular function in a small placebo-controlled study; sarilumab and rituximab had a neutral effect on CV events; and canakinumab, an IL-1 inhibitor administered at 150 mg for every 3 months had a significantly lower rate of myocardial infarction compared with that of the placebo [76,129–134]. Several studies have consistently reported that tocilizumab was associated with increased total cholesterol, HDL, LDL, and triglyceride levels, [74,91]. But the MEASURE study demonstrated that the concentration of proatherogenic small and dense LDL particles was not increased [135]. No studies have reported an increase in CV events with tocilizumab [91].

Small Molecule Inhibitors of Janus Kinase

Tofacitinib and baricitinib, newer small-molecule inhibitors of janus kinase (JAK), increase total and LDL cholesterol levels by 10–20% [136]. Increased dose-dependent LDL and HDL levels were reported with baricitinib use; the mean change was 13.15 mg/dL (95% CI: 8.89–17.42) and 5.40 mg/dL (95% CI: 3.07–7.74), respectively [130]. A recently published pooled cohort study of 3492 patients with RA, with more than 7860 patient-years of exposure to baricitinib, did not reveal a significant association between baricitinib treatment and the occurrence of CV events or congestive heart failure [137]. A meta-analysis including 20 studies investigated the influence of biologic agents and tofacitinib on the lipid profile of patients with RA and revealed increased cholesterol (OR 4.64; 95% CI 2.71, 7.95, $p < 0.001$), HDL (OR 2.25; 95% CI 1.14, 4.44, $p = 0.020$), and LDL (OR 4.80; 95% CI 3.27, 7.05, $p < 0.001$) levels; however, despite this effect on lipid levels, better inflammation control with those medications appears to result in lower mortality and reduced incidence of CV events [138].

With the exception of the ENTRACTE trial, which compared tocilizumab and etanercept, no head-to-head study has been conducted on the impact of biological agents on CV risk and safety. The ENTRACTE trial reported no significant difference in CV events between the tocilizumab and etanercept groups [85]. Observational studies have reported a higher incidence of myocardial infarction among older patients with anti-TNF inhibitors than with abatacept and tocilizumab, and no difference in CV risk was observed when comparing tocilizumab with abatacept [76,139].

Statins

The risk of RA may be lower in patients with a longer duration or high intensity of statin use [139]. Treatment with statins is beneficial in lowering CV risk in patients with RA due to their lipid-lowering and other pleiotropic effects that slow down coronary non-calcified plaque progression and suppress the effects of inflammation on plaque progression and CAC [78,118,140–143].

4. Discussion

4.1. Chronic Inflammation

RA has a complex etiology that involves a combination of genetic susceptibility and environmental triggers. The most prominent genetic risk is the presence of the human leukocyte antigen DRB1*04:01 gene, which encodes a shared epitope—a 5-amino acid sequence—inducing the binding of post-translationally modified (citrullinated) proteins. Another genetic risk factor is PTPN22, which increases citrullination [38]. The major environmental risk factors include tobacco smoking, being of female sex, being of advanced age, and certain foods [38–40]. Autoimmune processes include the recognition of synovial tissue self-antigens, such as type II collagen, proteoglycans, and cartilage protein gp39 [41–43]. The activation and combination of these two major mechanisms are crucial for joint destruction and bone erosion in RA. Initially, the joint's intimal lining expands, causing synoviocyte activation and proliferation. These cells start releasing pro-inflammatory cytokines (such as TNF-α, IL-1, and IL-6), metalloproteinases, prostaglandins, and leukotrienes. Synovial invasion into the adjacent articular structures damages the cartilage and bone, manifesting as joint swelling. Subsequently, synovial layer proliferation contributes to the activation of neutrophils and T- and B-lymphocytes, leading to their infiltration into the joints. This infiltration results in the secretion of cytokines and proteinases that further damage the extracellular matrix. Effector CD4+ T cells play a crucial role in disease progression and are characterized by an imbalance between Th1/Th17 and regulatory T cells [44,45]. As the pathogenic processes of atherosclerosis and synovial inflammation in RA share a common pathway, the understanding of these processes represents a cornerstone of CV risk management in patients with RA. Sustained synovial secretion of inflammatory mediators leads to chronic low-grade activation and dysfunction of the vascular endothelium, promoting the accelerated development of atherosclerosis in RA [46].

Citrullinated synovial proteins induce the production of anti-CCP autoantibodies, largely linked to RA. These antibodies are associated with more severe forms of RA [47,48] and have been extensively studied in the context of CV. According to López-Longo et al., anti-CCP antibody titer levels > 25 units/mL carry a higher risk of ischemic heart disease (6.5 vs. 2.6%, OR: 2.58, 95% CI: 1.17–5.65) without affecting mortality [49]. Previous studies clarified the association of citrullinated proteins and anti-CCP antibodies with early subclinical atherosclerosis and atherosclerotic plaque promotion. This association involves the interaction of anti-CCP antibodies with citrullinated fibrinogen in plaques, inducing inflammation and contributing to heart failure. Additionally, anti-CCP antibodies targeting citrullinated sarcomeric proteins, namely fibrinogen and vimentin, can lead to heart issues independently of coronary artery disease [50–52]. However, these studies had important limitations, such as the inability to demonstrate a direct anti-CCP complex in plaque [50] and many false-positive fluorodeoxyglucose uptake results [51]. Several studies addressing anti-CCP positivity reported that it was associated with higher total mortality and increased fatal CV outcomes but not with heart failure or recurrent ischemia [52–55]; study limitations are listed in Table S1. Conversely, other large studies did not find a significant association between anti-CCP and rheumatoid factor positivity and CV morbidity and mortality, [56,57], which we consider to have greater relevance. Moreover, other antibodies present in RA are possibly associated with CVD risk, including antibodies against anti-CarP and malondialdehyde–acetaldehyde adducts [53]. Genetic susceptibility and environmental triggers also lead to constant activation and clonal expansion of specific CD4 + CD28 null T cell subsets, which play a crucial role in the pathogenesis of RA. The loss of CD28, a co-stimulatory molecule required for normal T cell activation, correlates with seropositivity and extra-articular RA manifestations [58]. Increased expression of perforin and killer cell immunoglobulin-like receptors in these cells, with potential direct cytotoxic effects on endothelial cells and their dysfunction, can cause early atherosclerosis, plaque rupture, and thrombosis [59–61]. This expression strongly stimulates the activity and recruitment of macrophages and T cells to the plaque, contributing to reactive oxygen species production, inhibiting collagen production, stimulating matrix metalloproteinases, and inducing tissue factor expression [62]. According to Liuzzo et al. [63], the level of CD4 + CD28 null T-cells in patients' blood was an independent predictor of future acute coronary events in patients with RA (OR: 3.01, 95% CI: 1.1–8.25, $p = 0.023$). The activated endothelium promotes the binding of neutrophils, monocytes, and platelets, which is further potentiated by neutrophils, IL-8, and monocyte CCL2 chemokines. Adherent neutrophils and monocytes promote further activation of the vascular endothelium with PAR-1, creating a vicious cycle that leads to endothelial dysfunction. Neutrophils exposed to activated platelets form intravascular neutrophil extracellular traps, which—by expression of endothelium-activating proteases, histones, and tissue factors—promote the development of intravascular pro-inflammatory and pro-thrombotic milieus [14]. This finding is substantiated by numerous published studies and reviews.

Many studies have focused on the role of inflammatory cytokines in atherogenesis and CV disease development, as well as their use for risk stratification. Newer studies reported that CRP and fibrinogen are less likely to be causally associated with atherogenesis, but pro-inflammatory cytokines (IL-6, IL-18, and TNF-α) could be directly etiologically associated with atherogenesis by regulation of inflammatory cascades [64,65]. In a prospective study with 1514 participants and a meta-analysis of 29 studies with approximately 17,000 participants, Kaptoge et al. [66] studied the roles of five pro-inflammatory cytokines, IL-6 and IL-18, MMP-9, sCD40L, and TNF-α in coronary heart disease and concluded that higher baseline levels of IL-6, IL-18, and TNF-α were associated with a 10–25% higher risk of non-fatal myocardial infarction and CV death, whereas sCD40L and MMP-9 did not show any such association.

Chronic inflammation also has pro-coagulant effects mediated by several mechanisms, including increased expression of adhesion molecules for tissue factors, reduced synthesis of nitrogen oxide and thrombomodulin, and increased pro-coagulant properties of the endothelium [67]. Endothelial dysfunction is further mediated by the induction of NADPH oxidases and dysfunction of antioxidant systems [68]. Significantly increased levels of tissue factors, fibrinogen, von Willebrand factor, factor (F) VIII, activated FXIIa, and markers of thrombin synthesis have been observed in patients with RA with high inflammatory activity [67,69]. Platelets activated by cytokine-sensitized endothelial neutrophils or monocytes or by anti-CCP antibody exposure are key elements in the development of acute CV syndromes and in atherosclerotic plaque formation, recruiting leukocytes to the sites of endothelial damage and inflammation, activating complement and other inflammatory receptors, and releasing cytokines and chemokines [70]. Together, these mechanisms shift the hemostatic balance to a prothrombotic state in RA [52]. A meta-analysis by Zhou et al. [71] confirmed that platelet counts are elevated in patients with RA and could serve to assess disease activity. CV risk estimation in the general population is based on different risks that underestimate the CV risk in patients with RA. It is hypothesized that chronic inflammation is the key determinant contributing to these underestimations. This is further supported by studies like the HOOM and CARRÉ studies, which are in line with the Framingham score or SCORE system, as suggested by several studies [72]. Nonetheless, these studies have limitations in terms of the methods used to estimate CV risk.

IL-6 and TNF-α are independently associated with a higher coronary calcium score and increased CV risk, favoring the hypothesis that RA-related increased CV risk is associated with higher levels of inflammatory cytokines and their deleterious effects on endothelial cells [52,73,74]. This finding is supported by several published studies. The effect manifests at a very early stage in RA, mostly targeting the carotid and coronary arteries, and is associated with a significant proportion of acute CV events [46]. High-grade inflammation associated with increased CV morbidity and mortality, with CRP levels and ESR as independent markers, was reported in a population-based study spanning a 20-year follow-up period, which is in concordance with several earlier research findings [57,75–77]. The use of CRP, or highly sensitive CRP, as a predictor of CV risk in modified CV risk calculators was not adopted in standard cardiology practice [78].

Endothelial dysfunction in RA is the result of complex interactions among modifiable CV risk factors, genetic predisposition, chronic inflammation, pro-oxidative stress, pro-thrombotic status, and metabolic abnormalities (insulin resistance and dyslipidemia) [78,79]. It is present in a very early stage of RA, even before or within one year of the clinical onset of RA—as well as in arterial wall atherosclerosis—with an increased risk of coronary heart disease and myocardial infarction [80,81]. According to Gonzalez-Gay et al. [81], endothelial dysfunction is worsened by long-standing RA of >20 years compared with RA of <7 years; however, the success of inflammation control was not investigated. A recently described case of critical limb ischemia in a 27-year-old man with an 8-year history of psoriasis (a chronic inflammatory disease similar to RA), and without any CV risk factors, points to inflammation as the main cause of endothelial dysfunction and vascular damage, regardless of the presence of traditional or inherited CV risk factors. However, notably, this is a single case, and the outcomes of inflammation management and articular involvement were not described [82]. Endothelial dysfunction in RA can be assessed by measuring circulating soluble adhesive molecules such as E-selectin, P-selectin, ICAM-1, VCAM-1, and flow-mediated arterial dilatation, all of which are suggested for use in CV risk assessment; this observation is supported by a meta-analysis of 20 studies including 852 patients with RA [83].

Duplex atherosclerosis screening is mostly used for detecting atherosclerotic plaques that are predictive of CV disease [83]. Although carotid intima–media thickness measurements were used in previous investigations to assess CV burden in RA, they are no longer recommended as per ESC guidelines [17,27]. However, the detection of carotid plaque formation has a predictive value with a pronounced effect in early-stage RA and in men with a higher inflammation burden [17,84].

Flow-mediated dilatation, augmentation index, pulse wave velocity, CAC score, SPECT/CT, PET/CT, and PET/MRI are also used to assess atherosclerotic burden; however, non-imaging methods have many limitations and confounding factors [36]. The CAC score, a measure of coronary artery calcification and subclinical atherosclerosis, is closely related to the degree of atherosclerotic plaque burden and is a strong predictor of CV events [36]. Paccou et al. [85] conducted a comparison between asymptomatic patients with RA and healthy controls and reported higher prevalence and severity of both coronary artery calcification and abdominal aorta calcification in patients with RA. CAC was independently associated with older age and hypertension, whereas abdominal aorta calcification was independently associated with older age and erosive arthritis. However, there are some reservations concerning this method; for example, non-calcified plaques cannot be detected. Accelerated atherosclerosis in RA, in addition to epicardial artery disease, can cause microvascular dysfunction. This dysfunction plays a crucial role in regulating myocardial perfusion and contributes to the accelerated development of CV disease (Figure 2).

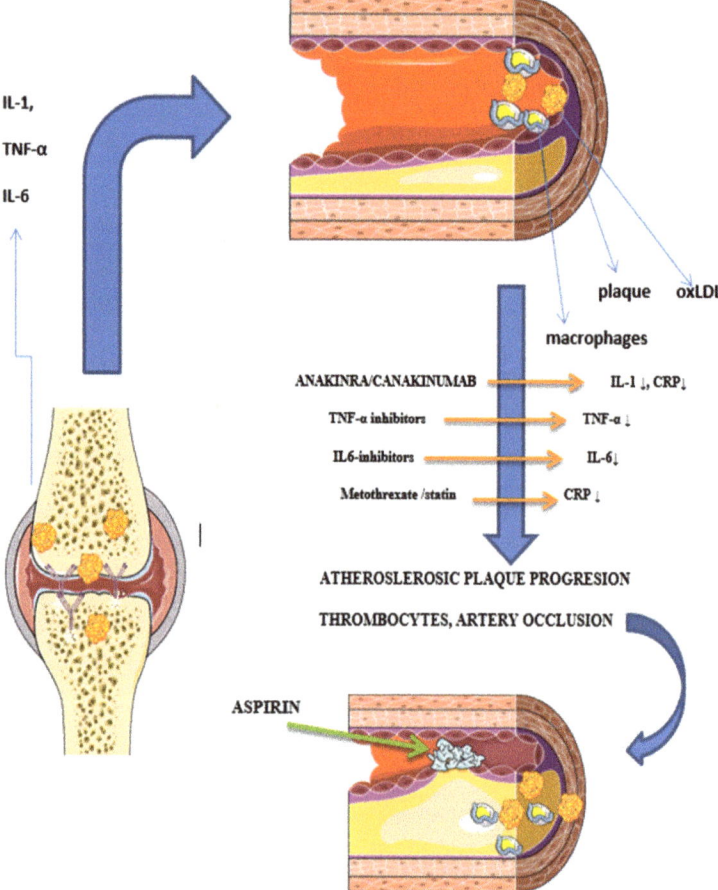

Figure 2. Role of proinflammatory cytokines and medication in vascular damage.

Proinflammatory cytokines interleukin 1 (IL-1), tumour necrosis factor alpha (TNF-α) and interleukin 6 (IL-6) are interconnected in signalling pathways and they are targets for drugs that are used to treat rheumatic diseases and have gained interest as potential drugs for secondary prevention of ASCVD in RA. ASCVD and rheumatoid synovitis both develop via similar inflammatory mechanisms. The first stage involves endothelial dysfunction, whith inflammatory cells infiltration in the joint capsule and the beginning of plaque formation in the artery's sub-intima. The decreased anti-oxidative activity in RA patients also encourages LDL oxidation and foam cell production.. *Methotrexate:* Enhances macrophage cholesterol efflux and prevents foams cell differentiation and activation. Up-regulates free radical scavenging; improves endothelial function. *TNF-α inhibitors:* TNF-α promotes numerous inflammatory responses associated with atherosclerosis, including induction of vascular adhesion and monocyte/macrophage proliferation. TNF-α impacts lipid metabolism by stimulating liver triglyceride production. Atherosclerosis development and RA inflammation are both slowed down by inhibiting these processes. *Tocilizumab (IL-6):* Decreases inflammatory proteins such as serum amyloid A, and restores the anti-atherogenic function of HDL by increasing HDL cholesterol efflux capacity. *Canakinumab IL-1β:* significantly reduced hsC-reactive protein levels from baseline, as compared with placebo, without reducing the LDL cholesterol level. *Statins:* decrease LDL cholesterol by inhibiting HMG-CoA and lowering hsCRP.

4.2. Influence of Medications

4.2.1. NSAIDs

NSAIDs and COX2 inhibitors have good anti-inflammatory and analgesic effects; they can paradoxically increase the risk of acute CV diseases, especially stroke and myocardial infarction. In particular, NSAIDs such as diclofenac and rofecoxib inhibit prostacyclin synthesis [32,85–92]. This is supported by strong evidence, as in the study by Gargiulo et al. [90]. Other adverse effects include an increased risk of atrial fibrillation and heart failure, induction, or aggravation of arterial hypertension (due to their effect on sodium and water retention), as well as induction of acute or chronic kidney damage and gastrointestinal complications—especially in elderly patients with multiple comorbidities [90–94]. Inhibition of different isoenzymes of COX and a decrease in prostaglandins at the inflammatory sites increase thromboxane A2 (COX-1) and decrease prostaglandin I2 (COX-2) production, which may lead to vasoconstriction, platelet activation, hypertension, accelerated atherosclerosis, renal sodium retention with peripheral edema, and heart failure [92]. Many trials and meta-analyses supported those conclusions: COX-2 inhibitors increased the risk of CV events by 42% [88,94], highly increased the risk of CV-related mortality (adjusted OR 0.54, 95% CI 0.34–0.86) [94], increased the risk of first-time myocardial infarction within 180 days of initiation of NSAIDs [95], and were associated with a higher relative risk of myocardial infarction with diclofenac and rofecoxib [96]. The VIGOR and APPROVe trials led to rofecoxib withdrawal due to the high risk of thrombotic events, which was supported by a meta-analysis of 28 RA studies published by Roubille et al. This study reported an 18% increased risk of all CV events (RR, 1.18; 95% CI 1.01 to 1.38; $p = 0.04$) and strokes with a greater effect with COX-2 inhibitors (RR, 1.36; 95% CI 1.10 to 1.67; $p = 0.004$) than with nonselective NSAIDs (RR, 1.08; 95% CI 0.94 to 1.24; $p = 0.28$) [88,91]. The highest increase in CV events occurred with rofecoxib (RR, 1.58; 95% CI 1.24 to 2.00; $p < 0.001$), which led to rofecoxib withdrawal, but other NSAIDs did not show significant effects on the risk of myocardial infarction, heart failure, or major adverse cardiac events; however, very few events were included in the analysis and did not provide strong evidence [89]. An analysis of 19 studies with patients with RA and osteoarthritis reported a significantly increased risk of CV events with diclofenac and rofecoxib and a non-significant increased risk with celecoxib. Etoricoxib and rofecoxib significantly increased the risk of hypertension, as did naproxen for stroke; however, not all NSAIDs were included in the investigation and analyzed for cardiovascular side effects [89]. NSAIDs should be prescribed at the lowest effective doses and for the shortest possible duration with caution when prescribing to patients with CV disease or in the presence of CV risk factors. They should be avoided in patients with treatment-resistant hypertension, high CV risk, and severe chronic kidney disease; naproxen or celecoxib are the preferred choices in these diseases [72,91,93]. For patients with pre-existing hypertension, who are on renin-angiotensin system blockers, dose increases or additions of a different drug class should be considered. Gastric prophylaxis is also recommended, especially if NSAIDs are combined with glucocorticoids in the elderly and in patients with a moderate to high risk of peptic ulcer disease [93]. The use of acetylsalicylic acid for the primary prevention of CV disease in patients with RA is not recommended [17,78].

4.2.2. Glucocorticoids

Glucocorticoids have potent anti-inflammatory and immunosuppressive effects and are widely used in RA treatment. The addition of low-dose glucocorticoids (below 7.5 mg/daily prednisone) to DMARDs in early RA slows the radiological progression of bone destruction [92,98]. Long-term use of glucocorticoids at high and low doses significantly increases CV risk, with an unfavorable impact on lipid metabolism, obesity, insulin production, insulin resistance, and blood pressure [22,36,99]. Although a meta-analysis of six randomized controlled trials with 689 patients with RA reported good glucocorticoid safety profiles, numerous studies have found an increased incidence of all-cause and CV mortality, hypertension, hyperglycemia, diabetes, osteoporosis, and myocardial infarction with dose- and time-dependent glucocorticoid usage [22,92,100]. Many registries and large meta-analyses support the conclusions of the effects of glucocorticoids on CV risk and mortality, with some dose-dependent effects. These include the Scotland National Health Service RA database, the General Practice Research Database, and a meta-analysis of 28 studies by Roubille et al. [88]. An older meta-analysis of 37 studies reported poor associations between low-dose glucocorticoids (<10 mg/day) and CV risk factors, beneficial effects on lipid profiles, an increase in insulin resistance or glycemia, and no effect on blood pressure, with a trend of increasing major CV events, myocardial infarction, stroke, and mortality [100]. According to current guidelines, glucocorticoids should be used at the lowest possible dose, continuation should be regularly reassessed, and remission withdrawal should be considered [101,102].

4.2.3. Classical DMARDs

Considering DMARDs, a meta-analysis of observational and prospective studies reported on the beneficial effects of MTX, sulfasalazine, and hydroxychloroquine on CV risk [36,84,100,103–105]. MTX is an antifolate immunosuppressive drug that inhibits neutrophil chemotaxis and synthesis of proinflammatory cytokines and exerts antiatherogenic and cardioprotective effects [102–105]. According to an analysis of 8 prospective studies, 2 retrospective studies, and 694 publications, with 66,334 participants and 6235 events, MTX was associated with a 21% lower overall risk for CV events (95% CI: 0.73–0.87, $p < 0.001$) and an 18% lower risk for myocardial infarction (95% CI: 0.71–0.96, $p = 0.01$) [103]. A study on CAC, using computed tomography, reported a lower coronary calcification burden with MTX use in patients with RA [85]. Another meta-analysis of 28 studies reported an overall 21% CV risk reduction with MTX (RR, 0.72; 95% CI: 0.57–0.91; $p = 0.007$) as well as an 18% myocardial infarction risk reduction, a trend towards a decreasing risk of heart failure, and no effect on strokes and major adverse cardiac events—although the last may be due to the lower number of events resulting in insufficient statistical power to detect a significant effect [88]. An older meta-analysis of 18 studies also reported a reduced risk of CV events in patients with RA treated with MTX: a reduction in overall mortality of 41% and 70% in two studies; a reduction in CV-related morbidity of 89%, 35%, 17%, and 15% in four studies; an 18% risk reduction for myocardial infarction in one study (with a selection bias due to the exclusion of fatal events); and a trend towards risk reduction in three studies. One study showed a 20% reduction in the risk of hospitalization with congestive heart failure (significant bias), and another study showed an 11% reduction in the risk of stroke and a trend towards it [106,107]. Several studies have reported that MTX increases total cholesterol, LDL, HDL, and triglyceride levels in RA, with a possible explanation that it reflects the normalization of lipid levels due to the suppression of inflammation, without increasing CV risk [74]. Hydroxychloroquine has antirheumatic effects by targeting autoantigen processing in macrophages, suppressing T-lymphocytes, and neutralizing the prothrombotic effects of antiphospholipid antibodies [91,104]. Hydroxychloroquine improves lipid and glycemic indices, reduces the risk of thromboembolic events, enhances the elasticity of peripheral arteries and systemic vascular resistance, and reduces CV risk [72,91,104,108]. However, considerations of methodology, transparency, and reproducibility that affect the credibility of the conclusions were asserted in the latter meta-analysis [109]. Several case reports have asserted the consideration of hydroxychloroquine cardiotoxicity (restrictive cardiomyopathy and conduction disorders); however, in those cases, patients had prolonged use of large cumulative doses. The use of hydroxychloroquine is considered safe at therapeutic doses with periodic ECG monitoring [104]. Combination therapy with MTX, sulfasalazine, and hydroxychloroquine also decreases CV risk by improving inflammation reduction, increasing HDL, lowering LDL, and improving the ratio of total cholesterol to HDL, as against MTX monotherapy or in combination with etanercept. However, the study only included patients with early RA with high disease activity and who were naïve to DMARDs [110]. In contrast, azathioprine, cyclosporine, and leflunomide increased the risk of CV events by 80% compared to MTX monotherapy [111,112]. Leflunomide has potent anti-inflammatory and immunomodulatory effects but increases the risk of hypertension, which has been reported in 2.1–10.6% of cases in different studies [91,113]. Cyclosporine is used for the treatment of severe early RA and has many adverse effects, including vasoconstriction, thrombosis, and hypertension; blood pressure and renal function monitoring are advised when using cyclosporine [91,113]. Azathioprine is a purine analog with rare adverse effects, which include angina, renal and subclavian vein thrombosis, hypotension, and cardiogenic shock [91,113].

4.2.4. Biologic Agents

Biologics are used to treat many different autoimmune diseases by targeting inflammatory cytokines (TNF-α and IL-6) and cytokine receptors, interrupting the inflammatory vicious cycle, and are recommended even in early RA with low-severity inflammatory arthritis [91,112]. By suppressing inflammation and maintaining low disease activity, they significantly reduce CV risk and the incidences of myocardial infarction, heart failure, and cerebrovascular events in patients with RA [91,113–116]. Anti-TNF agents neutralize soluble- and/or membrane-bound TNF and act as monoclonal antibodies or soluble receptors [91].

In a large cohort study of 2757 patients with RA treated with infliximab, etanercept, or adalimumab, a significant increase in heart failure was reported in patients with high disease activity and concomitant glucocorticoid or COX inhibitor therapy, while anti-TNF therapy did not significantly contribute to the risk; only sporadic cases of acute coronary syndromes, arrhythmias, and AV block for infliximab were reported [115]. In a large, retrospective study, Solomon et al. reported that anti-TNF-α therapy may be associated with a reduced CV risk compared with classic DMARD therapy. The incidence rates per 100 person-years for the composite cardiovascular end point for classic DMARD and anti-TNF therapy were 3.05 (95% CI, 2.54–3.65) and 2.52 (95% CI, 2.12–2.98), respectively [113]. Jacobsson et al., in a prospective cohort study with 983 participants [116]; Ljung et al., in a prospective cohort study with 6864 patients with RA [117]; and an earlier meta-analysis of 20 studies by Westlake et al. reported similar conclusions [106]. In addition to the anti-inflammatory effect of anti-TNF-α therapy and the consequential improvement of joint function, they may indirectly lead to increased levels of physical activity, which will subsequently decrease the incidence of other cardiovascular risk factors, such as diabetes mellitus and hypertension [114]. Karpouzas et al. reported slower non-calcified coronary plaque progression with longer biologics usage independent of inflammation, prednisone dose, and statin use [118].

A recently published meta-analysis of 26 longitudinal studies addressing anti-TNF therapy influence on BMI found a small increase in body weight and BMI—which was on average 0.90 kg, 2.34 kg, and 2.27 kg for infliximab, etanercept, and adalimumab, respectively at 4 and 104 weeks of follow-up [119]. The ATTACH study reported that the use of anti-TNF therapy increased mortality or worsened heart failure in patients with moderate to severe chronic heart failure, especially those with an ischemic etiology, but the RENAISSANCE and RECOVER clinical trials did not confirm this for etanercept [120]. A possible reduction in insulin resistance with anti-TNF therapy was reported in a meta-analysis of 12 studies; however, the heterogeneity of the studies was high [121]. A meta-analysis of studies considering the impact of biologics (tocilizumab, abatacept, rituximab, and TNF inhibitors) on CV risk and safety reported fewer CV events with rituximab and neutral effects of others compared to classic DMARDs, but significant heterogeneity on CV outcomes was reported [122]. A large meta-analysis, which included 43 biological registers and 27 publications, addressed the issue of biologics safety and effect on mortality, and it reported that overall mortality and CV events were significantly reduced in patients treated with anti-TNFs: RR = 0.60 [95% CI 0.38–0.94] and RR = 0.62 [95% CI 0.44–0.88], respectively, with no effect on neoplasm risk; however, serious infections significantly increased during anti-TNF treatment (RR = 1.48 [1.18–1.85]) compared to classical DMARD treatment [123]. Another meta-analysis of 28 studies of patients with RA reported that anti-TNF treatment was significantly associated with an overall CV risk reduction of approximately 30% [88]. Cheung et al. analyzed the effect of anti-TNF therapy on subclinical atherosclerosis, and six studies measured at least one parameter before and after treatment (24th and 52nd weeks): intima–media thickness, pulse wave velocity, and augmentation index; they found that anti-TNF therapy had no effect on all three parameters at the 24th week and on intima–media thickness at the 52nd week [124]. An older meta-analysis of 32 studies by Daien et al. reported increased total cholesterol and HDL levels and unchanged LDL levels with long-term anti-TNF therapy, with uncertain effects on CV risk [125]; however, the total cholesterol/HDL ratio was not significantly altered by anti-TNF therapy [74]. These anti-TNF therapeutic effects may reflect the normalization of lipid levels to those prior to RA due to suppression of inflammation [74,114]. A meta-analysis by Zhao et al., which included 6321 patients with RA from 11 randomized clinical trials, reported strong evidence of an increased incidence of hypertension associated with some anti-TNF therapies (OR = 1.8896, 95% CI: 1.35–2.65) as well as an increasing incidence of hypertension with longer therapy duration, especially for certolizumab but not for etanercept, tofacitinib, infliximab, and golimumab [126]. Results from a new Korean observational study with 996 patients with RA did not find an increased incidence of HA with biologics compared with classical DMARDs in general, but MTX had a lower incidence of hypertension, which could be explained by the hypothesis that MTX restores vasodilation-related adenosine levels in the body [127]. A neutral effect of anti-TNF agents on HA incidence was reported by Desai et al. from a large cohort study with 4822 patients using TNF-α inhibitors and 2400 using classical DMARDs [128]. Despite some methodological limitations, these studies strongly support the increased beneficial effects of anti-TNF agents compared to classical RA medications, probably due to more efficient inflammation control and successful achievement of long-term RA remission.

The effect of non-anti-TNF agents—abatacept, tocilizumab, sarilumab, anakinra, and rituximab—on CV risk has also been evaluated. Abatacept was found to have 20% greater CV risk reduction than anti-TNF agents; tocilizumab had the same effect on CV risk as MTX monotherapy; anakinra showed improved vascular and left ventricular function in a small placebo-controlled study; sarilumab and rituximab had a neutral effect on CV events; and canakinumab, an IL-1 inhibitor of 150 mg administered every 3 months, was associated with a significantly lower rate of myocardial infarction than the placebo [76,129–134]. Several studies have consistently reported that tocilizumab was associated with increased total cholesterol, HDL, LDL, and triglyceride levels [74,91]. The MEASURE study found that tocilizumab + MTX treatment did not increase the concentration of proatherogenic small and dense LDL particles, while antiatherogenic small and medium HDL particles were increased and structurally altered to a less inflammatory state than with MTX alone [135]. There have been no reports of an increase in CV events with tocilizumab [91]. These medications, especially abatacept and anakinra, are also strongly recommended for CVD prevention in RA.

4.2.5. Small Molecule Inhibitors of JAK

Tofacitinib and baricitinib, newer small-molecule inhibitors of JAK, increase total and LDL cholesterol levels by 10–20% [136]. For baricitinib, a meta-analysis of six studies with 3552 patients reported significantly increased dose-dependent LDL and HDL with baricitinib use; the mean change was 13.15 mg/dL (95% CI: 8.89–17.42) and 5.40 mg/dL (95% CI: 3.07–7.74), respectively. Although the increased relative risk of CV events was not statistically significant, an association may exist [130]. A recently published pooled cohort study of 3492 patients with RA, with more than 7860 patient-years of exposure to baricitinib did not reveal a significant association between baricitinib treatment and the occurrence of CV events or congestive heart failure [137]. The influence of biologic agents and tofacitinib, a JAK inhibitor, on the lipid profile of patients with RA was analyzed in a meta-analysis of 20 articles by Soto et al.; they reported increased cholesterol (OR 4.64; CI 95% 2.71, 7.95, $p < 0.001$), HDL (OR 2.25; 95% CI 1.14, 4.44, $p = 0.020$), and LDL (OR 4.80; 95% CI 3.27, 7.05, $p < 0.001$) levels, but despite this effect, better inflammation control with those medications appears to result in lower mortality and incidence of cardiovascular events. However, other biologic or non-biologic agents were not included in the analysis [138].

Other than the ENTRACTE trial, which compared tocilizumab and etanercept, no head-to-head study has been conducted on the impact of biological agents on CV risk and safety. The ENTRACTE trial reported no significant difference in CV events between the tocilizumab and etanercept groups [85]. Some observational studies have reported a higher incidence of myocardial infarction among older patients with anti-TNF inhibitors than with abatacept and tocilizumab and no difference in CV risk when comparing tocilizumab with abatacept [76,139].

4.2.6. Statins role in CVD prevention

The use of statins in the management of CVDs seems to have a neutral effect on RA development, and the risk of RA may be lower in patients with a longer duration or greater intensity of statin use [139]. Treatment with statins is beneficial in lowering CV risk in patients with RA due to their lipid-lowering and other pleiotropic effects that slow down coronary non-calcified plaque progression and suppress the effects of inflammation on plaque progression and CAC [77,118,141,142]. A meta-analysis of 11 relevant studies reported a standardized mean difference in DAS28 of -0.55 (95% CI: -0.83 to -0.26, $p = 0.0002$), supporting the positive effect of statins on RA [143]. However, the indiscriminate use of statins is not recommended in all patients with RA, and CV risk assessment and appropriate statin use according to the guidelines for primary and secondary CVD prevention in this population is necessary [17].

4.3. The Role of Inflammatory Markers in RA Activity and CV Risk Assessment

Biomarkers are used in disease diagnosis, treatment, and monitoring of disease progression and complications. They are also used to determine regression or remission of the disease. Although they are not always sufficiently sensitive and specific in certain situations, they still serve as a useful tool for monitoring the disease. Notably, RA activity reflects CV risk.

CRP is one of the most used markers worldwide and is routinely evaluated as a marker of systemic inflammation in RA [144]. Due to its limited specificity, CRP is most often utilized in conjunction with another blood biomarker. A low level of this biomarker indicates disease stability and the effectiveness of therapy. When using highly specific therapy directed against precisely defined inflammatory cytokines, monitoring the serum levels can facilitate the assessment of the treatment success and disease stability. In the early stages of inflammation, IL-6 is a key proinflammatory factor that causes a variety of cells to produce and secrete acute-phase proteins. Infection-related neutrophil generation and activation, B-cell proliferation and differentiation, immunoglobulin synthesis, and T-cell proliferation and differentiation are all stimulated by IL-6. The onset of inflammation and the change from acute to chronic inflammation are both significantly influenced by IL-6 levels [145]. Serum IL-6 levels stand as a reflective biomarker of RA disease activity [146].

TNF- is crucial to understanding the pathogenesis of RA. The expression of serum TNF- may make early RA more inflammatory [147]. As a result, it is necessary to test patients with RA for this cytokine to keep track of disease activity, which may be helpful for patients who are undergoing anti-TNF therapy. The inflammatory response is further enhanced by TNF-α, which is a potent inducer of other proinflammatory cytokines and chemokines [148]. Rheumatoid factors and anti-CCP, which are diagnostic markers of RA, can be used to track the progression of the disease.

5. Conclusions

In conclusion, to prevent CV disease in patients with RA, two main complementary strategies were considered. They were strict inflammation control with as few flares as possible and the management of modifiable risk factors.

Since CV morbidity and mortality in RA are alarmingly high, it is crucial to comprehend the mechanisms that cause and control atherosclerosis so that highly specific treatment plans can be created to reduce the CV health burden that patients with RA bear. The development of atherogenic foam cells is aided by proinflammatory cytokines, including IL-6 and TNF-α. The creation of a proatherogenic environment favors the development of atherosclerotic diseases because of endothelial dysfunction and RA-derived autoantibodies, which increase the inflammatory potential of macrophages. Understanding the potential interactions between inflammation and traditional cardiovascular (CV) risk factors in driving atherosclerosis in rheumatoid arthritis (RA) is a crucial area of investigation that requires further exploration.

Achieving and maintaining long-term RA remission using novel therapeutic agents is crucial. Early recognition and strict control of modifiable risk factors based on these guidelines are paramount. Effective patient education, implementation of these measures, increased surveillance, early active identification of risk factors by general practitioners and specialists, an interdisciplinary approach, and accessibility of the health care system play key roles in achieving these goals.

Supplementary Materials: The following supporting information can be downloaded at https://www.mdpi.com/article/10.3390/medicina59091550/s1, Table S1: articles characteristics and comments included in review.

Author Contributions: D.B.: primary investigator and cardiology data analysis; I.B.: database screening and cardiology data analysis; S.Š.: cardiology data analysis; D.K.: cardiology data analysis; S.N.: rheumatology data analysis. All authors have read and agreed to the published version of the manuscript.

Funding: This research received no external funding.

Data Availability Statement: The list and data from all used articles in this review can be provided upon request.

Acknowledgments: The authors would like to acknowledge: D. Dukić and M. Dukić for the statistical data analysis.

Conflicts of Interest: The authors declare no conflict of interest.

References

1. Mitchell, D.M.; Spitz, P.W.; Young, D.Y.; Bloch, D.A.; McShane, D.J.; Fries, J.F. Survival, prognosis, and causes of death in rheumatoid-arthritis. *Arthritis Rheum.* **1986**, *29*, 706–714. [CrossRef] [PubMed]
2. Scott, D.L.; Coulton, B.L.; Symmons, D.P.M. Long-term outcome of threating rheumatoid arthritis—Results after 20 years. *Lancet* **1987**, *1*, 1108–1111. [CrossRef]
3. Arnett, F.C.; Edworthy, S.M.; Bloch, D.A.; Mcshane, D.J.; Fries, J.F.; Cooper, N.S.; Healey, L.A.; Kaplan, S.R.; Liang, M.H.; Luthra, H.S.; et al. The american rheumatism association 1987 revised criteria for the classification of rheumatoid arthritis. *Arthritis Rheum.* **1988**, *31*, 315–324. [CrossRef] [PubMed]
4. Aletaha, D.; Neogi, T.; Silman, A.J.; Funovits, J.; Felson, D.T.; Bingham, C.O., 3rd; Birnbaum, N.S.; Burmester, G.R.; Bykerk, V.P.; Cohen, M.D.; et al. 2010 Rheumatoid arthritis classification criteria: An American College of Rheumatology/European League Against Rheumatism collaborative initiative. *Ann. Rheum. Dis.* **2010**, *69*, 1580–1588. [CrossRef]
5. Lee, D.M.; Weinblatt, M.E. Rheumatoid arthritis. *Lancet* **2001**, *358*, 903–911. [CrossRef]
6. Symmons, D.P. Epidemiology of rheumatoid arthritis: Determinants of onset, persistence and outcome. *Best Pract. Res. Clin. Rheumatol.* **2002**, *16*, 707–722. [CrossRef] [PubMed]
7. Sakai, R.; Hirano, F.; Kihara, M.; Yokoyama, W.; Yamazaki, H.; Harada, S.; Nanki, T.; Koike, R.; Miyasaka, N.; Harigai, M. High prevalence of cardiovascular comorbidities in patients with rheumatoid arthritis from a population-based cross-sectional study of a Japanese health insurance database. *Mod. Rheumatol.* **2016**, *26*, 522–528. [CrossRef]
8. Koivuniemi, R.; Paimela, L.; Leirisalo-Repo, M. Causes of death in patients with rheumatoid arthritis from 1971 to 1991 with special reference to autopsy. *Clin. Rheumatol.* **2009**, *28*, 1443–1447. [CrossRef]
9. Maradit-Kremers, H.; Nicola, P.J.; Crowson, C.S.; Ballman, K.V.; Gabriel, S.E. Cardiovascular death in rheumatoid arthritis: A population-based study. *Arthritis Rheum.* **2005**, *52*, 722–732. [CrossRef]
10. Sokka, T.; Abelson, B.; Pincus, T. Mortality in rheumatoid arthritis: 2008 update. *Clin. Exp. Rheumatol.* **2009**, *26*, S35–S61.
11. Meune, C.; Touzé, E.; Trinquart, L.; Allanore, Y. High risk of clinical cardiovascular events in rheumatoid arthritis: Levels of associations of myocardial infarction and stroke through a systematic review and meta-analysis. *Arch. Cardiovasc. Dis.* **2010**, *103*, 253–261. [CrossRef]
12. Meune, C.; Touzé, E.; Trinquart, L.; Allanore, Y. Trends in cardiovascular mortality in patients with rheumatoid arthritis over 50 years: A systematic review and meta-analysis of cohort studies. *Rheumatology* **2009**, *48*, 1309–1313. [CrossRef]
13. Aviña-Zubieta, J.A.; Choi, H.K.; Sadatsafavi, M.; Etminan, M.; Esdaile, J.M.; Lacaille, D. Risk of cardiovascular mortality in patients with rheumatoid arthritis: A meta-analysis of observational studies. *Arthritis Rheum.* **2008**, *59*, 1690–1697. [CrossRef]
14. Meyer, P.W.; Anderson, R.; Ker, J.A.; Ally, M.T. Rheumatoid arthritis and risk of cardiovascular disease. *Cardiovasc. J. Afr.* **2018**, *29*, 317–321. [CrossRef] [PubMed]
15. Siebert, S.; Lyall, D.M.; Mackay, D.F.; Porter, D.; McInnes, I.B.; Sattar, N.; Pell, J.P. Characteristics of rheumatoid arthritis and its association with major comorbid conditions: Cross-sectional study of 502 649 UK Biobank participants. *RMD Open* **2016**, *2*, e000267. [CrossRef]
16. Van Doornum, S.; McColl, G.; Wicks, I.P. Accelerated atherosclerosis—An extraarticular feature of rheumatoid arthritis? *Arthritis Rheum.* **2002**, *46*, 862–873. [CrossRef]
17. Visseren, F.L.; Mach, F.; Smulders, Y.M.; Carballo, D.; Koskinas, K.C.; Bäck, M.; Benetos, A.; Biffi, A.; Boavida, J.-M.; Capodanno, D.; et al. 2021 ESC Guidelines on cardiovascular disease prevention in clinical practice: Developed by the Task Force for cardiovascular disease prevention in clinical practice with representatives of the European Society of Cardiology and 12 medical societies With the special contribution of the European Association of Preventive Cardiology (EAPC). *Eur. Heart J.* **2021**, *42*, 3227–3337. [PubMed]
18. Panoulas, V.F.; Metsios, G.S.; Pace, A.V.; John, H.; Treharne, G.J.; Banks, M.J.; Kitas, G.D. Hypertension in rheumatoid arthritis. *Rheumatology* **2008**, *4*, 1286–1298. [CrossRef] [PubMed]
19. Innala, L.; Sjöberg, C.; Möller, B.; Ljung, L.; Smedby, T.; Södergren, A.; Magnusson, S.; Rantapää-Dahlqvist, S.; Wållberg-Jonsson, S. Co-morbidity in patients with early rheumatoid arthritis—Inflammation matters. *Thromb. Haemost.* **2016**, *18*, 33. [CrossRef]
20. Grosso, G.; Erba, G.; Valena, C.; Riva, M.; Betelli, M.; Allevi, E.; Bonomi, F.; Barbarossa, S.; Ricci, M.; Facchetti, R.; et al. THU0145 Cardiovascular Risk Factor Profile in an Italian Cohort of Patients with Rheumatoid Arthritis: Results of a Three Year Follow-up. *Ann. Rheum. Dis.* **2015**, *74*, 244. [CrossRef]
21. Gherghe, A.M.; Dougados, M.; Combe, B.; Landewé, R.; Mihai, C.; Berenbaum, F.; Mariette, X.; Wolterbeek, R.; van der Heijde, D. Cardiovascular and selected comorbidities in early arthritis and early spondyloarthritis, a comparative study: Results from the ESPOIR and DESIR cohorts. *RMD Open* **2015**, *1*, e000128. [CrossRef]
22. Boyer, J.-F.; Gourraud, P.-A.; Cantagrel, A.; Davignon, J.-L.; Constantin, A. Traditional cardiovascular risk factors in rheumatoid arthritis: A meta-analysis. *Jt. Bone Spine* **2011**, *78*, 179–183. [CrossRef]
23. Heliövaara, M.; Aho, K.; Aromaa, A.; Knekt, P.; Reunanen, A. Smoking and risk of rheumatoid arthritis. *J. Rheumatol.* **1993**, *20*, 1830–1835.
24. La Hoz, J.C.-D.; Amaya-Amaya, J.; Molano-González, N.; Gutiérrez-Infante, F.; Anaya, J.M.; Rojas-Villarraga, A. FRI0055 The influence of cigarette smoking on disease activity and joint erosions in rheumatoid arthritis: A systematic review and meta-analysis. *Ann. Rheum. Dis.* **2013**, *72*, A387. [CrossRef]

25. Klareskog, L.; Stolt, P.; Lundberg, K.; Källberg, H.; Bengtsson, C.; Grunewald, J.; Rönnelid, J.; Harris, H.E.; Ulfgren, A.K.; Rantapää-Dahlqvist, S.; et al. A new model for an etiology of rheumatoid arthritis: Smoking may trigger HLA–DR (shared epitope)–restricted immune reactions to autoantigens modified by citrullination. *Arthritis Rheum.* **2006**, *54*, 38–46. [CrossRef]
26. Welsing, P.M.J.; Van Gestel, A.M.; Swinkels, H.L.; Kiemeney, L.A.L.M.; Van Riel, P.L.C.M. The relationship between disease activity, joint destruction, and functional capacity over the course of rheumatoid arthritis. *Arthritis Rheum.* **2001**, *44*, 2009–2017. [CrossRef]
27. Piepoli, M.F.; Hoes, A.W.; Agewall, S.; Albus, C.; Brotons, C.; Catapano, A.L.; Cooney, M.T.; Corrà, U.; Cosyns, B.; Deaton, C.; et al. Task Force 2016 European Guidelines on cardiovascular disease prevention in clinical practice: The Sixth Joint Task Force of the European Society of Cardiology and Other Societies on Cardiovascular Disease Prevention in Clinical Practice (constituted by representatives of 10 societies and by invited experts). *Eur. J. Prev. Cardiol.* **2016**, *23*, NP1–NP96.
28. Baghdadi, L.R.; Woodman, R.J.; Shanahan, E.M.; Mangoni, A.A. The Impact of Traditional Cardiovascular Risk Factors on Cardiovascular Outcomes in Patients with Rheumatoid Arthritis: A Systematic Review and Meta-Analysis. *PLoS ONE* **2015**, *10*, e0117952. [CrossRef] [PubMed]
29. Jiang, P.; Li, H.; Li, X. Diabetes mellitus risk factors in rheumatoid arthritis: A systematic review and meta-analysis. *Clin. Exp. Rheumatol.* **2015**, *33*, 115–121. [PubMed]
30. Guin, A.; Sinhamahapatra, P.; Misra, S.; Mazumder, S.R.C.; Chatterjee, S.; Ghosh, A. Incidence and effect of insulin resistance on progression of atherosclerosis in rheumatoid arthritis patients of long disease duration. *Biomed. J.* **2019**, *42*, 394–402. [CrossRef]
31. Dougados, M.; Soubrier, M.; Antunez, A.; Balint, P.; Balsa, A.; Buch, M.H.; Casado, G.; Detert, J.; El-Zorkany, B.; Emery, P.; et al. Prevalence of comorbidities in rheumatoid arthritis and evaluation of their monitoring: Results of an international, cross-sectional study (COMORA). *Ann. Rheum. Dis.* **2020**, *73*, 62–68. [CrossRef] [PubMed]
32. Stavropoulos-Kalinoglou, A.; Metsios, G.S.; Koutedakis, Y.; Nevill, A.M.; Douglas, K.M.; Jamurtas, A.; van Zanten, J.J.C.S.V.; Labib, M.; Kitas, G.D. Redefining overweight and obesity in rheumatoid arthritis patients. *Ann. Rheum. Dis.* **2007**, *66*, 1316–1321. [CrossRef] [PubMed]
33. Castro, L.L.; Lanna, C.C.D.; Rocha, M.P.; Ribeiro, A.L.P.; Telles, R.W. Recognition and control of hypertension, diabetes, and dyslipidemia in patients with rheumatoid arthritis. *Rheumatol. Int.* **2018**, *38*, 1437–1442. [CrossRef] [PubMed]
34. Beinsberger, J.; Heemskerk, J.W.; Cosemans, J.M. Chronic arthritis and cardiovascular disease: Altered blood parameters give rise to a prothrombotic propensity. *Semin. Arthritis Rheum.* **2014**, *44*, 345–352. [CrossRef]
35. Nowak, B.; Madej, M.; Łuczak, A.; Małecki, R.; Wiland, P. Disease Activity, Oxidized-LDL Fraction and Anti-Oxidized LDL Antibodies Influence Cardiovascular Risk in Rheumatoid Arthritis. *Adv. Clin. Exp. Med.* **2016**, *25*, 43–50. [CrossRef]
36. Giles, J.T.; Wasko, M.C.M.; Chung, C.P.; Szklo, M.; Blumenthal, R.S.; Kao, A.; Bokhari, S.; Zartoshti, A.; Stein, C.M.; Bathon, J.M. Exploring the Lipid Paradox Theory in Rheumatoid Arthritis: Associations of Low Circulating Low-Density Lipoprotein Concentration With Subclinical Coronary Atherosclerosis. *Arthritis Rheumatol.* **2011**, *71*, 1426–1436. [CrossRef]
37. McGrath, C.M.; Young, S.P. Lipid and Metabolic Changes in Rheumatoid Arthritis. *Curr. Rheumatol. Rep.* **2015**, *17*, 57. [CrossRef]
38. Gregersen, P.K.; Silver, J.; Winchester, R.J. The shared epitope hypothesis. an approach to understanding the molecular genetics of susceptibility to rheumatoid arthritis. *Arthritis Rheum.* **1987**, *30*, 1205–1213. [CrossRef]
39. McInnes, I.B.; Schett, G. Mechanisms of Disease: The Pathogenesis of Rheumatoid Arthritis. *N. Engl. J. Med.* **2011**, *365*, 2205–2219. [CrossRef]
40. Wang, D.; Zhang, J.; Lau, J.; Wang, S.; Taneja, V.; Matteson, E.L.; Vassallo, R. Mechanisms of lung disease development in rheumatoid arthritis. *Nat. Rev. Rheumatol.* **2019**, *15*, 581–596. [CrossRef]
41. Londei, M.; Savill, C.M.; Verhoef, A.; Brennan, F.; Leech, Z.A.; Duance, V.; Maini, R.N.; Feldmann, M. Persistence of collagen type II-specific T-cell clones in the synovial membrane of a patient with rheumatoid arthritis. *Proc. Natl. Acad. Sci. USA* **1987**, *86*, 636–640. [CrossRef] [PubMed]
42. Glant, T.T.; Radacs, M.; Nagyeri, G.; Olasz, K.; Laszlo, T.; Boldizsar, F.; Hegyi, A.; Finnegan, A.; Mikecz, K. Proteoglycan-induced arthritis and recombinant human proteoglycan aggrecan G1 domain-induced arthritis in BALB/c mice resembling two subtypes of rheumatoid arthritis. *Arthritis Rheum.* **2011**, *63*, 1312–1321. [CrossRef] [PubMed]
43. Verheijden, G.F.M.; Rijnders, A.W.M.; Bos, E.; Roo, C.J.J.C.-D.; van Staveren, C.J.; Miltenburg, A.M.M.; Meijerink, J.H.; Elewaut, D.; de Keyser, F.; Veys, E.; et al. Human cartilage glycoprotein-39 as a candidate autoantigen in rheumatoid arthritis. *Arthritis Rheum.* **2011**, *40*, 1115–1125. [CrossRef] [PubMed]
44. Smolen, J.S.; Aletaha, D.; Barton, A.; Burmester, G.R.; Emery, P.; Firestein, G.S.; Kavanaugh, A.; McInnes, I.B.; Solomon, D.H.; Strand, V.; et al. Rheumatoid arthritis. *Nat. Rev. Dis. Primers* **2018**, *4*, 23. [CrossRef]
45. Burmester, G.R.; Feist, E.; Dörner, T. Emerging cell and cytokine targets in rheumatoid arthritis. *Nat. Rev. Rheumatol.* **2014**, *10*, 77–88. [CrossRef]
46. Carbone, F.; Bonaventura, A.; Liberale, L.; Paolino, S.; Torre, F.; Dallegri, F.; Montecucco, F.; Cutolo, M. Atherosclerosis in Rheumatoid Arthritis: Promoters and Opponents. *Clin. Rev. Allergy Immunol.* **2020**, *58*, 1–14. [CrossRef]
47. Mewar, D.; Coote, A.; Moore, D.J.; Marinou, I.; Keyworth, J.; Dickson, M.C.; Montgomery, D.S.; Binks, M.H.; Wilson, A.G. Independent associations of anti-cyclic citrullinated peptide antibodies and rheumatoid factor with radiographic severity of rheumatoid arthritis. *Thromb. Haemost.* **2006**, *8*, R128. [CrossRef]

48. Sokolove, J.; Bromberg, R.; Deane, K.D.; Lahey, L.J.; Derber, L.A.; Chandra, P.E.; Edison, J.D.; Gilliland, W.R.; Tibshirani, R.J.; Norris, J.M.; et al. Autoantibody Epitope Spreading in the Pre-Clinical Phase Predicts Progression to Rheumatoid Arthritis. *PLoS ONE* **2012**, *7*, e35296. [CrossRef]
49. López-Longo, F.J.; Oliver-Miñarro, D.; de la Torre, I.; de Rábago, E.G.-D.; Sánchez-Ramón, S.; Rodríguez-Mahou, M.; Paravisini, A.; Monteagudo, I.; González, C.-M.; GarCía-Castro, M.; et al. Association between anti-cyclic citrullinated peptide antibodies and ischemic heart disease in patients with rheumatoid arthritis. *Arthritis Rheum.* **2009**, *61*, 419–424. [CrossRef]
50. Sokolove, J.; Brennan, M.J.; Sharpe, O.; Lahey, L.J.; Kao, A.H.; Krishnan, E.; Edmundowicz, D.; Lepus, C.M.; Wasko, M.C.; Robinson, W.H. Brief Report: Citrullination Within the Atherosclerotic Plaque: A Potential Target for the Anti-Citrullinated Protein Antibody Response in Rheumatoid Arthritis. *Arthritis Rheum.* **2013**, *65*, 1719–1724. [CrossRef]
51. Geraldino-Pardilla, L.; Zartoshti, A.; Ozbek, A.B.; Giles, J.T.; Weinberg, R.; Kinkhabwala, M.; Bokhari, S.; Bathon, J.M. Arterial Inflammation Detected With F-18-Fluorodeoxyglucose-Positron Emission Tomography in Rheumatoid Arthritis. *Arthritis Rheumatol.* **2018**, *70*, 30–39. [CrossRef]
52. DeMizio, D.J.; Geraldino-Pardilla, L.B. Autoimmunity and Inflammation Link to Cardiovascular Disease Risk in Rheumatoid Arthritis. *Rheumatol. Ther.* **2020**, *7*, 19–33. [CrossRef]
53. Liang, K.P.; Maradit-Kremers, H.; Crowson, C.S.; Snyder, M.R.; Therneau, T.M.; Roger, V.L.; Gabriel, S.E. Autoantibodies and the Risk of Cardiovascular Events. *J. Rheumatol.* **2009**, *36*, 2462–2469. [CrossRef] [PubMed]
54. Humphreys, J.H.; AB van Nies, J.; Chipping, J.; Marshall, T.; Mil, A.H.v.d.H.-V.; Symmons, D.P.; Verstappen, S.M. Rheumatoid factor and anti-citrullinated protein antibody positivity, but not level, are associated with increased mortality in patients with rheumatoid arthritis: Results from two large independent cohorts. *Thromb. Haemost.* **2014**, *16*, 1–8. [CrossRef]
55. McCoy, S.S.; Crowson, C.S.; Maradit-Kremers, H.; Therneau, T.M.; Roger, V.L.; Matteson, E.L.; Gabriel, S.E. Longterm outcomes and treatment after myocardial infarction in patients with rheumatoid arthritis. *J. Rheumatol.* **2013**, *40*, 605–610. [CrossRef]
56. Mackey, R.H.; Kuller, L.H.; Deane, K.D.; Walitt, B.T.; Chang, Y.F.; Holers, V.M.; Robinson, W.H.; Tracy, R.P.; Hlatky, M.A.; Eaton, C.B.; et al. Rheumatoid Arthritis, Anti-Cyclic Citrullinated Peptide Positivity, and Cardiovascular Disease Risk in the Women's Health Initiative. *Arthritis Rheumatol.* **2015**, *67*, 2311–2322. [CrossRef]
57. Innala, L.; Möller, B.; Ljung, L.; Magnusson, S.; Smedby, T.; Södergren, A.; Öhman, M.-L.; Rantapää-Dahlqvist, S.; Wållberg-Jonsson, S. Cardiovascular events in early RA are a result of inflammatory burden and traditional risk factors: A five year prospective study. *Thromb. Haemost.* **2010**, *13*, R131. [CrossRef]
58. Pawlik, A.; Ostanek, L.; Brzosko, I.; Brzosko, M.; Masiuk, M.; Machalinski, B.; Gawronska-Szklarz, B. The expansion of CD4+CD28-T cells in patients with rheumatoid arthritis. *Thromb. Haemost.* **2003**, *5*, R210–R213. [CrossRef]
59. Winchester, R.; Giles, J.T.; Nativ, S.; Downer, K.; Zhang, H.-Z.; Bag-Ozbek, A.; Zartoshti, A.; Bokhari, S.; Bathon, J.M. Association of Elevations of Specific T Cell and Monocyte Subpopulations in Rheumatoid Arthritis with Subclinical Coronary Artery Atherosclerosis. *Arthritis Rheumatol.* **2016**, *68*, 92–102. [CrossRef]
60. Nakajima, T.; Goek, O.; Zhang, X.Y.; Kopecky, S.L.; Frye, R.L.; Goronzy, J.J.; Weyand, C.M. De novo expression of killer immunoglobulin-like receptors and signaling proteins regulates the cytotoxic function of CD4 T cells in acute coronary syndromes. *Circ. Res.* **2003**, *93*, 106–113. [CrossRef] [PubMed]
61. Dumitriu, I.E.; Baruah, P.; Finlayson, C.J.; Loftus, I.M.; Antunes, R.F.; Lim, P.; Bunce, N.; Kaski, J.C. High Levels of Costimulatory Receptors OX40 and 4-1BB Characterize CD4 (+) CD28 (null) T Cells in Patients with Acute Coronary Syndrome. *Circ. Res.* **2010**, *110*, 857–869. [CrossRef]
62. López-Mejías, R.; Castañeda, S.; González-Juanatey, C.; Corrales, A.; Ferraz-Amaro, I.; Genre, F.; Remuzgo-Martínez, S.; Rodriguez-Rodriguez, L.; Blanco, R.; Llorca, J.; et al. Cardiovascular risk assessment in patients with rheumatoid arthritis: The relevance of clinical, genetic and serological markers. *Autoimmun. Rev.* **2016**, *15*, 1013–1030. [CrossRef]
63. Liuzzo, G.; Biasucci, L.M.; Brugaletta, S.; Digianuario, G.; Pinnelli, M.; Giubilato, G.; Giubilato, S.; Colafrancesco, V.; Rebuzzi, A.G.; Crea, F. An unusual population of T-lymphocytes, (CD4+CD28null) T-cells, is associated with the recurrence of acute coronary events in patients with unstable angina. *Circulation* **2005**, *112*, U586.
64. Libby, P. Inflammatory Mechanisms: The Molecular Basis of Inflammation and Disease. *Nutr. Rev.* **2007**, *65*, 140–146. [CrossRef]
65. Swerdlow, D.I.; Holmes, M.V.; Kuchenbaecker, K.B.; Engmann, J.E.L.; Shah, T.; Sofat, R.; Guo, Y.R.; Chung, C.; Peasey, A.; Ster, R.P.; et al. The interleukin-6 receptor as a target for prevention of coronary heart disease: A mendelian randomisation analysis. *Lancet* **2012**, *379*, 1214–1224. [PubMed]
66. Kaptoge, S.; Seshasai, S.R.K.; Jørgensen, T.; Danesh, J.; Gao, P.; Freitag, D.F.; Butterworth, A.S.; Borglykke, A.; Di Angelantonio, E.; Gudnason, V.; et al. Inflammatory cytokines and risk of coronary heart disease: New prospective study and updated meta-analysis. *Eur. Heart J.* **2014**, *35*, 578–589. [CrossRef]
67. van den Oever, I.A.M.; Sattar, N.; Nurmohamed, M.T. Thromboembolic and cardiovascular risk in rheumatoid arthritis: Role of the haemostatic system. *Ann. Rheum. Dis.* **2014**, *73*, 954–957. [CrossRef] [PubMed]
68. Small, H.Y.; Migliarino, S.; Czesnikiewicz-Guzik, M.; Guzik, T.J. Hypertension: Focus on autoimmunity and oxidative stress. *Free Radic. Biol. Med.* **2018**, *125*, 104–115. [CrossRef]
69. Peters, M.J.L.; Nurmohamed, M.T.; van Eijk, I.C.; Verkleij, C.J.N.; Marx, P.F. Thrombin-activatable fibrinolysis inhibitor and its relation with inflammation in rheumatoid arthritis. *Ann. Rheum. Dis.* **2009**, *68*, 1232–1233. [CrossRef] [PubMed]
70. Habets, K.L.; Trouw, L.A.; Levarht, E.N.; Korporaal, S.J.; Habets, P.A.; de Groot, P.; Huizinga, T.W.; Toes, R.E. Anti-citrullinated protein antibodies contribute to platelet activation in rheumatoid arthritis. *Thromb. Haemost.* **2015**, *17*, 209. [CrossRef]

71. Zhou, Z.W.; Chen, H.M.; Ju, H.X.; Sun, M.Z.; Jin, H. Platelet indices in patients with chronic inflammatory arthritis: A systematic review and meta-analysis. *Platelets* **2020**, *31*, 834–844. [CrossRef] [PubMed]
72. Agca, R.; Hopman, L.H.; Laan, K.J.; van Halm, V.P.; Peters, M.J.; Smulders, Y.M.; Dekker, J.M.; Nijpels, G.; Stehouwer, C.D.; Voskuyl, A.E.; et al. Cardiovascular Event Risk in Rheumatoid Arthritis Compared with Type 2 Diabetes: A 15-year Longitudinal Study. *J. Rheumatol.* **2020**, *47*, 316–324. [CrossRef] [PubMed]
73. Cugno, M.; Marzano, A.V.; Asero, R.; Tedeschi, A. Activation of blood coagulation in chronic urticaria: Pathophysiological and clinical implications. *Intern. Emerg. Med.* **2010**, *5*, 97–101. [CrossRef]
74. Choy, E.; Ganeshalingam, K.; Semb, A.G.; Szekanecz, Z.; Nurmohamed, M. Cardiovascular risk in rheumatoid arthritis: Recent advances in the understanding of the pivotal role of inflammation, risk predictors and the impact of treatment. *Rheumatology* **2014**, *53*, 2143–2154. [CrossRef] [PubMed]
75. Myasoedova, E.; Crowson, C.S.; Kremers, H.M.; Roger, V.L.; Fitz-Gibbon, P.D.; Therneau, T.M.; Gabriel, S.E. Lipid paradox in rheumatoid arthritis: The impact of serum lipid measures and systemic inflammation on the risk of cardiovascular disease. *Ann. Rheum. Dis.* **2011**, *70*, 482–487. [CrossRef]
76. Ridker, P.M.; Everett, B.M.; Thuren, T.; MacFadyen, J.G.; Chang, W.H.; Ballantyne, C.; Fonseca, F.; Nicolau, J.; Koenig, W.; Anker, S.D.; et al. Antiinflammatory Therapy with Canakinumab for Atherosclerotic Disease. *N. Engl. J. Med.* **2017**, *377*, 1119–1131. [CrossRef]
77. Goodson, N.J.; Brookhart, A.M.; Symmons, D.P.M.; Silman, A.J.; Solomon, D.H. Non-steroidal anti-inflammatory drug use does not appear to be associated with increased cardiovascular mortality in patients with inflammatory polyarthritis: Results from a primary care based inception cohort of patients. *Ann. Rheum. Dis.* **2009**, *68*, 367–372. [CrossRef]
78. Gonzalez-Gay, M.A.; Gonzalez-Juanatey, C.; Martin, J. Rheumatoid Arthritis: A Disease Associated with Accelerated Atherogenesis. *Semin. Arthritis Rheum.* **2005**, *35*, 8–17. [CrossRef]
79. Kerola, A.M.; Kerola, T.; Kauppi, M.J.; Kautiainen, H.; Virta, L.J.; Puolakka, K.; Nieminen, T.V. Cardiovascular comorbidities antedating the diagnosis of rheumatoid arthritis. *Ann. Rheum. Dis.* **2013**, *72*, 1826–1829. [CrossRef]
80. Södergren, A.; Karp, K.; Boman, K.; Eriksson, C.; Lundström, E.; Smedby, T.; Söderlund, L.; Rantapää-Dahlqvist, S.; Wållberg-Jonsson, S. Atherosclerosis in early rheumatoid arthritis: Very early endothelial activation and rapid progression of intima media thickness. *Arthritis Res. Ther.* **2010**, *12*, R158. [CrossRef]
81. González-Gay, M.A.; González-Juanatey, C.; Miranda-Filloy, J.A.; García-Unzueta, M.T.; Llorca, J. Lack of association between flow-mediated endothelium-dependent vasodilatation and biomarkers of endothelial dysfunction in patients with severe rheumatoid arthritis. *Rheumatol. Int.* **2012**, *32*, 4071–4072. [CrossRef] [PubMed]
82. Maga, M.; Laczak, P.; Kaczmarczyk, P.; Wandzilak, M.; Maga, P. Images in Vascular Medicine: Successful endovascular treatment of psoriasis-induced critical limb ischemia. *Vasc. Med.* **2021**, *26*, 350–351. [CrossRef]
83. Di Minno, M.N.D.; Ambrosino, P.; Lupoli, R.; Di Minno, A.; Tasso, M.; Peluso, R.; Tremoli, E. Clinical assessment of endothelial function in patients with rheumatoid arthritis: A meta-analysis of literature studies. *Eur. J. Intern. Med.* **2015**, *26*, 835–842. [CrossRef] [PubMed]
84. Ambrosino, P.; Tasso, M.; Lupoli, R.; Di Minno, A.; Baldassarre, D.; Tremoli, E.; Di Minno, M.N.D. Non-invasive assessment of arterial stiffness in patients with rheumatoid arthritis: A systematic review and meta-analysis of literature studies. *Ann. Med.* **2015**, *47*, 457–467. [CrossRef]
85. Paccou, J.; Renard, C.; Liabeuf, S.; Kamel, S.; Fardellone, P.; Massy, Z.A.; Brazier, M.; Mentaverri, R. Coronary and Abdominal Aorta Calcification in Rheumatoid Arthritis: Relationships with Traditional Cardiovascular Risk Factors, Disease Characteristics, and Concomitant Treatments. *J. Rheumatol.* **2014**, *41*, 2137–2144. [CrossRef] [PubMed]
86. McGettigan, P.; Henry, D. Cardiovascular risk and inhibition of cyclooxygenase—A systematic review of the observational studies of selective and nonselective inhibitors of cyclooxygenase. *JAMA—J. Am. Med. Assoc.* **2006**, *296*, 1633–1644. [CrossRef] [PubMed]
87. Kearney, P.M.; Baigent, C.; Godwin, J.; Halls, H.; Emberson, J.R.; Patrono, C. Faculty Opinions recommendation of Do selective cyclo-oxygenase-2 inhibitors and traditional non-steroidal anti-inflammatory drugs increase the risk of atherothrombosis? Meta-analysis of randomised trials. *BMJ-Br. Med. J.* **2006**, *332*, 1302–1305. [CrossRef] [PubMed]
88. Roubille, C.; Richer, V.; Starnino, T.; McCourt, C.; McFarlane, A.; Fleming, P.; Siu, S.; Kraft, J.; Lynde, C.; Pope, J.; et al. The effects of tumour necrosis factor inhibitors, methotrexate, non-steroidal anti-inflammatory drugs and corticosteroids on cardiovascular events in rheumatoid arthritis, psoriasis and psoriatic arthritis: A systematic review and meta-analysis. *Ann. Rheum. Dis.* **2015**, *74*, 480–489. [CrossRef]
89. Cabassi, A.; Tedeschi, S.; Perlini, S.; Verzicco, I.; Volpi, R.; Gonzi, G.; Del, S. Canale Non-steroidal anti-inflammatory drug effects on renal and cardiovascular function: From physiology to clinical practice. *Eur. J. Prev. Cardiol.* **2020**, *27*, 850–867. [CrossRef]
90. Gargiulo, G.; Capodanno, D.; Longo, G.; Capranzano, P.; Tamburino, C. Updates on NSAIDs in patients with and without coronary artery disease: Pitfalls, interactions and cardiovascular outcomes. *Expert Rev. Cardiovasc. Ther.* **2014**, *12*, 1185–1203. [CrossRef]
91. Gasparyan, A.Y.; Ayvazyan, L.; Cocco, G.; Kitas, G.D. Adverse Cardiovascular Effects of Antirheumatic Drugs: Implications for Clinical Practice and Research. *Curr. Pharm. Des.* **2012**, *18*, 1543–1555. [CrossRef]

92. Szeto, C.-C.; Sugano, K.; Wang, J.-G.; Fujimoto, K.; Whittle, S.; Modi, G.K.; Chen, C.-H.; Park, J.-B.; Tam, L.-S.; Vareesangthip, K.; et al. Non-steroidal anti-inflammatory drug (NSAID) therapy in patients with hypertension, cardiovascular, renal or gastrointestinal comorbidities: Joint APAGE/APLAR/APSDE/APSH/APSN/PoA recommendations. *Gut* **2020**, *69*, 617–629. [CrossRef]
93. Zheng, L.; Du, X. Non-steroidal Anti-inflammatory Drugs and Hypertension. *Cell Biochem. Biophys.* **2014**, *69*, 209–211. [CrossRef] [PubMed]
94. Caldwell, B.; Aldington, S.; Weatherall, M.; Shirtcliffe, P.; Beasley, R. Risk of cardiovascular events and celecoxib: A systematic review and meta-analysis. *J. R. Soc. Med.* **2006**, *99*, 132–140. [CrossRef] [PubMed]
95. Helin-Salmivaara, A.; Virtanen, A.; Vesalainen, R.; Grönroos, J.M.; Klaukka, T.; Idänpään-Heikkilä, J.E.; Huupponen, R. NSAID use and the risk of hospitalization for first myocardial infarction in the general population: A nationwide case-control study from Finland. *Eur. Heart J.* **2006**, *27*, 1657–1663. [CrossRef] [PubMed]
96. Schneeweiss, S.; Solomon, D.H.; Wang, P.S.; Rassen, J.; Brookhart, M.A. Simultaneous assessment of short-term gastrointestinal benefits and cardiovascular risks of selective cyclooxygenase 2 inhibitors and nonselective nonsteroidal anti-inflammatory drugs—An instrumental variable analysis. *Arthritis Rheum.* **2006**, *54*, 3390–3398. [CrossRef]
97. Fabule, J.; Adebajo, A. Comparative evaluation of cardiovascular outcomes in patients with osteoarthritis and rheumatoid arthritis on recommended doses of nonsteroidal anti-inflammatory drugs. *Ther. Adv. Musculoskelet. Dis.* **2014**, *6*, 111–130. [CrossRef]
98. del Rincón, I.; Battafarano, D.F.; Restrepo, J.F.; Erikson, J.M.; Escalante, A. Glucocorticoid Dose Thresholds Associated With All-Cause and Cardiovascular Mortality in Rheumatoid Arthritis. *Arthritis Rheumatol.* **2014**, *66*, 264–272. [CrossRef]
99. Soubrier, M.; Chamoux, N.B.; Tatar, Z.; Couderc, M.; Dubost, J.J.; Mathieu, S. Cardiovascular risk in rheumatoid arthritis. *Jt. Bone Spine* **2014**, *81*, 298–302. [CrossRef]
100. Ravindran, V.; Rachapalli, S.; Choy, E.H. Safety of medium- to long-term glucocorticoid therapy in rheumatoid arthritis: A meta-analysis. *Rheumatology* **2009**, *48*, 807–811. [CrossRef]
101. Ruyssen-Witrand, A.; Fautrel, B.; Saraux, A.; Le Loët, X.; Pham, T. Cardiovascular risk induced by low-dose corticosteroids in rheumatoid arthritis: A systematic literature review. *Jt. Bone Spine* **2011**, *78*, 23–30. [CrossRef] [PubMed]
102. Agca, R.; Heslinga, S.C.; Rollefstad, S.; Heslinga, M.; McInnes, B.; Peters, M.J.L.; Kvien, T.K.; Dougados, M.; Radner, H.; Atzeni, F.; et al. EULAR recommendations for cardiovascular disease risk management in patients with rheumatoid arthritis and other forms of inflammatory joint disorders: 2015/2016 update. *Ann. Rheum. Dis.* **2017**, *76*, 17–28. [CrossRef] [PubMed]
103. Suissa, S.; Bernatsky, S.; Hudson, M. Antirheumatic drug use and the risk of acute myocardial infarction. *Arthritis Rheum.* **2006**, *55*, 531–536. [CrossRef] [PubMed]
104. Rempenault, C.; Combe, B.; Barnetche, T.; Gaujoux-Viala, C.; Lukas, C.; Morel, J.; Hua, C. Metabolic and cardiovascular benefits of hydroxychloroquine in patients with rheumatoid arthritis: A systematic review and meta-analysis. *Ann. Rheum. Dis.* **2018**, *77*, 98–103. [CrossRef] [PubMed]
105. Widdifield, J.; Abrahamowicz, M.; Paterson, J.M.; Huang, A.; Thorne, J.C.; Pope, J.E.; Kuriya, B.; Beauchamp, M.-E.; Bernatsky, S. Associations Between Methotrexate Use and the Risk of Cardiovascular Events in Patients with Elderly-onset Rheumatoid Arthritis. *J. Rheumatol.* **2019**, *46*, 467–474. [CrossRef] [PubMed]
106. Westlake, S.L.; Colebatch, A.N.; Baird, J.; Curzen, N.; Kiely, P.; Quinn, M.; Choy, E.; Ostor, A.J.K.; Edwards, C.J. Tumor necrosis factor antagonists and the risk of cardiovascular disease in patients with rheumatoid arthritis: A systematic literature review. *Rheumatology* **2011**, *50*, 518–531. [CrossRef]
107. Micha, R.; Imamura, F.; von Ballmoos, M.W.; Solomon, D.H.; Hernán, M.A.; Ridker, P.M.; Mozaffarian, D. Systematic Review and Meta-Analysis of Methotrexate Use and Risk of Cardiovascular Disease. *Am. J. Cardiol.* **2011**, *108*, 1362–1370. [CrossRef]
108. Morris, S.J.; Wasko, M.C.M.; Antohe, J.L.; Sartorius, J.A.; Kirchner, H.L.; Dancea, S.; Bili, A. Hydroxychloroquine use associated with improvement in lipid profiles in rheumatoid arthritis patients. *Arthritis Care Res.* **2011**, *63*, 530–534. [CrossRef]
109. Li, H.-Z.; Xu, X.-H.; Lin, N.; Lu, H.-D. Metabolic and cardiovascular benefits of hydroxychloroquine in patients with rheumatoid arthritis: A systematic review and meta-analysis. *Ann. Rheum. Dis.* **2019**, *78*, e21. [CrossRef] [PubMed]
110. Charles-Schoeman, C.; Wang, X.; Lee, Y.Y.; Shahbazian, A.; Navarro-Millán, I.; Yang, S.; Chen, L.; Cofield, S.S.; Moreland, L.W.; O'Dell, J.; et al. Association of Triple Therapy With Improvement in Cholesterol Profiles Over Two-Year Followup in the Treatment of Early Aggressive Rheumatoid Arthritis Trial. *Arthritis Rheumatol.* **2016**, *68*, 577–586. [CrossRef]
111. Solomon, D.H.; Avorn, J.; Katz, J.N.; Weinblatt, M.E.; Setoguchi, S.; Levin, R.; Schneeweiss, S. Immunosuppressive medications and hospitalization for cardiovascular events in patients with rheumatoid arthritis. *Arthritis Rheum.* **2006**, *54*, 3790–3798. [CrossRef] [PubMed]
112. Smolen, J.S.; Landewé, R.; Breedveld, F.C.; Buch, M.; Burmester, G.; Dougados, M.; Emery, P.; Gaujoux-Viala, C.; Gossec, L.; Nam, J.; et al. EULAR recommendations for the management of rheumatoid arthritis with synthetic and biological disease-modifying antirheumatic drugs: 2013 update. *Ann. Rheum. Dis.* **2014**, *73*, 492–509. [CrossRef] [PubMed]
113. Solomon, D.H.; Curtis, J.R.; Saag, K.G.; Lii, J.; Chen, L.; Harrold, L.R.; Herrinton, L.J.; Graham, D.J.; Kowal, M.K.; Kuriya, B.; et al. Cardiovascular Risk in Rheumatoid Arthritis: Comparing TNF-α Blockade with Nonbiologic DMARDs. *Am. J. Med.* **2013**, *126*, 730.e9–730.e17. [CrossRef] [PubMed]
114. Toussirot, E. Effects of TNF alpha inhibitors on adiposity and other cardiovascular risk factors: Implications for the cardiovascular prognosis in patients with rheumatoid arthritis. *Expert Opin. Drug Saf.* **2015**, *14*, 525–532. [CrossRef]

115. Barnabe, C.; Martin, B.-J.; Ghali, W.A. Systematic review and meta-analysis: Anti-tumor necrosis factor α therapy and cardiovascular events in rheumatoid arthritis. *Arthritis Care Res.* **2011**, *63*, 522–529. [CrossRef]
116. Jacobsson, L.T.H.; Turesson, C.; Gülfe, A.; Kapetanovic, M.C.; Petersson, I.F.; Saxne, T.; Geborek, P. Treatment with tumor necrosis factor blockers is associated with a lower incidence of first cardiovascular events in patients with rheumatoid arthritis. *J. Rheumatol.* **2005**, *32*, 1213–1218.
117. Ljung, L.; Rantapää-Dahlqvist, S.; Jacobsson, L.T.H.; Askling, J. Response to biological treatment and subsequent risk of coronary events in rheumatoid arthritis. *Ann. Rheum. Dis.* **2016**, *75*, 2087–2094. [CrossRef]
118. Karpouzas, G.A.; Ormseth, S.R.; Hernandez, E.; Budoff, M.J. Impact of Cumulative Inflammation, Cardiac Risk Factors, and Medication Exposure on Coronary Atherosclerosis Progression in Rheumatoid Arthritis. *Arthritis Rheumatol.* **2020**, *72*, 400–408. [CrossRef]
119. Singh, S.; Fumery, M.; Singh, A.G.; Singh, N.; Prokop, L.J.; Dulai, P.S.; Sandborn, W.J.; Curtis, J.R. Comparative Risk of Cardiovascular Events With Biologic and Synthetic Disease-Modifying Antirheumatic Drugs in Patients With Rheumatoid Arthritis: A Systematic Review and Meta-Analysis. *Arthritis Care Res.* **2020**, *72*, 561–576. [CrossRef]
120. Chung, E.S.; Packer, M.; Lo, K.H.; Fasanmade, A.A.; Willerson, J.T.; Investigators, A. Randomized, double-blind, placebo-controlled, trial of infliximab, a chimeric monoclonal antibody to tumor necrosis factor-alpha, in patients with moderate-to-severe heart failure—Results of the Anti-TNF Therapy Against Congestive Heart Failure (ATTACH) trial. *Circulation* **2003**, *107*, 3133–3140.
121. Leporini, C.; Russo, E.; D'angelo, S.; Arturi, F.; Tripepi, G.; Peluso, R.; Grembiale, R.D.; Olivieri, I.; De Sarro, G.; Ursini, F. Insulin-Sensiting Effects of Tumor Necrosis Factor Alpha Inhibitors in Rheumatoid Arthritis: A Systematic Review and Meta-Analysis. *Rev. Recent Clin. Trials* **2018**, *13*, 184–191. [CrossRef] [PubMed]
122. Castagné, B.; Viprey, M.; Martin, J.; Schott, A.-M.; Cucherat, M.; Soubrier, M. Cardiovascular safety of tocilizumab: A systematic review and network meta-analysis. *PLoS ONE* **2019**, *14*, e0220178. [CrossRef] [PubMed]
123. Divonne, M.d.L.F.; Gottenberg, J.E.; Salliot, C. Safety of biologic DMARDs in RA patients in real life: A systematic literature review and meta-analyses of biologic registers. *Jt. Bone Spine* **2017**, *84*, 133–140. [CrossRef] [PubMed]
124. Cheung, T.; Tsoi, M.; Cheung, B. SAT0099 Effect of TNF Inhibitors on Subclinical Atherosclerosis in Patients with Rheumatoid Arthritis: A Meta-Analysis. *Ann. Rheum. Dis.* **2015**, *74*, 685. [CrossRef]
125. Daien, C.I.; Duny, Y.; Barnetche, T.; Daures, J.P.; Combe, B.; Morel, J. Effect of TNF inhibitors on lipid profile in rheumatoid arthritis: A systematic review with meta-analysis. *Ann. Rheum. Dis.* **2012**, *71*, 862–868. [CrossRef]
126. Zhao, Q.W.; Hong, D.S.; Zhang, Y.; Sang, Y.L.; Yang, Z.H.; Zhang, X.G. Association Between Anti-TNF Therapy for Rheumatoid Arthritis and Hypertension A Meta-Analysis of Randomized Controlled Trials. *Medicine* **2015**, *94*, e731. [CrossRef]
127. Kim, S.K.; Kwak, S.G.; Choe, J.Y. Association between biologic disease modifying antirheumatic drugs and incident hypertension in patients with rheumatoid arthritis Results from prospective nationwide KOBIO Registry. *Medicine* **2020**, *99*, e19415. [CrossRef]
128. Desai, R.J.; Solomon, D.H.; Schneeweiss, S.; Danaei, G.; Liao, K.P.; Kim, S.C. Tumor Necrosis Factor-α Inhibitor Use and the Risk of Incident Hypertension in Patients with Rheumatoid Arthritis. *Epidemiology* **2016**, *27*, 414–422. [CrossRef]
129. Jin, Y.; Kang, E.H.; Brill, G.; Desai, R.J.; Kim, S.C. Cardiovascular (CV) Risk after Initiation of Abatacept versus TNF Inhibitors in Rheumatoid Arthritis Patients with and without Baseline CV Disease. *J. Rheumatol.* **2018**, *45*, 1240–1248. [CrossRef]
130. Schiff, M.H.; Kremer, J.M.; Jahreis, A.; Vernon, E.; Isaacs, J.D.; van Vollenhoven, R.F. Integrated safety in tocilizumab clinical trials. *Thromb. Haemost.* **2011**, *13*, R141. [CrossRef]
131. Fleischmann, R.; Lin, Y.; John, G.S.; van der Heijde, D.; Qiu, C.; Gomez-Reino, J.J.; Maldonado-Cocco, J.A.; Stanislav, M.; Seriolo, B.; Burmester, G.R. SAT0125 Long-Term Safety with Sarilumab Plus Conventional Synthetic Disease-Modifying Antirheumatic Drugs and Sarilumab Monotherapy in Rheumatoid Arthritis: An Integrated Analysis with 9000 Patient-Years of Follow-Up. *Ann. Rheum. Dis.* **2019**, *78*, 1130–1131. [CrossRef]
132. Ikonomidis, I.; Lekakis, J.P.; Nikolaou, M.; Paraskevaidis, I.; Andreadou, I.; Kaplanoglou, T.; Katsimbri, P.; Skarantavos, G.; Soucacos, P.N.; Kremastinos, D.T. Inhibition of Interleukin-1 by Anakinra Improves Vascular and Left Ventricular Function in Patients With Rheumatoid Arthritis. *Circulation* **2008**, *117*, 2662–2669. [CrossRef] [PubMed]
133. van Vollenhoven, R.F.; Emery, P.; O Bingham, C.; Keystone, E.C.; Fleischmann, R.M.; E Furst, D.; Tyson, N.; Collinson, N.; Lehane, P.B. Long-term safety of rituximab in rheumatoid arthritis: 9.5-year follow-up of the global clinical trial programme with a focus on adverse events of interest in RA patients. *Ann. Rheum. Dis.* **2013**, *72*, 1496–1502. [CrossRef]
134. Day, A.L.; Singh, J.A. Cardiovascular Disease Risk in Older Adults and Elderly Patients with Rheumatoid Arthritis: What Role Can Disease-Modifying Antirheumatic Drugs Play in Cardiovascular Risk Reduction? *Drugs Aging* **2019**, *36*, 493–510. [CrossRef]
135. McInnes, I.B.; Thompson, L.; Giles, J.T.; Bathon, J.M.; E Salmon, J.; Beaulieu, A.D.; E Codding, C.; Carlson, T.H.; Delles, C.; Lee, J.S.; et al. Effect of interleukin-6 receptor blockade on surrogates of vascular risk in rheumatoid arthritis: MEASURE, a randomised, placebo-controlled study. *Ann. Rheum. Dis.* **2015**, *74*, 694–702. [CrossRef] [PubMed]
136. Tanaka, Y.; Suzuki, M.; Nakamura, H.; Toyoizumi, S.; Zwillich, S.H. Tofacitinib Study Investigators Phase II study of tofacitinib (CP-690,550) combined with methotrexate in patients with rheumatoid arthritis and an inadequate response to methotrexate. *Arthritis Care Res.* **2011**, *63*, 1150–1158. [CrossRef]
137. Taylor, P.C.; Weinblatt, M.E.; Burmester, G.R.; Rooney, T.P.; Witt, S.; Walls, C.D.; Issa, M.; Salinas, C.A.; Saifan, C.; Zhang, X.; et al. Cardiovascular Safety During Treatment With Baricitinib in Rheumatoid Arthritis. *Arthritis Rheumatol.* **2019**, *71*, 1042–1055. [CrossRef]

138. Souto, A.; Salgado, E.; Maneiro, J.R.; Mera, A.; Carmona, L.; Gómez-Reino, J.J. Lipid profile changes in patients with chronic inflammatory arthritis treated with biologic agents and tofacitinib in randomized clinical trials: A systematic review and meta-analysis. *Arthritis Rheumatol.* **2015**, *67*, 117–127. [CrossRef]
139. Zhang, J.; Xie, F.; Yun, H.; Chen, L.; Muntner, P.; Levitan, E.B.; Safford, M.M.; Kent, S.T.; Osterman, M.T.; Lewis, J.D.; et al. Comparative effects of biologics on cardiovascular risk among older patients with rheumatoid arthritis. *Ann. Rheum. Dis.* **2016**, *75*, 1813–1818. [CrossRef]
140. Myasoedova, E.; Karmacharya, P.; Garcia, A.D.; Davis, J.; Murad, M.H.; Crowson, C. Effect of statin use on the risk of rheumatoid arthritis: A systematic review and meta-analysis. *Semin Arthritis Rheum.* **2020**, *50*, 1348–1356. [CrossRef]
141. Soulaidopoulos, S.; Nikiphorou, E.; Dimitroulas, T.; Kitas, G.D. The Role of Statins in Disease Modification and Cardiovascular Risk in Rheumatoid Arthritis. *Front. Med.* **2018**, *5*, 24. [CrossRef]
142. Danninger, K.; Hoppe, U.C.; Pieringer, H. Do statins reduce the cardiovascular risk in patients with rheumatoid arthritis? *Int. J. Rheum. Dis.* **2014**, *17*, 606–611. [CrossRef]
143. Xing, B.; Yin, Y.-F.; Zhao, L.-D.; Wang, L.; Zheng, W.-J.; Chen, H.; Wu, Q.-J.; Tang, F.-L.; Zhang, F.-C.; Shan, G.; et al. Effect of 3-Hydroxy-3-Methylglutaryl-Coenzyme A Reductase Inhibitor on Disease Activity in Patients with Rheumatoid Arthritis A Meta-Analysis. *Medicine* **2015**, *94*, e572. [CrossRef] [PubMed]
144. Marnell, L.; Mold, C.; Du Clos, T.W. C-reactive protein: Ligands, receptors and role in inflammation. *Clin. Immunol.* **2005**, *117*, 104–111. [CrossRef] [PubMed]
145. Iwase, S.; Nakada, T.-A.; Hattori, N.; Takahashi, W.; Takahashi, N.; Aizimu, T.; Yoshida, M.; Morizane, T.; Oda, S. Interleukin-6 as a diagnostic marker for infection in critically ill patients: A systematic review and meta-analysis. *Am. J. Emerg. Med.* **2019**, *37*, 260–265. [CrossRef]
146. Shimamoto, K.; Ito, T.; Ozaki, Y.; Amuro, H.; Tanaka, A.; Nishizawa, T.; Son, Y.; Inaba, M.; Nomura, S. Serum Interleukin 6 Before and After Therapy with Tocilizumab Is a Principal Biomarker in Patients with Rheumatoid Arthritis. *J. Rheumatol.* **2013**, *40*, 1074–1081. [CrossRef]
147. Rincón-López, E.M.; Gómez, M.L.N.; Matos, T.H.-S.; Aguilera-Alonso, D.; Moreno, E.D.; Saavedra-Lozano, J.; García, B.S.; Sebastián, M.d.M.S.; Morín, M.G.; Bieler, C.B.; et al. Interleukin 6 as a marker of severe bacterial infection in children with sickle cell disease and fever: A case–control study. *BMC Infect. Dis.* **2021**, *21*, 1–9. [CrossRef] [PubMed]
148. Inam Illahi, M.; Amjad, S.; Alam, S.M.; Ahmed, S.T.; Fatima, M.; Shahid, M.A. Serum tumor necrosis fac-tor-alpha as a competent biomarker for evaluation of disease activity in early rheumatoid arthritis. *Cureus* **2021**, *13*, e15314.

Disclaimer/Publisher's Note: The statements, opinions and data contained in all publications are solely those of the individual author(s) and contributor(s) and not of MDPI and/or the editor(s). MDPI and/or the editor(s) disclaim responsibility for any injury to people or property resulting from any ideas, methods, instructions or products referred to in the content.

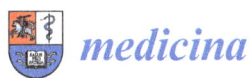

Article

Antibodies against Serum Anti-Melanoma Differentiation-Associated Gene 5 in Rheumatoid Arthritis Patients with Chronic Lung Diseases

Shomi Oka [1,2], Takashi Higuchi [1,3], Hiroshi Furukawa [1,2,*], Kota Shimada [4,5], Akira Okamoto [6,†], Atsushi Hashimoto [4,7], Akiko Komiya [2,8], Koichiro Saisho [9,10], Norie Yoshikawa [9], Masao Katayama [11], Toshihiro Matsui [2,4], Naoshi Fukui [2,12], Kiyoshi Migita [13,14] and Shigeto Tohma [1,2]

[1] Department of Rheumatology, National Hospital Organization Tokyo National Hospital, 3-1-1 Takeoka, Kiyose 204-8585, Japan
[2] Clinical Research Center for Allergy and Rheumatology, National Hospital Organization Sagamihara National Hospital, 18-1 Sakuradai, Minami-ku, Sagamihara 252-0392, Japan
[3] Department of Nephrology, Ushiku Aiwa General Hospital, 896 Shishiko-cho, Ushiku 300-1296, Japan
[4] Department of Rheumatology, National Hospital Organization Sagamihara National Hospital, 18-1 Sakuradai, Minami-ku, Sagamihara 252-0392, Japan
[5] Department of Rheumatic Diseases, Tokyo Metropolitan Tama Medical Center, 2-8-29 Musashi-dai, Fuchu 183-8524, Japan
[6] Department of Rheumatology, National Hospital Organization Himeji Medical Center, 68 Hon-machi, Himeji 670-8520, Japan
[7] Department of Internal Medicine, Sagami Seikyou Hospital, 6-2-11 Sagamiohno, Minami-ku, Sagamihara 252-0303, Japan
[8] Department of Clinical Laboratory, National Hospital Organization Sagamihara National Hospital, 18-1 Sakuradai, Minami-ku, Sagamihara 252-0392, Japan
[9] Department of Orthopedics/Rheumatology, National Hospital Organization Miyakonojo Medical Center, 5033-1 Iwayoshi-cho, Miyakonojo 885-0014, Japan
[10] Tanimura Hospital, 10-2 Kitakoji, Nobeoka 882-0041, Japan
[11] Department of Internal Medicine, National Hospital Organization Nagoya Medical Center, 4-1-1 Sannomaru, Naka-ku, Nagoya 460-0001, Japan
[12] Department of Life Sciences, Graduate School of Arts and Sciences, The University of Tokyo, 3-8-1 Komaba, Meguro-ku, Tokyo 153-8902, Japan
[13] Clinical Research Center, National Hospital Organization Nagasaki Medical Center, 2-1001-1 Kubara, Omura 856-8562, Japan
[14] Department of Gastroenterology and Rheumatology, Fukushima Medical University School of Medicine, 1 Hikarigaoka, Fukushima 960-1295, Japan
* Correspondence: furukawa-tky@umin.org
† Deceased.

Abstract: Chronic lung diseases (CLD), including interstitial lung disease (ILD) and airway diseases (ADs), are common complications of rheumatoid arthritis (RA). Rheumatoid factor (RF) and anti-citrullinated peptide antibodies are reported to be associated with CLD in RA patients. The presence of anti-melanoma differentiation-associated gene 5 (MDA5) antibodies (Abs) is associated with clinically amyopathic dermatomyositis developing into rapidly progressive ILD. However, few studies on anti-MDA5 Abs in RA have been published. Here, we analyzed the association of anti-MDA5 Abs with CLD complications in RA. Anti-MDA5 Abs were quantified in sera from RA patients with or without CLD. Anti-MDA5 Ab levels were higher in RA patients with ADs than without (mean ± SDM, 4.4 ± 2.4 vs. 4.0 ± 4.2, $p = 0.0001$). AUC values of anti-MDA5 Ab and RF ROC curves were similar in RA patients with or without CLD (0.578, 95%CI 0.530–0.627 and 0.579, 95%CI 0.530–0.627, respectively, $p = 0.9411$). Multiple logistic regression analysis of anti-MDA5 Abs and clinical characteristics yielded an MDA5-index with a higher AUC value than anti-MDA5 Ab alone (0.694, 95%CI 0.648–0.740, $p = 5.08 \times 10^{-5}$). Anti-MDA5 Abs were associated with ADs in RA patients and could represent a biomarker for CLD, similar to RF. The involvement of anti-MDA5 Abs in the pathogenesis of ADs in RA is proposed.

Keywords: rheumatoid arthritis; anti-melanoma differentiation-associated gene 5 antibodies; airway diseases; chronic lung disease

1. Introduction

Rheumatoid arthritis (RA) is an autoimmune disease characterized by the destruction of synovial joints. Chronic lung diseases (CLD) are frequently present in RA, and include interstitial lung disease (ILD), airway diseases (ADs) and emphysema. The complication of ILD or ADs confers a dismal prognosis for RA patients [1–5]. Usual interstitial pneumonia (UIP) is especially associated with very poor prognosis in RA patients [6]. It is therefore important to clarify the pathogenesis of ILD and ADs in RA patients.

Krebs von den lungen-6 (KL-6) and surfactant protein-D (SP-D) are biomarkers for idiopathic pulmonary fibrosis, and also for ILD in RA [7,8]. It has also been reported that KL-6 and SP-D are increased in ADs and emphysema [9,10]. Rheumatoid factors (RFs) are antibodies (Abs) against the Fc portion of immunoglobulin G. Anti-citrullinated peptide antibodies (ACPAs) are Abs against citrullinated peptides generated by posttranslational modification of arginine residues. RF and ACPA are used as rheumatoid arthritis classification criteria [11]. RFs are associated with ILD in RA [12,13]. ACPAs are also associated with ILD in RA [12,14,15]. The presence of RF is associated with mortality of RA patients [16]. RF and ACPA are considered to be biomarkers for ILD in RA [17].

Anti-melanoma differentiation-associated gene 5 (MDA5) Abs are directed against RNA helicase. Their presence is associated with clinically amyopathic dermatomyositis developing into rapidly progressive ILD with a poor prognosis [18–21]. It has been reported that anti-MDA5 Abs are not present in RA patients [22]. However, few validation studies on anti-MDA5 Abs in RA with CLD have been conducted. In the present study, we investigated the association of anti-MDA5 Abs with CLD in RA patients.

2. Materials and Methods

2.1. Patients

RA patients (n = 558) were recruited at Himeji Medical Center, Miyakonojo Medical Center, Nagasaki Medical Center, Nagoya Medical Center, Sagamihara Hospital and Tokyo Hospital. All patients fulfilled the rheumatoid arthritis classification criteria [11], or American College of Rheumatology criteria for RA [23]. They were diagnosed as having UIP, nonspecific interstitial pneumonia (NSIP), ADs, emphysema, or no CLD, based on the predominant findings of chest computed tomography; the findings of ADs are centrilobular or peribronchial nodules, branching linear structures, bronchial dilatation, bronchial wall thickening, or atelectasis [9]. The CLD(+) group includes UIP, NSIP, ADs, and emphysema and ILD groups include UIP and NSIP patients. Sera were collected from these RA patients and assessed for anti-MDA5 Abs. This study was reviewed and approved by the Research Ethics Committees of Tokyo Hospital (190010) and Sagamihara Hospital and the Central Institutional Review Board of the National Hospital Organization. Written informed consent was obtained from all patients. This study was conducted in accordance with the principles expressed in the Declaration of Helsinki.

2.2. Detection of Anti-MDA5 Abs

Anti-MDA5 Abs were detected using Mesacup anti-MDA5 tests, according to the manufacturer's instructions (Medical & Biological Laboratories, Tokyo, Japan, User's manual, https://www.info.pmda.go.jp/downfiles/ivd/PDF/130249_22700EZX00013000_A_01_01.pdf, accessed on 20 January 2023). Sera were diluted 1:100 with the dilution buffer of the kit. An index value was calculated according to the manufacturer's instructions as follows: index value = (optical density value of sample—optical density value of blank)/(optical density value of positive control—optical density value of blank) × 100. The cut-off value was set to 8.156, based on the 98th percentile among 52 healthy controls (mean age ± SDM:

35.4 ± 11.1, male number: 2 [3.8%]). RF was also measured with an N-latex RF kit (Siemens Healthcare Diagnostics, München, Germany), which measured IgM class RFs; the cut-off value was 15 U/mL. ACPA IgG was detected with Mesacup-2 test CCP; the cut-off value was 4.5 U/mL. KL-6 was measured with the Picolumi KL-6 Electrochemiluminescence immunoassay system (EIDIA Co., Ltd., Tokyo, Japan); the cut-off value was 500 U/mL. SP-D was measured with SP-D Yamasa EIA II kits (Yamasa Corporation, Choshi, Japan); the cut-off value was 110 ng/mL. The results of RF, ACPA, KL-6, and SP-D for some of the RA patients have been reported previously [10]. Steinbrocker stages were classification criteria of RA progression stages from I to IV and were evaluated as previously described [24].

2.3. Statistical Analysis

The clinical characteristics of the subsets of RA patients were compared with RA patients without CLD by Mann–Whitney U tests or Fisher's exact tests. The presence of Abs was compared in RA patients without CLD by Mann–Whitney U tests or Fisher's exact tests. Multiple logistic regression analysis was conducted to create an MDA5-index with covariates with $p_{adjusted} < 0.1$ (anti-MDA5 Abs, age [years], Steinbrocker stage [1–4], and smoking status [current smoker: 2, past smoker: 1, never smoker: 0]). ROC curves for Abs were used to compare RA patients with or without CLD. Area under the curve (AUC) values for ROC curves with 95% confidence intervals (CI) were calculated and compared with the AUC value of 0.5 or other ROC curves by Chi-square analysis. The optimized cut-off levels based on the highest Youden's index were estimated.

3. Results

3.1. Clinical Manifestations of Patients with RA

The clinical manifestations of the RA patients investigated here are described in Tables 1 and 2. The mean age, male:female ratio, age at onset, percentage of smokers or past smokers, KL-6 levels and SP-D levels were higher, and the Steinbrocker stage lower, in RA patients with ILD than in those without CLD. The mean age, age at onset, KL-6 levels and SP-D levels were higher in RA patients with ADs. The mean age, male:female ratio, age at onset, percentage of smokers or past smokers, KL-6 levels and SP-D levels were higher, and the Steinbrocker stage lower, in RA patients with emphysema.

Table 1. Characteristics and anti-MDA5 Ab of RA patients.

	ILD	p	UIP	p	NSIP	p	ADs	p	Emphysema	p
Number	138		63		75		166		39	
Mean age, years (SD)	68.6 (9.1)	4.48×10^{-7}	70.0 (10.0)	2.46×10^{-6}	67.5 (8.1)	0.0009	67.9 (10.5)	4.54×10^{-6}	66.8 (8.2)	0.0301
Male, n (%)	37 (26.8)	* 0.0307	23 (36.5)	* 0.0014	14 (18.7)	* 0.7239	28 (16.9)	* 1.0000	24 (61.5)	* 2.68×10^{-8}
Age at onset, years (SD)	56.5 (14.0)	9.64×10^{-7}	58.0 (15.7)	2.66×10^{-5}	55.2 (12.5)	0.0004	54.4 (15.5)	5.87×10^{-5}	57.4 (11.7)	0.0001
Steinbrocker stage III and IV, n (%)	58 (42.6)	* 0.0060	29 (47.5)	* 0.1473	29 (38.7)	* 0.0046	84 (53.2)	* 0.3444	13 (33.3)	* 0.0051
Smoker or past smoker, n (%)	56 (43.1)	* 0.0063	28 (47.5)	* 0.0072	28 (39.4)	* 0.1008	55 (37.4)	* 0.0816	30 (85.7)	* 1.37×10^{-10}
KL-6, U/mL (SD)	822.3 (776.2)	$<1 \times 10^{-16}$	904.7 (849.2)	1.04×10^{-14}	748.6 (703.0)	5.88×10^{-14}	370.3 (300.5)	0.0002	570.8 (455.3)	4.23×10^{-7}
SP-D, ng/mL (SD)	138.2 (152.2)	2.82×10^{-13}	149.6 (105.5)	1.41×10^{-11}	127.4 (186.4)	1.67×10^{-7}	78.7 (78.3)	0.0072	94.4 (68.4)	6.84×10^{-5}
Anti-MDA5 Ab, index value (SD)	4.4 (4.4)	0.4479	4.7 (4.6)	0.1289	4.2 (4.2)	0.8204	4.4 (2.4)	0.0001	4.1 (1.9)	0.0273
RF, U/mL (SD)	475.5 (1124.6)	0.0060	454.9 (888.5)	0.0032	492.9 (1295.9)	0.0472	208.0 (324.1)	0.1693	835.1 (1947.1)	0.0007
ACPA, U/mL (SD)	339.6 (714.2)	0.8122	260.7 (273.2)	0.8615	403.8 (927.8)	0.8428	271.0 (346.6)	0.5776	433.1 (393.8)	0.0052

RA: rheumatoid arthritis, ILD: including interstitial lung disease, UIP: usual interstitial pneumonia, NSIP: nonspecific interstitial pneumonia, ADs: airway diseases, CLD: chronic lung disease, MDA5: melanoma differentiation-associated gene 5, Ab: antibody, RF: rheumatoid factor, ACPA: anti-citrullinated peptide antibody. ILD group includes UIP and NSIP groups. Data are presented as the mean value or number of each group. Statistical differences were tested in comparison with the CLD(−) population by Fisher's exact test using 2 × 2 contingency tables or the Mann–Whitney U test. * Fisher's exact test was employed.

Table 2. Characteristics and anti-MDA5 Ab in RA patients with or without CLD.

	CLD(+)	p	CLD(−)
Number	343		215
Mean age, years (SD)	68.1 (9.7)	1.36×10^{-8}	62.4 (11.1)
Male, n (%)	89 (25.9)	* 0.0122	36 (16.7)
Age at onset, years (SD)	55.6 (14.5)	1.35×10^{-8}	48.6 (13.5)
Steinbrocker stage III and IV, n (%)	155 (46.5)	* 0.0087	125 (58.1)
Smoker or past smoker, n (%)	141 (45.2)	* 0.0001	57 (28.2)
KL-6, U/mL (SD)	601.6 (619.7)	1.33×10^{-15}	283.3 (274.3)
SP-D, ng/mL (SD)	109.5 (123.7)	2.09×10^{-10}	49.9 (39.4)
Anti-MDA5 Ab, index value (SD)	4.4 (3.3)		4.0 (4.2)
RF, U/mL (SD)	387.2 (1010.0)	0.0018	262.7 (609.5)
ACPA, U/mL (SD)	316.2 (530.1)	0.6626	275.3 (306.2)

RA: rheumatoid arthritis, ILD: interstitial lung disease, UIP: usual interstitial pneumonia, NSIP: nonspecific interstitial pneumonia, ADs: airway diseases, CLD: chronic lung disease, MDA5: melanoma differentiation-associated gene 5, Ab: antibody, RF: rheumatoid factor, ACPA: anti-citrullinated peptide antibody. ILD group includes UIP and NSIP groups. CLD(+) group includes UIP, NSIP, ADs, and emphysema groups. Data are presented as the mean value or number of each group. Statistical differences were tested in comparison with the CLD(−) population by Fisher's exact test using 2×2 contingency tables or the Mann–Whitney U test. * Fisher's exact test was employed.

3.2. Presence of Anti-MDA5 Abs in RA Patients

Anti-MDA5 Abs were quantified in the sera of RA patients, with the results shown in Tables 1 and 2. Anti-MDA5 Ab levels were significantly associated with ADs (mean ± SDM, 4.4 ± 2.4 vs. 4.0 ± 4.2, $p = 0.0001$), emphysema (4.1 ± 1.9 vs. 4.0 ± 4.2, $p = 0.0273$) and CLD (4.4 ± 3.3 vs. 4.0 ± 4.2, $p = 0.0018$). RF and ACPA were also quantified in RA patient sera (Table 2). RF levels were associated with ILD (475.5 ± 1124.6 vs. 262.7 ± 609.5 [U/mL], $p = 0.0020$), emphysema (835.1 ± 1947.1 vs. 262.7 ± 609.5 [U/mL], $p = 0.0007$), and CLD (387.2 ± 1010.0 vs. 262.7 ± 609.5 [U/mL], $p = 0.0018$). ACPA levels were associated with RA in patients with emphysema (433.1 ± 393.8 vs. 275.3 ± 306.2 [U/mL], $p = 0.0052$). Assessments of positivity for anti-MDA5 Abs, RF, and ACPA were also conducted in the RA patients (Supplementary Table S1). Although similar tendencies were observed, no significant associations were detected. Anti-MDA5 Ab levels in RA were also compared with those in healthy controls (Supplementary Tables S2 and S3) and were higher than the controls. Thus, anti-MDA5 Ab titers were associated with ADs and CLD in RA but not with RA in general.

The ROC curve for anti-MDA5 Abs was compared in RA patients with and without CLD (Figure 1A). The AUC value of the ROC curves for anti-MDA5 Abs (0.578, 95% CI 0.530−0.627) was similar to RF ($p = 0.9411$, Figure 1B) but tended to be higher than ACPA ($p = 0.0665$, Figure 1C). Thus, anti-MDA5 Ab values have similar characteristics to RF for the diagnosis of CLD.

ROC curves for anti-MDA5 Abs (A), RF (B), ACPA (C) and multiple logistic regression analysis with anti-MDA5 Abs, age (years), Steinbrocker stage (1–4), and smoking status (current smoker: 2, past smoker: 1, never smoker: 0) (D) were generated to compare CLD(+) and CLD(−) RA. The area under the curve (AUC) values of the ROC curves with 95% confidence intervals and the optimized cut-off levels with specificities and sensitivities are shown: MDA5: melanoma differentiation-associated gene 5, Ab: antibody, RF: rheumatoid factor, ACPA: anti-cyclic citrullinated peptide antibody, ROC: receiver operating characteristic, AUC: area under the curve, and CLD: chronic lung disease.

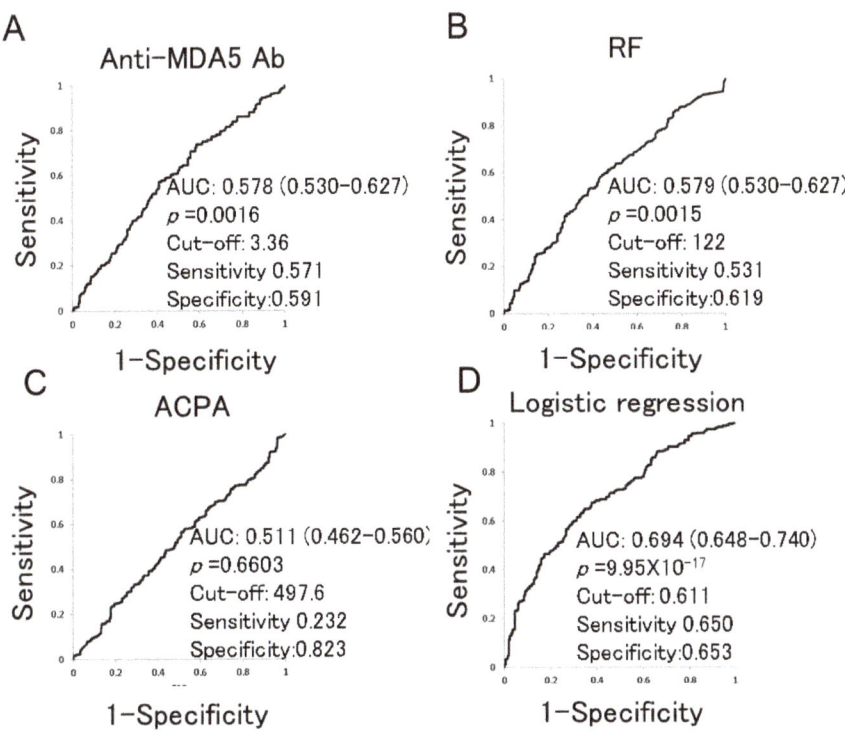

Figure 1. Receiver operating characteristic (ROC) curves using anti-MDA5 Abs (**A**), RF (**B**), ACPA (**C**), and multiple logistic regression analysis (**D**) for comparisons between CLD(+) and CLD(−) RA.

The results of multiple logistic regression analysis of anti-MDA5 Abs and patients' clinical characteristics are shown in Table 3. From these data, anti-MDA5 Abs, age, Steinbrocker stage, and smoking status were selected ($p_{\text{adjusted}} < 0.1$) to create an MDA5-index defined as: $0.0636 \times$ (anti-MDA5 Abs) $+ 0.0554 \times$ (age) $- 0.2037 \times$ (Steinbrocker stage) $+ 0.4615 \times$ (smoking status) $- 3.1211$. The ROC curve AUC value was 0.694 (95% CI 0.648–0.740, $p = 9.95 \times 10^{-17}$, Figure 1D), which was higher than for anti-MDA5 Abs ($p = 5.08 \times 10^{-5}$) or RF ($p = 0.0010$). Thus, multiple logistic regression analysis using anti-MDA5 Abs and certain clinical characteristics resulted in the generation of an MDA5-index with the highest AUC value.

Table 3. Multiple logistic regression analysis of Abs and clinical manifestations for RA with CLD.

Clinical Manifestations	Unconditioned			Conditioned on the Other Factors		
	OR	95%CI	p	OR$_{\text{adjusted}}$	95%CI	p_{adjusted}
Anti-MDA5 Ab (index value)	1.0309	(0.9782~1.0865)	0.2559	1.0608	(0.9919~1.1345)	0.0851
RF (IU/mL)	1.0002	(0.9999~1.0005)	0.1220	1.0002	(0.9999~1.0005)	0.2113
ACPA (U/mL)	1.0002	(0.9998~1.0007)	0.3153	1.0001	(0.9997~1.0006)	0.5674
Age, years	1.0542	(1.0357~1.0730)	4.88×10^{-9}	1.0592	(1.0298~1.0895)	6.24×10^{-5}
Male	1.7422	(1.1313~2.6831)	0.0117	1.2959	(0.7761~2.1639)	0.3217
Age at onset, years	1.0351	(1.0221~1.0482)	7.95×10^{-8}	0.9967	(0.9744~1.0195)	0.7758
Steinbrocker stage	0.7899	(0.6843~0.9117)	0.0013	0.8094	(0.6602~0.9924)	0.0420
Smoking status	1.5497	(1.1993~2.0025)	0.0008	1.5308	(1.1642~2.0129)	0.0023

RA: rheumatoid arthritis, CLD: chronic lung diseases, MDA5: melanoma differentiation-associated gene 5, Ab: antibody, RF: rheumatoid factor, ACPA: anti-citrullinated peptide antibody, OR: Odds ratio, CI: confidence interval. p, OR, 95%CI, p_{adjusted}, OR$_{\text{adjusted}}$ were calculated by logistic regression analysis on RA patients. Smoking status of RA patients were 0: never smoker, 1: past smoker, and 2: current smoker.

4. Discussion

In this study, anti-MDA5 Abs were found to be associated with ADs in RA patients. The AUC values of the ROC curves for anti-MDA5 Abs and RF were similar when comparing RA with and without CLD. An MDA5-index was generated from anti-MDA5 Abs, age, Steinbrocker stage, and smoking status with a ROC curve AUC value higher than for anti-MDA5 Abs or RF alone.

An association of RF with ILD has been previously reported in RA [12,13] and was confirmed in the present study. The association of ACPA with ILD was also reported in RA [12,14,15], but this was not confirmed here. On the other hand, we found that anti-MDA5 Abs were associated with ADs in RA, leading to the notion that anti-MDA5 Abs may be involved in the pathogenesis of ADs. In contrast, anti-MDA5 Abs, RF and ACPA were found to be associated with emphysema (but a possible confounding effect of smoking status could not be excluded). Thus, different specific roles of anti-MDA5 Abs, RF, and ACPA in the pathogenesis of CLD in RA patients should be investigated.

It was found that some clinical characteristics were associated with CLD in RA, though a causal relationship could not be confirmed in this study. These might be confounding factors. Using multiple logistic regression analyses of anti-MDA5 Abs and the clinical characteristics, we created an MDA5-index. This suggested that anti-MDA5 Abs could be used to generate a composite biomarker for CLD in RA. The cut-off level set in this study for anti-MDA5 Ab positivity (8.156) was lower than the kit manufacturer's recommended cut-off level (32) for clinically amyopathic dermatomyositis developing into rapidly progressive ILD. Anti-MDA5 Ab index levels >32 was observed in one RA patient without CLD in the present study. These data suggest that the characteristics of anti-MDA5 Abs regarding ADs in RA patients are different from clinically amyopathic dermatomyositis developing into rapidly progressive ILD. Thus, anti-MDA5 Abs could be used as an alternative biomarker for ADs or CLD in RA. However, results from anti-MDA5 Abs, RF and ACPA indicated that they are not better biomarkers for ILD in RA than KL-6 or SP-D.

Anti-MDA5 Abs have been detected in RA or idiopathic interstitial pneumonia patients developing rapidly progressive ILD [25–27]. They might also be detectable in ADs patients without RA. It was reported that pharmacological Janus kinase inhibition is effective against rapidly progressive ILD in dermatomyositis patients with anti-MDA5 Abs [28], suggesting that these drugs may also be useful for controlling ADs in RA patients. The titer of anti-MDA5 Abs was influenced by the treatment for ILD complicated with dermatomyositis [29] and the results of anti-MDA5 Ab levels in this study would be modified by the treatment for RA or RA disease activities.

To the best of our knowledge, this is the first report on anti-MDA5 Ab profiles in RA patents with CLD, describing an association of anti-MDA5 Abs with ADs. The independent association of anti-MDA5 Ab levels with CLD in RA was not confirmed in logistic regression analysis after adjustment. Because the study sample size was modest, larger-scale studies on anti-MDA5 Abs in RA should be performed to validate these results. The anti-MDA5 Ab profiles in patients with collagen vascular diseases other than RA or dermatomyositis should also be analyzed in future studies. The associations of anti-MDA5 Abs in other ethnic populations should be analyzed, since this study was performed only in Japanese populations. Anti-MDA5 Ab levels in RA should be compared with age-matched healthy controls, because age-matched controls were not available in this study.

Supplementary Materials: The following supporting information can be downloaded at: https://www.mdpi.com/article/10.3390/medicina59020363/s1, Figure S1: Distribution of anti-MDA5 Abs in 52 healthy controls. Table S1: The positivity of RF, ACPA, and anti-MDA5 Ab in the RA patients. Table S2: The comparison of anti-MDA5 Ab in the RA patients and controls.

Author Contributions: Conceptualization, H.F. and S.T.; validation, S.O. and H.F.; formal analysis, H.F.; investigation, S.O., T.H. and H.F.; resources, H.F., K.S. (Kota Shimada), A.O., A.H., A.K., K.S. (Koichiro Saisho), N.Y., M.K., T.M., N.F., K.M. and S.T.; data curation, H.F.; writing—original draft preparation, S.O.; writing—review and editing, H.F.; visualization, H.F.; supervision, S.T.; project administration, S.T.; funding acquisition, H.F., and S.T. All authors have read and agreed to the published version of the manuscript.

Funding: The work was supported by Health and Labour Science Research Grants from the Ministry of Health, Labour, and Welfare of Japan, Grants-in-Aid for Scientific Research (B,C) (22591090, 26293123, 15K09543, 18K08402) and for Young Scientists (B) (24791018) from the Japan Society for the Promotion of Science, Grants-in-Aid of the Practical Research Project for Allergic Diseases and Immunology (Research on Allergic Diseases and Immunology) from Japan Agency for Medical Research and Development, Grants-in-Aid for Clinical Research from National Hospital Organization, Research Grants from Daiwa Securities Health Foundation, Research Grants from Japan Research Foundation for Clinical Pharmacology, Research Grants from The Nakatomi Foundation, Research Grants from Takeda Science Foundation, Research Grants from Mitsui Sumitomo Insurance Welfare Foundation, and Bristol-Myers K.K. RA Clinical Investigation Grant from Bristol-Myers Squibb Co. Research grants were also received from the following pharmaceutical companies: Abbott Japan Co., Ltd., Astellas Pharma Inc., Chugai Pharmaceutical Co., Ltd., Eisai Co., Ltd., Mitsubishi Tanabe Pharma Corporation, Merck Sharp and Dohme Inc., Pfizer Japan Inc., Takeda Pharmaceutical Company Limited, and Teijin Pharma Limited.

Institutional Review Board Statement: This study was reviewed and approved by the Research Ethics Committees of Tokyo Hospital (190010, 29 May 2019) and Sagamihara Hospital and the Central Institutional Review Board of the National Hospital Organization.

Informed Consent Statement: Written informed consent was obtained from all patients. This study was conducted in accordance with the principles expressed in the Declaration of Helsinki.

Data Availability Statement: The data that support the findings of this study are not publicly available due to privacy and ethical restrictions. The data are available from the corresponding author upon reasonable request.

Conflicts of Interest: HF has the following conflicts, and the following funders are supported wholly or in part by the indicated pharmaceutical companies. The Japan Research Foundation for Clinical Pharmacology is run by Daiichi Sankyo, the Takeda Science Foundation is supported by an endowment from Takeda Pharmaceutical Company and the Nakatomi Foundation was established by Hisamitsu Pharmaceutical Co., Inc. The Daiwa Securities Health Foundation was established by Daiwa Securities Group Inc. and Mitsui Sumitomo Insurance Welfare Foundation was established by Mitsui Sumitomo Insurance Co., Ltd. HF was supported by research grants from Bristol-Myers Squibb Co. HF received honoraria from Ajinomoto Co., Inc., Daiichi Sankyo Co., Ltd., Dainippon Sumitomo Pharma Co., Ltd., Pfizer Japan Inc., and Takeda Pharmaceutical Company, Luminex Japan Corporation Ltd., and Ayumi Pharmaceutical Corporation. ST was supported by research grants from nine pharmaceutical companies: Abbott Japan Co., Ltd., Astellas Pharma Inc., Chugai Pharmaceutical Co., Ltd., Eisai Co., Ltd., Mitsubishi Tanabe Pharma Corporation, Merck Sharp and Dohme Inc., Pfizer Japan Inc., Takeda Pharmaceutical Company Limited, and Teijin Pharma Limited. ST received honoraria from Asahi Kasei Pharma Corporation, Astellas Pharma Inc., AbbVie GK., Chugai Pharmaceutical Co., Ltd., Ono Pharmaceutical Co., Ltd., Mitsubishi Tanabe Pharma Corporation, and Pfizer Japan Inc. The other authors have no financial or commercial conflict of interest to declare.

References

1. Hakala, M. Poor prognosis in patients with rheumatoid arthritis hospitalized for interstitial lung fibrosis. *Chest* **1988**, *93*, 114–118. [CrossRef] [PubMed]
2. Turesson, C.; Jacobsson, L.T. Epidemiology of extra-articular manifestations in rheumatoid arthritis. *Scand. J. Rheumatol.* **2004**, *33*, 65–72. [CrossRef] [PubMed]
3. Koduri, G.; Norton, S.; Young, A.; Cox, N.; Davies, P.; Devlin, J.; Dixey, J.; Gough, A.; Prouse, P.; Winfield, J.; et al. Interstitial lung disease has a poor prognosis in rheumatoid arthritis: Results from an inception cohort. *Rheumatology* **2010**, *49*, 1483–1489. [CrossRef] [PubMed]

4. Vergnenegre, A.; Pugnere, N.; Antonini, M.T.; Arnaud, M.; Melloni, B.; Treves, R.; Bonnaud, F. Airway obstruction and rheumatoid arthritis. *Eur. Respir. J.* **1997**, *10*, 1072–1078. [CrossRef] [PubMed]
5. Swinson, D.R.; Symmons, D.; Suresh, U.; Jones, M.; Booth, J. Decreased survival in patients with co-existent rheumatoid arthritis and bronchiectasis. *Br. J. Rheumatol.* **1997**, *36*, 689–691. [CrossRef] [PubMed]
6. Kim, E.J.; Elicker, B.M.; Maldonado, F.; Webb, W.R.; Ryu, J.H.; Van Uden, J.H.; Lee, J.S.; King, T.E., Jr.; Collard, H.R. Usual interstitial pneumonia in rheumatoid arthritis-associated interstitial lung disease. *Eur. Respir. J.* **2010**, *35*, 1322–1328. [CrossRef]
7. Ohnishi, H.; Yokoyama, A.; Kondo, K.; Hamada, H.; Abe, M.; Nishimura, K.; Hiwada, K.; Kohno, N. Comparative study of KL-6, surfactant protein-A, surfactant protein-D, and monocyte chemoattractant protein-1 as serum markers for interstitial lung diseases. *Am. J. Respir. Crit. Care. Med.* **2002**, *165*, 378–381. [CrossRef] [PubMed]
8. Nakajima, H.; Harigai, M.; Hara, M.; Hakoda, M.; Tokuda, H.; Sakai, F.; Kamatani, N.; Kashiwazaki, S. KL-6 as a novel serum marker for interstitial pneumonia associated with collagen diseases. *J. Rheumatol.* **2000**, *27*, 1164–1170. [PubMed]
9. Oka, S.; Furukawa, H.; Shimada, K.; Sugii, S.; Hashimoto, A.; Komiya, A.; Fukui, N.; Suda, A.; Tsunoda, S.; Ito, S.; et al. Association of Human Leukocyte Antigen Alleles with Chronic Lung Diseases in Rheumatoid Arthritis. *Rheumatology* **2016**, *55*, 1301–1307. [CrossRef] [PubMed]
10. Oka, S.; Higuchi, T.; Furukawa, H.; Shimada, K.; Okamoto, A.; Hashimoto, A.; Komiya, A.; Saisho, K.; Yoshikawa, N.; Katayama, M.; et al. Serum rheumatoid factor IgA, anti-citrullinated peptide antibodies with secretory components, and anti-carbamylated protein antibodies associate with interstitial lung disease in rheumatoid arthritis. *BMC Musculoskelet Disord.* **2022**, *23*, 46. [CrossRef]
11. Aletaha, D.; Neogi, T.; Silman, A.J.; Funovits, J.; Felson, D.T.; Bingham, C.O., 3rd; Birnbaum, N.S.; Burmester, G.R.; Bykerk, V.P.; Cohen, M.D.; et al. 2010 Rheumatoid arthritis classification criteria: An American College of Rheumatology/European League Against Rheumatism collaborative initiative. *Arthritis Rheum* **2010**, *62*, 2569–2581. [CrossRef] [PubMed]
12. Mori, S.; Koga, Y.; Sugimoto, M. Different risk factors between interstitial lung disease and airway disease in rheumatoid arthritis. *Respir. Med.* **2012**, *106*, 1591–1599. [CrossRef] [PubMed]
13. Kakutani, T.; Hashimoto, A.; Tominaga, A.; Kodama, K.; Nogi, S.; Tsuno, H.; Ogihara, H.; Nunokawa, T.; Komiya, A.; Furukawa, H.; et al. Related factors, increased mortality and causes of death in patients with rheumatoid arthritis-associated interstitial lung disease. *Mod. Rheumatol.* **2020**, *30*, 458–464. [CrossRef] [PubMed]
14. Zhu, J.; Zhou, Y.; Chen, X.; Li, J. A metaanalysis of the increased risk of rheumatoid arthritis-related pulmonary disease as a result of serum anticitrullinated protein antibody positivity. *J. Rheumatol.* **2014**, *41*, 1282–1289. [CrossRef] [PubMed]
15. Joshua, V.; Hensvold, A.H.; Reynisdottir, G.; Hansson, M.; Cornillet, M.; Nogueira, L.; Serre, G.; Nyren, S.; Karimi, R.; Eklund, A.; et al. Association between number and type of different ACPA fine specificities with lung abnormalities in early, untreated rheumatoid arthritis. *RMD Open* **2020**, *6*, e001278. [CrossRef] [PubMed]
16. Ajeganova, S.; Humphreys, J.H.; Verheul, M.K.; van Steenbergen, H.W.; van Nies, J.A.; Hafström, I.; Svensson, B.; Huizinga, T.W.; Trouw, L.A.; Verstappen, S.M.; et al. Anticitrullinated protein antibodies and rheumatoid factor are associated with increased mortality with different causes of death in patients with rheumatoid arthritis: A longitudinal study in three European cohorts. *Ann. Rheum. Dis.* **2016**, *75*, 1924–1932. [CrossRef]
17. Doyle, T.J.; Patel, A.S.; Hatabu, H.; Nishino, M.; Wu, G.; Osorio, J.C.; Golzarri, M.F.; Traslosheros, A.; Chu, S.G.; Frits, M.L.; et al. Detection of Rheumatoid Arthritis-Interstitial Lung Disease Is Enhanced by Serum Biomarkers. *Am. J. Respir. Crit. Care Med.* **2015**, *191*, 1403–1412. [CrossRef]
18. Sato, S.; Hirakata, M.; Kuwana, M.; Suwa, A.; Inada, S.; Mimori, T.; Nishikawa, T.; Oddis, C.V.; Ikeda, Y. Autoantibodies to a 140-kd polypeptide, CADM-140, in Japanese patients with clinically amyopathic dermatomyositis. *Arthritis Rheum.* **2005**, *52*, 1571–1576. [CrossRef]
19. Sato, S.; Hoshino, K.; Satoh, T.; Fujita, T.; Kawakami, Y.; Kuwana, M. RNA helicase encoded by melanoma differentiation-associated gene 5 is a major autoantigen in patients with clinically amyopathic dermatomyositis: Association with rapidly progressive interstitial lung disease. *Arthritis Rheum.* **2009**, *60*, 2193–2200. [CrossRef]
20. Chen, Z.; Cao, M.; Plana, M.N.; Liang, J.; Cai, H.; Kuwana, M.; Sun, L. Utility of anti-melanoma differentiation-associated gene 5 antibody measurement in identifying patients with dermatomyositis and a high risk for developing rapidly progressive interstitial lung disease: A review of the literature and a meta-analysis. *Arthritis Care Res.* **2013**, *65*, 1316–1324. [CrossRef]
21. So, H.; Wong, V.T.L.; Lao, V.W.N.; Pang, H.T.; Yip, R.M.L. Rituximab for refractory rapidly progressive interstitial lung disease related to anti-MDA5 antibody-positive amyopathic dermatomyositis. *Clin. Rheumatol.* **2018**, *37*, 1983–1989. [CrossRef] [PubMed]
22. Wang, K.; Zhao, J.; Wu, W.; Xu, W.; Sun, S.; Chen, Z.; Fu, Y.; Guo, L.; Du, H.; Ye, S. RNA-Containing Immune Complexes Formed by Anti-Melanoma Differentiation Associated Gene 5 Autoantibody Are Potent Inducers of IFN-α. *Front. Immunol.* **2021**, *12*, 743704. [CrossRef] [PubMed]
23. Arnett, F.C.; Edworthy, S.M.; Bloch, D.A.; McShane, D.J.; Fries, J.F.; Cooper, N.S.; Healey, L.A.; Kaplan, S.R.; Liang, M.H.; Luthra, H.S.; et al. The American Rheumatism Association 1987 revised criteria for the classification of rheumatoid arthritis. *Arthritis Rheum.* **1988**, *31*, 315–324. [CrossRef] [PubMed]
24. Steinbrocker, O.; Traeger, C.H.; Batterman, R.C. Therapeutic criteria in rheumatoid arthritis. *J. Am. Med. Assoc.* **1949**, *140*, 659–662. [CrossRef] [PubMed]

25. Matsumoto, H.; Sato, S.; Fujita, Y.; Yashiro-Furuya, M.; Matsuoka, N.; Asano, T.; Kobayashi, H.; Watanabe, H.; Migita, K. Rheumatoid Arthritis Complicated with Anti-melanoma Differentiation-associated Gene 5 Antibody-positive Interstitial Pneumonia. *Intern. Med.* **2019**, *58*, 737–742. [CrossRef]
26. González-Moreno, J.; Raya-Cruz, M.; Losada-Lopez, I.; Cacheda, A.P.; Oliver, C.; Colom, B. Rapidly progressive interstitial lung disease due to anti-MDA5 antibodies without skin involvement: A case report and literature review. *Rheumatol. Int.* **2018**, *38*, 1293–1296. [CrossRef] [PubMed]
27. Koga, T.; Kaieda, S.; Okamoto, M.; Masuda, K.; Fujimoto, K.; Sakamoto, S.; Nakamura, M.; Tominaga, M.; Kawayama, T.; Hoshino, T.; et al. Successful Treatment of Rapidly Progressive Unclassifiable Idiopathic Interstitial Pneumonia with Anti-melanoma Differentiation-associated Gene-5 Antibody by Intensive Immunosuppressive Therapy. *Intern. Med* **2018**, *57*, 1039–1043. [CrossRef] [PubMed]
28. Kurasawa, K.; Arai, S.; Namiki, Y.; Tanaka, A.; Takamura, Y.; Owada, T.; Arima, M.; Maezawa, R. Tofacitinib for refractory interstitial lung diseases in anti-melanoma differentiation-associated 5 gene antibody-positive dermatomyositis. *Rheumatology* **2018**, *57*, 2114–2119. [CrossRef]
29. Nishioka, A.; Tsunoda, S.; Abe, T.; Yoshikawa, T.; Takata, M.; Kitano, M.; Matsui, K.; Nakashima, R.; Hosono, Y.; Ohmura, K.; et al. Serum neopterin as well as ferritin, soluble interleukin-2 receptor, KL-6 and anti-MDA5 antibody titer provide markers of the response to therapy in patients with interstitial lung disease complicating anti-MDA5 antibody-positive dermatomyositis. *Mod. Rheumatol.* **2019**, *29*, 814–820. [CrossRef]

Disclaimer/Publisher's Note: The statements, opinions and data contained in all publications are solely those of the individual author(s) and contributor(s) and not of MDPI and/or the editor(s). MDPI and/or the editor(s) disclaim responsibility for any injury to people or property resulting from any ideas, methods, instructions or products referred to in the content.

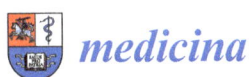

Article

Risk of Spine Surgery in Patients with Rheumatoid Arthritis: A Secondary Cohort Analysis of a Nationwide, Population-Based Health Claim Database

Chien-Han Chen [1], Chia-Wen Hsu [2] and Ming-Chi Lu [3,4,*]

[1] Division of Obstetrics and Gynecology, Dalin Tzu Chi Hospital, Buddhist Tzu Chi Medical Foundation, Dalin, Chiayi 62247, Taiwan; dm500307@tzuchi.com.tw
[2] Department of Medical Research, Dalin Tzu Chi Hospital, Buddhist Tzu Chi Medical Foundation, Dalin, Chiayi 62247, Taiwan; chiawen0114@yahoo.com.tw
[3] Division of Allergy, Immunology and Rheumatology, Dalin Tzu Chi Hospital, Buddhist Tzu Chi Medical Foundation, Dalin, Chiayi 62247, Taiwan
[4] School of Medicine, Tzu Chi University, Hualien City 97004, Taiwan
* Correspondence: dm252940@tzuchi.com.tw

Abstract: *Background and Objectives*: To study the risk of spine surgery, including cervical and lumbar spine surgeries in patients with rheumatoid arthritis (RA) compared with those without a diagnosis of RA. *Materials and Methods*: This is a secondary data analysis using population-based health claim data. We identified newly diagnosed adult patients with RA between January 2000 and December 2012, according to the International Classification of Diseases, Ninth revision, clinical modification code 714.0 from Taiwan's National Health Insurance Research Database. Using data frequency-matched by 10-year age intervals, sex and index year with the RA cohort at a ratio of 5:1, we assembled a comparison cohort. All patients were followed until the study outcomes occurred (overall spine surgery, cervical spine surgery, or lumbar spine surgery) or the end of follow-up. Adjusted incidence rate ratios (aIRR) were calculated using Poisson regression analysis with age group, socioeconomic status, geographical region, and osteoporosis included as potential confounders. *Results*: We identified 1287 patients with RA and 6435 patients without RA. The incidence of overall spine surgery (aIRR = 2.13, 95% confidence interval (CI) = 1.49–3.04) and lumbar spine surgery (aIRR = 2.14, 95% CI = 1.46–3.15) were all significantly higher in the RA cohort. Moreover, females over 45 years of age were particularly at risk for lumbar spine surgery. In RA patients, older age and the combination with the diagnosis of osteoporosis had an elevated risk for overall and lumbar spine surgery. *Conclusion:* Patients with RA had an increased risk of receiving spine surgery. Physicians should be vigilant for possible spinal problems in women and older patients with RA.

Keywords: rheumatoid arthritis; surgery; spine; lumbar vertebrae

Citation: Chen, C.-H.; Hsu, C.-W.; Lu, M.-C. Risk of Spine Surgery in Patients with Rheumatoid Arthritis: A Secondary Cohort Analysis of a Nationwide, Population-Based Health Claim Database. *Medicina* **2022**, *58*, 777. https://doi.org/10.3390/medicina58060777

Academic Editor: Daniela Opris-Belinski

Received: 17 May 2022
Accepted: 6 June 2022
Published: 8 June 2022

Publisher's Note: MDPI stays neutral with regard to jurisdictional claims in published maps and institutional affiliations.

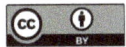

Copyright: © 2022 by the authors. Licensee MDPI, Basel, Switzerland. This article is an open access article distributed under the terms and conditions of the Creative Commons Attribution (CC BY) license (https://creativecommons.org/licenses/by/4.0/).

1. Introduction

Rheumatoid arthritis (RA) is a common systemic inflammatory autoimmune disease characterized by painful peripheral joints. The chronic inflammation can lead to joint destruction that can severely impair physical function in patients with RA. The worldwide prevalence of RA is 0.5–1.0% with a female-to-male ratio of approximately 2.5:1 [1]. The most common age of RA occurrence is 40–70 years old, and the incidence of RA increases with age [2]. The prevalence of RA in Taiwan was around 0.26–0.93% and patients with RA show a higher mortality rate compared with controls [3,4].

In addition to involving peripheral joints, RA could also affect the spine. Patients with RA can have some unique cervical spine disorders, including C1-2 instability, basilar invagination, and subaxial subluxation [5]. However, whether these cervical spine abnormalities would cause an increased risk of receiving cervical spine surgery in patients with RA is not clear. It should be noted that patients with RA had increased prevalence of spondylolisthesis and vertebral fracture compared with controls [6]. The increased rates of spondylolistheses might be attributed to the facet erosion and osteoporosis, and female patients with RA and those with elevated serum levels of C-reactive protein were at risk for developing lumbar spondylolisthesis [7,8]. Studies using magnetic resonance imaging (MRI) showed that lumbar endplate and facet erosion are common in patients with RA [9]. However, whether these conditions were associated with an elevated risk of receiving lumbar spine surgeries in patients with RA is still unknown. Therefore, the aim of this secondary cohort study was to investigate the risk of receiving overall spine surgery, cervical spine surgery, and lumbar spine surgery in patients with RA compared with those without RA using data from a nationwide health claim database.

2. Materials and Methods

2.1. Identification of the Rheumatoid Arthritis and Comparison Cohort

This is a secondary data analysis using population-based health claim data. The study protocol was reviewed and approved by the institutional review board of the Dalin Tzu Chi Hospital, Buddhist Tzu Chi Medical Foundation, Taiwan (No. B10004021, 21 December 2018). As the NHIRD files contain only deidentified secondary data, the requirement for obtaining informed consent from individual patients was waived. The source of our data is the claim data from the Taiwan's National Health Insurance Research Database (NHIRD).

The selection of patients in the RA cohort and the comparison cohort followed the protocol of our previous study, with some modifications [10]. Patients with newly diagnosed RA classified according to the International Classification of Diseases, ninth revision, clinical modification (ICD-9-CM) code 714.0 were identified from the 2000–2012 catastrophic illness datafile, which is a subset of the NHIRD. In Taiwan, to receive a waiver for medical co-payment, patients with RA can apply for a catastrophic illness certificate from the National Health Insurance Administration. The certification is issued to patients after their medical records, laboratory data, and imaging findings have been reviewed by at least two rheumatologists based on the American Rheumatism Association 1987 revised criteria [11]. In this study, the date of the application of the catastrophic illness certificate was defined as the index date for the RA.

A random sample of the outpatient datafile of the 2000 Longitudinal Health Insurance Database (LHID 2000) was used to assemble the comparison cohort. The LHID 2000 is a subfile of the NHIRD with health claim records between 1 January 2000 and 31 December 2012. Based on frequency matching for six 10-year age intervals, sex, and index year, five patients for each RA patient were selected.

Patients aged 20 to 80 years on the index date were included in the study. Patients who had been diagnosed with ankylosing spondylitis (ICD-9-CM code 720.0), or had received any spine surgery before the index data were excluded in both the RA and the comparison cohorts. Osteoporosis (ICD-9-CM code 733.0) was also included as a potential confounder in the regression analysis.

2.2. Identification of Cervical and Lumbar Spine Surgery

Patients in the RA and comparison cohorts were followed until the study outcomes had occurred or the end of follow-up period. Three study outcome variables were evaluated: overall spine surgery, cervical spine surgery, and lumbar spine surgery. Surgery codes were used to identify spine surgery from inpatient order datafiles. The codes included 64012B for costo-transversectomy; 64269B or 64270B for corrective osteotomy; 64144B or 64276B for curettage or excision of single or multiple vertebral body; 64160B for open reduction for fracture of spine; 64042C for close reduction for fracture of spine; 64279B for revisional diskectomy, cervical, thoracic, and lumbar; 64280B for revisional posterior spinal fusion with instrumentation, 83002C or 83003C for laminectomy; 83033C for laminoplasty; 83022C for cervical spine discectomy; 83024C for lumbar spine diskectomy; 83043B, 83044B, 83045B, 83046B, 83095B, 83096B, and 83097B for spine fusion;. Spine surgeries due to cancer (ICD-

9-CM codes 140–239) and infection (ICD-9-CM codes 001–139), osteomyelitis (ICD-9-CM code 730), and intraspinal abscess (ICD-9-CM code 324) were excluded.

As the location of the surgery for most spine surgeries, except discectomy, is not specified by procedure codes, spine surgeries were classified into those related to the cervical or lumbar vertebrae based on the following ICD-9-CM diagnostic and procedure codes: ICD-9-CM procedure code 81.01, 81.02 and 81.03 for cervical spinal fusion; 81.04, and 81.05 for lumbar fusion, and 81.06, 81.07 and 81.08 for lumbar and lumbosacral fusion. Only spine surgeries that occurred 90 days after the index date were included in our analyses. A 90-day interval was used to lower the possibility of including spine surgeries that were not related to RA.

2.3. Statistical Analysis

The basic characteristics of the patients in the RA cohort and the comparison cohort were compared with the chi-square test for categorical variables and the t-test for continuous variables, as appropriate. The patients' socioeconomic status was trichotomized into three groups based on their payroll-related insured amount, with cutoff points at TWD 19,000 and TWD 24,000 [12].

Incidence rate per 1000 person-years was calculated for the RA and the comparison cohorts, separately for each of the three outcome variables. Incidence rate ratios (IRR) and adjusted IRR with 95% confidence interval (CI) were calculated using generalized linear model with Poisson log-linear link function and person-years as the offset variable. Additional subgroup analyses were performed stratifying by sex or age groups (20–44, 45–59, and 60–80 years). All statistical analyses were conducted using IBM SPSS Statistics for Windows, version 24.0 (IBM Corp, Armonk, NY, USA). Two-tailed p values < 0.05 were considered statistically significant.

3. Results

The study flow chart is shown in Figure 1.

Table 1 shows the basic characteristics of the patients in the RA cohort and the comparison cohort. A total of 1287 patients with newly diagnosed RA and 6435 patients without RA were selected from the database. The overall mean age was 53.4 years, with a standard deviation of 13.4 years. There were no significant differences between the two groups in sex (78.8% were females, $p > 0.999$) and age intervals ($p > 0.999$). In addition, there were no significant differences between the two cohorts in the distribution of geographic region ($p = 0.455$), but socioeconomic status was significantly higher in the RA cohort ($p < 0.001$). The prevalence of osteoporosis was also significantly higher in the RA cohort ($p < 0.001$).

The IRRs and adjusted IRR (aIRR) of overall spine surgery, cervical spine surgery, and lumbar spine surgery for the RA cohort and the comparison cohort, stratified by sex are shown in Table 2. For overall spine surgery, patients with RA (aIRR = 2.13; 95% confidence interval (CI) 1.49–3.04) and female patients with RA (aIRR = 2.43; 95% CI 1.65–3.58), but not male patients with RA showed a significantly higher incidence compared with the comparison cohort.

In addition, we stratified the location of spine surgeries into cervical and lumbar spine surgery. The location of spine surgery was determined using both ICD-9-CM diagnostic codes and procedure codes. After excluding those surgeries related to cancer, infection, osteomyelitis, and intraspinal abscess, we identified 50 spine surgeries in patients with RA, and 7 were located in the cervical spine, 42 in the lumbar spine and 1 in the thoracic spine. In the comparison cohort, 99 spine surgeries were identified, including 16 cervical spine surgeries, 82 lumbar spine surgeries, and 1 thoracic spine surgery. Two patients were receiving concurrent cervical and lumbar spine surgeries during the same admission course. We found that there was no significantly increased risk of cervical spine surgeries in patients with RA, either male or female patients. For lumbar spine surgery, patients with RA (aIRR = 2.14; 95% CI 1.46–3.15) and female patients with RA (aIRR = 2.44; 95%

CI 1.61–3.69), but not male patients with RA, showed a significantly higher incidence compared with the comparison cohort.

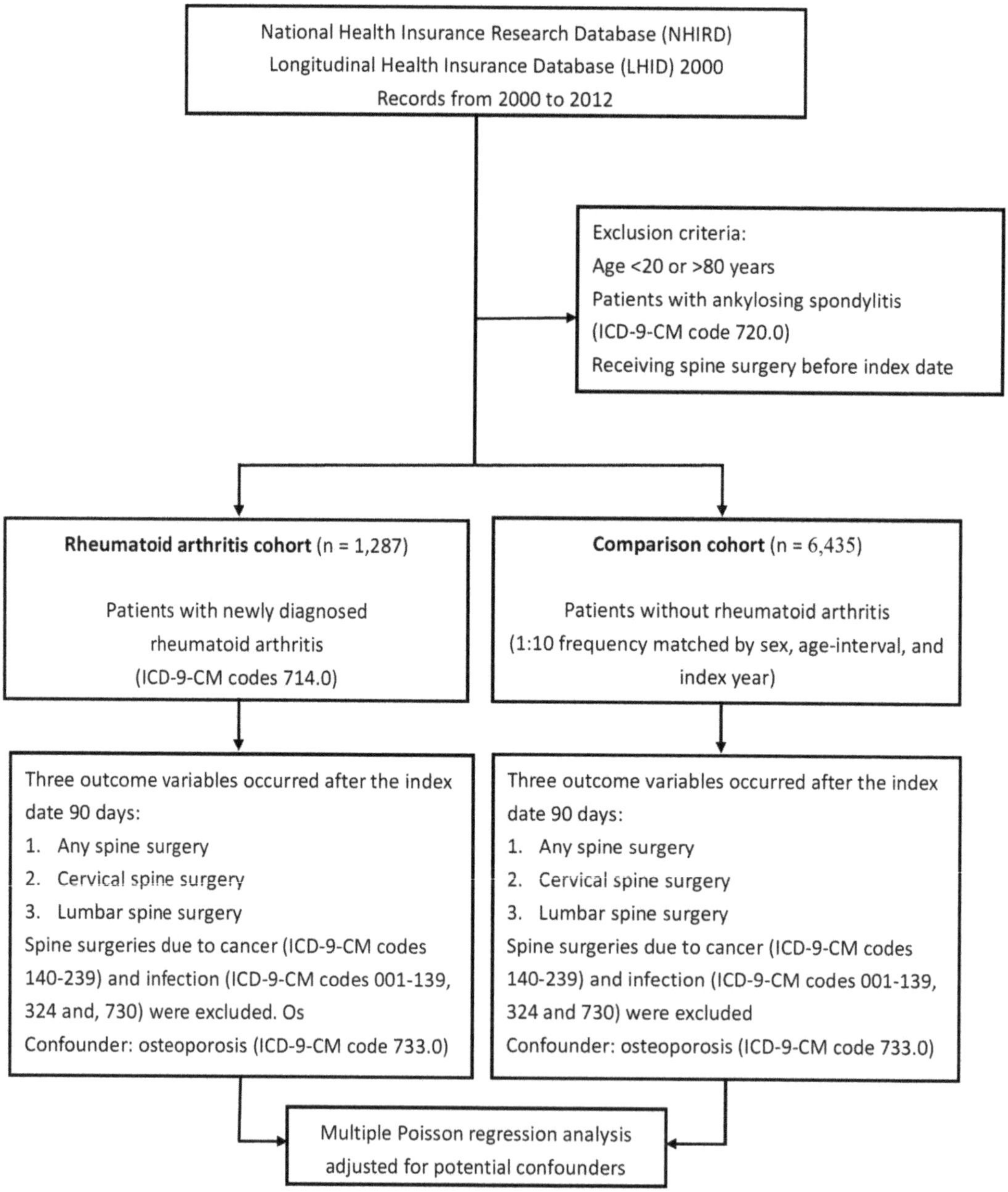

```
┌─────────────────────────────────────────────────┐
│   National Health Insurance Research Database (NHIRD)   │
│   Longitudinal Health Insurance Database (LHID) 2000    │
│              Records from 2000 to 2012                  │
└─────────────────────────────────────────────────┘
                        │
                        │      ┌──────────────────────────────────┐
                        │      │ Exclusion criteria:              │
                        ├─────▶│ Age <20 or >80 years             │
                        │      │ Patients with ankylosing spondylitis │
                        │      │ (ICD-9-CM code 720.0)            │
                        │      │ Receiving spine surgery before index date │
                        │      └──────────────────────────────────┘
            ┌───────────┴───────────┐
            ▼                       ▼
┌───────────────────────┐   ┌───────────────────────────┐
│ Rheumatoid arthritis  │   │ Comparison cohort (n = 6,435) │
│ cohort (n = 1,287)    │   │                           │
│                       │   │ Patients without rheumatoid arthritis │
│ Patients with newly   │   │ (1:10 frequency matched by sex, age-interval, and │
│ diagnosed rheumatoid  │   │ index year)               │
│ arthritis             │   │                           │
│ (ICD-9-CM codes 714.0)│   │                           │
└───────────────────────┘   └───────────────────────────┘
```

Figure 1. The flow chart for the study.

Three outcome variables occurred after the index date 90 days:
1. Any spine surgery
2. Cervical spine surgery
3. Lumbar spine surgery

Spine surgeries due to cancer (ICD-9-CM codes 140-239) and infection (ICD-9-CM codes 001-139, 324 and, 730) were excluded. Os Confounder: osteoporosis (ICD-9-CM code 733.0)

Three outcome variables occurred after the index date 90 days:
1. Any spine surgery
2. Cervical spine surgery
3. Lumbar spine surgery

Spine surgeries due to cancer (ICD-9-CM codes 140-239) and infection (ICD-9-CM codes 001-139, 324 and 730) were excluded Confounder: osteoporosis (ICD-9-CM code 733.0)

Multiple Poisson regression analysis adjusted for potential confounders

Table 1. Basic characteristics of the patients in the rheumatoid arthritis cohort and the comparison cohort (n = 7722).

Variable	n (%)				p
	RA Cohort 1287 (16.7)		Comparison Cohort 6435 (83.3)		
Sex					>0.999
male	273	(21.2)	1365	(21.2)	
female	1014	(78.8)	5070	(78.8)	
Age group (years)					>0.999
20.0–29.9	58	(4.5)	290	(4.5)	
30.0–39.9	141	(11.0)	705	(11.0)	
40.0–49.9	297	(23.1)	1485	(23.1)	
50.0–59.9	376	(29.2)	1880	(29.2)	
60.0–69.9	235	(18.3)	1175	(18.3)	
70.0–80.0	180	(14.0)	900	(14.0)	
Mean age (SD), years	53.4	(13.4)	53.4	(13.4)	0.959
Mean follow up duration (SD), years	6.04	(3.63)	5.71	(3.86)	0.004
Osteoporosis	132	(10.3)	218	(3.4)	<0.001
Socioeconomic status (n = 7701)					<0.001
low	595	(46.6)	3714	(57.8)	
middle	456	(35.7)	1800	(28.0)	
high	225	(17.7)	911	(14.2)	
Geographic region (n = 7462)					0.455
northern	723	(58.4)	3740	(60.1)	
central	226	(18.2)	1030	(16.6)	
southern	262	(21.1)	1328	(21.3)	
eastern	28	(2.3)	125	(2.0)	

Socioeconomic status was estimated by insurance premiums based on salary. Low: ≤19,000 New Taiwan dollars (TWD); middle: 19,001–24,000 TWD; and high: >24,000 TWD. IQR: interquartile range; RA: rheumatoid arthritis; SD: standard deviation. p values were obtained by the chi-square test for categorical variables and the t-test for continuous variables, as appropriate.

Table 2. The incidence rate and incidence risk ratio of spine surgery in the rheumatoid arthritis cohort and the comparison cohort (n = 7722).

Outcome Variable	RA Cohort (n = 1287)			Comparison Cohort (n = 6435)			IRR (95% CI) p	Adjusted IRR * (95% CI) p
	No. of Patient	Person-Years	IR	No. of Patient	Person-Years	IR		
Spine surgery								
total	50	7572	6.60	97	35,821	2.71	2.44 (1.73–3.43) <0.001	2.13 (1.49–3.04) <0.001
male	5	1531	3.27	23	7541	3.05	1.07 (0.41–2.82) 0.890	1.03 (0.38–2.81) 0.950
female	45	6041	7.45	74	28,280	2.62	2.85 (1.96–4.12) <0.001	2.43 (1.65–3.58) <0.001
Cervical								
total	7	7572	0.92	16	35,821	0.45	2.07 (0.85–5.03) 0.108	1.79 (0.68–4.71) 0.238
male	1	1531	0.65	7	7541	0.93	0.70 (0.09–5.72) 0.742	0.89 (0.11–7.44) 0.915
female	6	6041	0.99	9	28,280	0.32	3.12 (1.11–8.77) 0.031	2.27 (0.74–6.98) 0.153
Lumbar								
total	42	7572	5.55	82	35,821	2.29	2.42 (1.67–3.52) <0.001	2.14 (1.46–3.15) <0.001
male	4	1531	2.61	18	7541	2.39	1.10 (0.37–3.24) 0.870	0.99 (0.32–3.05) 0.989
female	38	6041	6.29	64	28,280	2.26	2.78 (1.86–4.15) <0.001	2.44 (1.61–3.69) <0.001

CI: confidence interval; IR: incidence rate per 1000 person-years; IRR: incidence rate ratio; RA: rheumatoid arthritis.
* Adjusted for age group, socioeconomic status, geographic region, and osteoporosis.

IRs and IRRs of overall spine surgery, cervical spine surgery, and lumbar spine surgery for the RA cohort and the comparison cohort, stratified by three age groups (20–44 years, 45–59 years, and 60–80 years) are shown in Table 3. In overall spine surgery, while the IRRs were significant for all three age groups, the magnitude was the largest in the youngest age group (aIRR = 5.73; 95% CI 1.55–21.21) in the RA cohort compared with the comparison cohort. For cervical spine surgery, the risk of was elevated in the youngest age group with marginal significance (aIRR = 8.98; 95% CI 0.84–96.26, p = 0.070). For lumbar spine surgery, the risk ratio was significantly elevated in the age group 45–59 years (aIRR = 2.32; 95% CI 1.30–4.13) and the 60–80 years (aIRR = 1.90, 95% CI 1.10–3.29).

Table 3. The incidence rate and incidence risk ratio of spine surgery in the RA cohort and the comparison cohort (n = 7722).

Outcome Variable	RA Cohort (n = 1287)			Comparison Cohort (n = 6435)			IRR (95% CI)	Adjusted IRR * (95% CI)
	No. of Patient	Person-Years	IR	No. of Patient	Person-Years	IR	p	p
Spine surgery								
Age group, years								
20–44.9	7	2050	3.41	4	9827	0.41	8.39 (2.46–28.66) 0.001	5.73 (1.55–21.21) 0.009
45–59.9	20	3362	5.95	43	15,938	2.70	2.20 (1.30–3.75) 0.003	2.22 (1.29–3.84) 0.004
60–80.0	23	2160	10.65	50	10,056	4.97	2.14 (1.31–3.51) 0.003	1.78 (1.06–2.98) 0.029
Cervical								
Age group, years								
20–44.9	4	2050	1.95	1	9827	0.10	19.17 (2.14–171.55) 0.008	8.98 (0.84–96.26) 0.070
45–59.9	2	3362	0.59	6	15,938	0.38	1.58 (0.32–7.83) 0.575	2.07 (0.40–10.70) 0.387
60–80.0	1	2160	0.46	9	10,056	0.89	0.52 (0.07–4.08) 0.532	0.50 (0.06–4.07) 0.516
Lumbar								
Age group, years								
20–44.9	3	2050	1.46	3	9827	0.31	4.79 (0.97–23.75) 0.055	4.58 (0.91–23.13) 0.066
45–59.9	18	3362	5.35	37	15,938	2.32	2.31 (1.31–4.05) 0.004	2.32 (1.30–4.13) 0.004
60–80.0	21	2160	9.72	42	10,056	4.18	2.33 (1.38–3.93) 0.002	1.90 (1.10–3.29) 0.022

CI: confidence interval; IR: incidence rate per 1000 person-years; IRR: incidence rate ratio. * Adjusted for sex, socioeconomic status, geographic region, and osteoporosis.

In Table 4, we analyzed the risks of overall spine surgery and lumbar spine surgery in patients with RA. In overall spine surgery, the IRRs were significantly elevated in age group 60–80 years (aIRR = 3.06; 95% CI 1.22–7.69) compared with age group 20–44 years and in those with the diagnosis of osteoporosis (aIRR = 3.06; 95% CI 1.22–7.69) compared with those without osteoporosis for patients with RA. In lumbar spine surgery, the IRRs were also significant elevated in age group 60–80 years (aIRR = 5.36; 95% CI 1.56–18.40) compared with age group 20–44 years and in those with the diagnosis of osteoporosis (aIRR = 2.80; 95% CI 1.46–5.36) compared with those without osteoporosis for patients with RA.

Table 4. The risk factors for spine surgery and lumbar spine surgery in the RA cohort (n = 1287).

Variable	Overall Spine Surgery aIRR * (95% CI)	p	Lumbar Spine Surgery aIRR * (95% CI)	p
Sex (female/male)				
male	Ref		Ref	
female	2.16 (0.85–5.51)	0.107	2.27 (0.80–6.45)	0.123
Age group (years)				
20–44.9	Ref		Ref	
45–59.9	1.85 (0.74–4.63)	0.192	3.23 (0.94–11.05)	0.062
60–80	3.06 (1.22–7.69)	0.018	5.36 (1.56–18.40)	0.008
Osteoporosis				
No	Ref		Ref	
Yes	2.34 (1.25–4.38)	0.008	2.80 (1.46–5.36)	0.002
Socioeconomic status				
low	Ref		Ref	
Middle and high	1.07 (0.60–1.91)	0.816	1.07 (0.57–2.00)	0.836
Geographic region				
northern	Ref		Ref	
central, southern, and eastern	1.13 (0.64–2.00)	0.678	0.97 (0.52–1.80)	0.916

CI: confidence interval; aIRR: adjusted incidence rate ratio; * Adjusted for sex, age group, osteoporosis, socioeconomic status, and geographic region.

4. Discussion

Our cohort study showed that patients with RA exhibited a significantly increased risk of receiving spine surgery, especially over the lumbar spine but not the cervical spine. It should be noted that only seven cases receiving cervical spine surgery over 1287 patients with RA and 16 over 6435 controls were identified. The number of cases might be too small to reach statistical significance. According to a meta-analysis using 12 studies, long RA duration was a risk factor for cervical spine involvement [13]. RA cervical spine involvement in patients with RA has been reported to occur generally after 10 years of disease duration [14]. However, the mean follow-up period was only 6.04 years (standard deviation 3.63 years) for our patients with RA. Therefore, a larger sample and a longer follow-up duration are needed to further clarify the risk of cervical spine surgery in patients with RA.

In this study, we found that the risk of receiving lumbar spine surgery was significantly elevated in patients with RA, especially in female patients older than 45 years. Lumbar spine problems may have been overlooked in patients with RA [15]. In fact, abnormal radiologic findings in the lumbar spine were detected in 57% of patients with RA [16]. Suzuki et al. showed that patients with RA were more likely to have spondylolisthesis, vertebral fracture, and scoliosis compared with controls [6]. Our study also demonstrated that patients with RA had a higher risk of receiving lumbar spine surgery, even with adjustment for osteoporosis. Patients with RA receiving spine surgery had a three-fold increase in complications, such as radiographic evidence of nonunion, implant failure, symptomatic adjacent segment disease, and infection [17]. Female and older patients are already prone to having degenerative lumbar spondylolisthesis [18]. The participation of inflammation caused by RA might further accelerate the process [9].

There are several limitations in this study. First, due to the constraints imposed by the NHIRD database, the disease activity of RA, imaging, and serology reports were not available for analysis. Second, the identification of spine surgery was based on the diagnosis and procedure codes from the ICD-9-CM, which limits further investigation of the detailed surgery types. Third, as there is universal health coverage in Taiwan with low financial barrier for accessing medical care, including surgeries, our findings may not be generalizable to other populations based on different medical care systems. Finally, in addition to age, there are multiple other risk factors for developing spondylolisthesis including genetic, occupation, daily activity, sport, obesity and sedentary work [19,20]. This information was not available from the NHIRD database.

5. Conclusions

Patients with RA had an increased risk of receiving spine surgery, especially in the lumbar spine. Female and older patients with RA were at higher risk. Physicians should be vigilant for possible spinal problems in women and older patients with RA.

Author Contributions: Conceptualization, C.-H.C., C.-W.H. and M.-C.L.; methodology, C.-H.C., and C.-W.H.; software, M.-C.L.; validation, C.-H.C., C.-W.H. and M.-C.L.; formal analysis, C.-W.H.; investigation, C.-H.C., C.-W.H. and M.-C.L.; resources, M.-C.L.; data curation, M.-C.L.; writing—original draft preparation, C.-H.C. and C.-W.H.; writing—review and editing, M.-C.L.; visualization, M.-C.L.; supervision, M.-C.L.; project administration, M.-C.L.; funding acquisition, M.-C.L. All authors have read and agreed to the published version of the manuscript.

Funding: This work was supported by grants from Buddhist Tzu Chi Medical Foundation, Taiwan (No: TCMF-A 108-05).

Institutional Review Board Statement: The study was conducted in accordance with the Declaration of Helsinki, and approved by the Institutional Review Board (or Ethics Committee) of the Dalin Tzu Chi Hospital, Buddhist Tzu Chi Medical Foundation, Taiwan (No. B10004021, 21 December 2018).

Informed Consent Statement: The NHIRD files contain deidentified secondary data, the need for informed consent from individual subjects was waived.

Data Availability Statement: Availability of data and material: The data that support the findings of this study are available on request from the corresponding author. The data are not publicly available due to the Taiwan Personal Information Protection Act.

Acknowledgments: This study is based in part on data from the National Health Insurance Research Database provided by the National Health Insurance Administration, Ministry of Health and Welfare and managed by the National Health Research Institutes, Taiwan. The interpretation and conclusions contained herein do not represent those of the National Health Insurance Administration, Ministry of Health and Welfare or the National Health Research Institutes, Taiwan.

Conflicts of Interest: The authors declare no conflict of interest.

References

1. Scott, D.L.; Wolfe, F.; Huizinga, T.W. Rheumatoid arthritis. *Lancet* **2010**, *376*, 1094–1108. [CrossRef]
2. Lee, D.M.; Weinblatt, M.E. Rheumatoid arthritis. *Lancet* **2001**, *358*, 903–911. [CrossRef]
3. Chou, C.T.; Pei, L.; Chang, D.M.; Lee, C.F.; Schumacher, H.R.; Liang, M.H. Prevalence of rheumatic diseases in Taiwan: A population study of urban, suburban, rural differences. *J. Rheumatol.* **1994**, *21*, 302–306. [PubMed]
4. Kuo, C.F.; Luo, S.F.; See, L.C.; Chou, I.J.; Chang, H.C.; Yu, K.H. Rheumatoid arthritis prevalence, incidence, and mortality rates: A nationwide population study in Taiwan. *Rheumatol. Int.* **2013**, *33*, 355–360. [CrossRef] [PubMed]
5. Kim, H.J.; Nemani, V.M.; Riew, K.D.; Brasington, R. Cervical spine disease in rheumatoid arthritis: Incidence, manifestations, and therapy. *Curr. Rheumatol. Rep.* **2015**, *17*, 9. [CrossRef] [PubMed]
6. Suzuki, A.; Tamai, K.; Takahashi, S.; Yamada, K.; Inui, K.; Tada, M.; Okano, T.; Sugioka, Y.; Koike, T.; Nakamura, H. Do rheumatoid arthritis patients have low back pain or radiological lumbar lesions more frequently than the healthy population?—Cross-sectional analysis in a cohort study with age and sex-matched healthy volunteers. *Spine J.* **2020**, *20*, 1995–2002. [CrossRef] [PubMed]
7. Hagege, B.; Tubach, F.; Alfaiate, T.; Forien, M.; Dieudé, P.; Ottaviani, S. Increased rate of lumbar spondylolisthesis in rheumatoid arthritis: A case-control study. *Eur. J. Clin. Investig.* **2018**, *48*, e12991. [CrossRef] [PubMed]
8. Sugimura, Y.; Miyakoshi, N.; Miyamoto, S.; Kasukawa, Y.; Hongo, M.; Shimada, Y. Prevalence of and factors associated with lumbar spondylolisthesis in patients with rheumatoid arthritis. *Mod. Rheumatol.* **2016**, *26*, 342–346. [CrossRef] [PubMed]
9. Yamada, K.; Suzuki, A.; Takahashi, S.; Yasuda, H.; Tada, M.; Sugioka, Y.; Okano, T.; Koike, T.; Nakamura, H. MRI evaluation of lumbar endplate and facet erosion in rheumatoid arthritis. *J. Spinal Disord. Tech.* **2014**, *27*, E128–E135. [CrossRef] [PubMed]
10. Lu, M.C.; Koo, M.; Lai, N.S. Incident spine surgery in patients with ankylosing spondylitis: A secondary cohort analysis of a nationwide, population-based health claims database. *Arthritis Care Res.* **2018**, *70*, 1416–1420. [CrossRef] [PubMed]
11. Arnett, F.C.; Edworthy, S.M.; Bloch, D.A.; McShane, D.J.; Fries, J.F.; Cooper, N.S.; Healey, L.A.; Kaplan, S.R.; Liang, M.H.; Luthra, H.S.; et al. The American Rheumatism Association 1987 revised criteria for the classification of rheumatoid arthritis. *Arthritis Rheum.* **1988**, *31*, 315–324. [CrossRef] [PubMed]

12. Lu, M.C.; Hsu, B.B.; Koo, M.; Lai, N.S. Higher risk of incident ankylosing spondylitis in patients with uveitis: A secondary cohort analysis of a nationwide, population-based health claims database. *Scand. J. Rheumatol.* **2017**, *46*, 468–473. [CrossRef] [PubMed]
13. Zhu, S.; Xu, W.; Luo, Y.; Zhao, Y.; Liu, Y. Cervical spine involvement risk factors in rheumatoid arthritis: A meta-analysis. *Int. J. Rheum. Dis.* **2017**, *20*, 541–549. [CrossRef] [PubMed]
14. Del Grande, M.; Del Grande, F.; Carrino, J.; Bingham, C.O., III; Louie, G.H. Cervical spine involvement early in the course of rheumatoid arthritis. *Semin. Arthritis Rheum.* **2014**, *43*, 738–744. [CrossRef] [PubMed]
15. Joo, P.; Ge, L.; Mesfin, A. Surgical management of the lumbar spine in rheumatoid arthritis. *Global Spine J.* **2020**, *10*, 767–774. [CrossRef] [PubMed]
16. Kawaguchi, Y.; Matsuno, H.; Kanamori, M.; Ishihara, H.; Ohmori, K.; Kimura, T. Radiologic findings of the lumbar spine in patients with rheumatoid arthritis, and a review of pathologic mechanisms. *J. Spinal Disord. Tech.* **2003**, *16*, 38–43. [CrossRef] [PubMed]
17. Kang, C.N.; Kim, C.W.; Moon, J.K. The outcomes of instrumented posterolateral lumbar fusion in patients with rheumatoid arthritis. *Bone Joint J.* **2016**, *98*, 102–108. [CrossRef] [PubMed]
18. Jacobsen, S.; Sonne-Holm, S.; Rovsing, H.; Monrad, H.; Gebuhr, P. Degenerative lumbar spondylolisthesis: An epidemiological perspective: The Copenhagen Osteoarthritis Study. *Spine* **2007**, *32*, 120–125. [CrossRef] [PubMed]
19. Akkawi, I.; Zmerly, H. Degenerative Spondylolisthesis: A Narrative Review. *Acta Biomed.* **2022**, *92*, e2021313. [PubMed]
20. Jiang, H.; Yang, Q.; Jiang, J.; Zhan, X.; Xiao, Z. Association between COL11A1 (rs1337185) and ADAMTS5 (rs162509) gene polymorphisms and lumbar spine pathologies in Chinese Han population: An observational study. *BMJ Open* **2017**, *7*, e015644. [CrossRef] [PubMed]

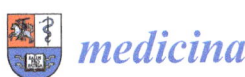

Review

Increased Risk of Common Orthopedic Surgeries for Patients with Rheumatic Diseases in Taiwan

Min-Chih Hsieh [1], Malcolm Koo [2,3], Chia-Wen Hsu [4] and Ming-Chi Lu [5,6,*]

[1] Division of Obstetrics and Gynecology, Dalin Tzu Chi Hospital, Buddhist Tzu Chi Medical Foundation, Dalin, Chiayi 622401, Taiwan
[2] Graduate Institute of Long-term Care, Tzu Chi University of Science and Technology, Hualien City 970302, Taiwan
[3] Dalla Lana School of Public Health, University of Toronto, Toronto, ON M5T 3M7, Canada
[4] Department of Medical Research, Dalin Tzu Chi Hospital, Buddhist Tzu Chi Medical Foundation, Dalin, Chiayi 622401, Taiwan
[5] Division of Allergy, Immunology and Rheumatology, Dalin Tzu Chi Hospital, Buddhist Tzu Chi Medical Foundation, Dalin, Chiayi 622401, Taiwan
[6] School of Medicine, Tzu Chi University, Hualien City 970374, Taiwan
* Correspondence: e360187@yahoo.com.tw

Abstract: *Background and Objectives:* Rheumatic diseases, including rheumatoid arthritis, ankylosing spondylitis, psoriasis, and systemic lupus erythematosus (SLE), are characterized by chronic arthritis or spondyloarthritis, which can lead to joint and spine destruction. Our previous studies showed that the risk of common orthopedic surgeries, including total knee replacement (TKR), total hip replacement (THR), or spine surgery, was increased in patients with rheumatoid arthritis, ankylosing spondylitis, psoriasis, and SLE. The aim of this review was to summarize the risk of TKR, THR, cervical spine, and lumbar spine surgery on the basis of studies conducted using data from Taiwan's National Health Insurance Research Database (NHIRD). *Materials and Methods:* The risk of TKR, THR, cervical spine surgery, and lumbar spine surgery in patients with rheumatoid arthritis, ankylosing spondylitis, psoriasis, and SLE was summarized from the results of our previous studies and unpublished findings based on NHIRD data. *Results:* Patients with rheumatoid arthritis and psoriasis and men with ankylosing spondylitis showed an increased risk of TKR. Patients with rheumatoid arthritis, ankylosing spondylitis, and women with SLE showed an increased risk of receiving THR. Only patients with ankylosing spondylitis had an increased risk of cervical spine surgery, and patients with rheumatoid arthritis or ankylosing spondylitis showed an increased risk of lumbar spine surgery. Although the risk of THR, TKR, or spine surgery in these patients has declined in the era of biologics use, direct evidence for the effects of biologics agents is not yet available. *Conclusions:* There was an increased risk of common orthopedic surgery in patients with rheumatoid arthritis, ankylosing spondylitis, psoriasis, and SLE. Clinicians should be vigilant to reduce the increased risk of TKR and THR in young and middle-aged patients with rheumatoid arthritis, THR in young patients with ankylosing spondylitis, and young female patients with SLE, as well as cervical spine surgery in young patients with ankylosing spondylitis.

Keywords: rheumatoid arthritis; systemic lupus erythematosus; ankylosing spondylitis; psoriasis; total knee replacement; total hip replacement; spine surgery

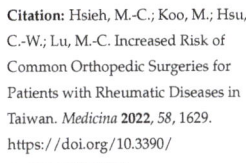

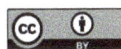

1. Introduction

Rheumatic diseases are a group of diseases characterized by chronic joint inflammation, leading to the destruction of the joints and spine. Rheumatic diseases are the major cause of disability worldwide, and the burden of rheumatic diseases is increasing [1]. Rheumatoid arthritis, ankylosing spondylitis, psoriasis, and systemic lupus erythematosus (SLE) are common rheumatic diseases that cause active arthritis and can lead to joint deformity.

Rheumatoid arthritis is a common systemic autoimmune disease characterized by chronic inflammation of the peripheral joints. Chronic inflammation in the peripheral joints can lead to joint destruction that results in discomfort and disability. In addition to the peripheral joints, rheumatoid arthritis can involve large joints, including the knee, hip, and cervical [2,3] or lumbar spine [4,5]. The prevalence of rheumatoid arthritis ranges from 0.5 to 1.0% around the world, with a female-to-male ratio of 2.5:1. Rheumatoid arthritis commonly occurs in people aged 40–70 years, with the incidence increasing with age [6]. The prevalence of rheumatoid arthritis in Taiwan was found to range from 0.26% to 0.93% [7], and patients with rheumatoid arthritis were associated with a higher mortality rate compared with controls [8].

Ankylosing spondylitis belongs to the spondyloarthritis family and is characterized by a bony fusion of the vertebral joints. The prevalence of ankylosing spondylitis ranged from 0.19% to 0.54% in Taiwan (7), with a male-to-female ratio of 2:1 [9]. Because of long-standing inflammation of the spine, patients with ankylosing spondylitis often develop spinal deformities that lead to spine instability and neurological deficits. Ankylosing spondylitis can also affect peripheral large joints, including knees and hips [10].

Psoriasis is a common chronic, immune-mediated skin disease presented as erythematous, thick, and scaly areas of the skin [11]. The prevalence of psoriasis was estimated to vary from 0.16% to 0.23% in Taiwan [12]. Around 20%–30% of patients with psoriasis could develop psoriatic arthritis [13], which can cause joint damage leading to deformity and may require surgery to alleviate pain and restore function [14]. However, a study based on the Taiwan National Health Insurance Research Database (NHIRD) showed that 8.2% of patients with psoriasis had psoriatic arthritis [15], and therefore, increased effort should be made to improve the diagnosis of psoriatic arthritis. Psoriatic arthritis can affect the spine, causing inflammatory neck and back pain, eventually leading to reduced spinal mobility [16].

SLE is a prototype of the systemic autoimmune disease, and it predominately affects women during their childbearing age [17]. The prevalence of SLE was 14.3 per 10,000 people in the female population in 2011 in Taiwan [18]. SLE typically involves the joints, skin, kidneys, lungs, nerve systems, and hematological systems. Patients with SLE showed increased morbidity and mortality. In the past, joint involvement in SLE was considered mild and only caused pain in the peripheral joints. However, current evidence shows that patients with SLE can have active, erosive arthritis, which leads to the deformity of joints [19,20]. Mertelsmann-Voss et al. reported that patients with SLE had an increased risk of receiving arthroplasty on the hip and knee joints in the United States [21].

2. Common Orthopedic Surgeries

Both total knee replacement (TKR) and total hip replacement (THR) are common orthopedic surgery for severe joint destruction from osteoarthritis, rheumatic diseases, or osteonecrosis, and their rates are increasing around the world [22,23]. In Taiwan, the rate of primary TKR was 28.5 per 100,000 people in 1998 and has increased to 56.8 per 100,000 people in 2009. The rate of primary THR was 17.5 per 100,000 people in 1998 and increased to 19.5 per 100,000 people in 2009 [24]. In addition, there was a high prevalence of spinal surgeries in Taiwan, and the common spine surgeries were discectomy, laminectomy, spinal fusion, and spinal fracture reduction [25,26]. Since rheumatic diseases are characterized by active inflammation of the joints or the spine, it is expected that patients with these rheumatic diseases might show an increased risk of receiving a joint replacement or spinal surgery. Our research group had previously published several articles on the risk of THR and TKR in patients with ankylosing spondylitis, psoriasis, and SLE [27–29] and the risk of spinal surgery in patients with rheumatoid arthritis and ankylosing spondylitis [30,31].

The aim of this review was to summarize our previous study results on the risks of TKR, THR, and cervical spine and lumbar surgery. All our studies were based on data from the NHIRD in Taiwan. We also included the results of unpublished data exploring the risk of spinal surgery in patients with SLE and psoriasis. Because the risk of spinal surgery did not differ in patients with SLE or psoriasis compared with the controls, the results of these analyses were not previously published. Although Lee et al. reported that patients with rheumatoid arthritis were 4.82 times more likely to receive THR (95% confidence interval [CI] 3.84–6.04) and 3.85 times more likely to undergo TKR (95% CI 3.48–4.25) compared with controls, risks of TKR and THR in patients with RA stratified by age or sex were unavailable in their report [32]. Therefore, in the present study, our own unpublished data were presented instead of those from Lee et al. for these risk estimates. As patients with SLE are predominantly female, only women were included in the analysis of SLE.

3. Risk of Total Knee Replacement in Patients with Rheumatic Diseases

Among patients with rheumatic diseases, the risk of overall TKR was highest in patients with rheumatoid arthritis (adjusted incidence rate ratio (aIRR) = 3.77; 95% confidence interval [CI] 2.82–5.04), followed by patients with psoriasis (aIRR = 1.38; 95% CI 1.09–1.75), but the risk of TKR was not significantly elevated in patients with ankylosing spondylitis or female patients with SLE (Table 1).

Table 1. A summary of the incidence rate ratio, 95% confidence interval, and p value of total knee replacement surgery in patients with rheumatoid arthritis, ankylosing spondylitis, psoriasis, and systemic lupus erythematosus.

	Rheumatoid Arthritis (n = 1557)	Ankylosing Spondylitis [28] (n = 3462)	Psoriasis [27] (n = 10,819)	Systemic Lupus Erythematosus [29] * (n = 557)
Overall	3.77 (2.82–5.04) <0.001	1.10 (0.78–1.54) 0.591	1.38 (1.09–1.75) 0.007	NA
Male	3.27 (1.53–7.02) 0.002	1.89 (1.04–3.41) 0.036	1.29 (0.87–1.92) 0.209	NA
Female	3.93 (2.87–5.39) <0.001	0.88 (0.59–1.34) 0.554	1.44 (1.08–1.93) 0.014	1.81 (0.69–4.75) 0.227
Age effect (only the significant age interval was shown)	20–44 years 74.18 (9.80–561.38) <0.001 45–59 years 6.86 (4.20–11.20) <0.001 60–80 years 1.68 (1.08–2.62) 0.02	NS	60–80 years 1.31 (1.00–1.71) 0.047	NS

Data were presented as an incidence rate ratio (IRR) and 95% confidence interval (CI), and p value; NA—not available; NS—no statistically significant association; * For systemic lupus erythematosus, only female patients were analyzed.

When stratified by sex, we found that both male (aIRR = 3.27; 95% CI 1.53–7.02) and female (aIRR = 3.93; 95% CI 2.87–5.39) patients with rheumatoid arthritis showed an elevated risk of receiving TKR. Only male patients showed an elevated risk of TKR (aIRR = 1.89; 95% CI 1.04–3.41), and female patients with psoriasis showed an elevated risk of TKR (aIRR = 1.44; 95% CI 1.08–1.93).

As for the effect of age, all age groups showed an increased risk of TKR in patients with rheumatoid arthritis. It is an unexpected finding that young patients with rheumatoid arthritis (20–44 years) showed a very high risk of receiving TKR (aIRR = 74.18; 95% CI 9.80–561.38). In psoriasis, the older age group (60–80 years) showed a significantly elevated risk (aIRR = 1.31; 95% CI 1.00–1.71) of receiving TKR.

Currently, the use of biologics along with early, aggressive treatment strategies has allowed patients with rheumatoid arthritis to better control their disease activities. The risk of receiving TKR and THR in patients with rheumatoid arthritis has decreased after the start of the era of biologics agents in Japan and Canada [33,34]. Finally, in patients with ankylosing spondylitis or SLE, the risk of TKR was not elevated when stratified by age group.

4. Risk of Total Hip Replacement in Patients with Rheumatic Diseases

The risk of THR was the highest in female patients with SLE (aIRR = 6.47; 95% CI 2.43–17.22), followed by patients with ankylosing spondylitis (aIRR = 5.91; 95% CI 3.39–10.30), and patients with rheumatoid arthritis (aIRR = 3.30; 95% CI 1.95–5.60) (Table 2). The risk of receiving THR did not increase in patients with psoriasis.

Table 2. A summary of the incidence rate ratio, 95% confidence interval, and p value of total hip replacement surgery in patients with rheumatoid arthritis, ankylosing spondylitis, psoriasis, and systemic lupus erythematosus.

	Rheumatoid Arthritis (n = 1287)	Ankylosing Spondylitis [28] (n = 3462)	Psoriasis [27] (n = 10,819)	Systemic Lupus Erythematosus [29] * (n = 557)
Overall	3.30 (1.95–5.60) <0.001	5.91 (3.39–10.30) <0.001	1.27 (0.88–1.84) 0.204	NA
Male	4.35 (1.69–11.23) 0.002	12.59 (5.54–28.58) <0.001	1.40 (0.90–2.19) 0.137	NA
Female	2.86 (1.50–30.18) 0.001	2.34 (0.95–5.73) 0.064	1.09 (0.55–2.19) 0.803	6.47 (2.43–17.22) <0.001
Age effect (only showed the significant age interval)	20–44 years 6.96 (1.61–30.18) 0.010 45–59 years 7.00 (2.78–17.62) <0.001	20–39 years 27.66 (6.13–124.81) <0.001 40–80 years 3.84 (2.00–7.36) <0.001	NS	20–44 years 7.70 (2.19–27.12) 0.001

Data were presented as an incidence rate ratio (IRR) and 95% confidence interval (CI), and p value; NA—not available; NS—no statistically significant association; * For systemic lupus erythematosus, only female patients were analyzed.

When stratified by sex, both male (aIRR = 4.35; 95% CI 1.69–11.23) and female (aIRR = 2.86; 95% CI 1.50–30.18) patients with rheumatoid arthritis showed an increased risk of receiving THR. In patients with ankylosing spondylitis, only male patients showed an increased risk of receiving THR.

As for the effect of age, both the young (aIRR = 6.96; 95% CI 1.61–30.18) and middle age (aIRR = 7.00; 95% CI 2.78–17.62) group patients with rheumatoid arthritis showed an elevated risk of receiving THR. In patients with ankylosing spondylitis, both the younger and older age groups showed an elevated risk of receiving THR, and the risk of THR in the young age group (20–39 years) was very high (aIRR = 27.66; 95% CI 6.13–124.81). In SLE, the younger age group (20–44 years) also showed an increased risk of THR (aIRR = 7.70; 95% CI 2.19–27.12), and the main cause of THR was osteonecrosis. The main reason for osteonecrosis in patients with SLE was high-dose steroid usage. Therefore, rheumatologists should be vigilant regarding the use of steroids for SLE treatment.

In the era of biologics use, the risk of THR has begun to decrease in patients with rheumatoid arthritis [33,34]. For patients with ankylosing spondylitis, the need for THR has also changed [35] and decreased in those under 60 years of age [36]. However, Stovall et al. indicated that the risk of THR/TKR was not reduced with any combinations of NSAIDs, DMARDs, or tumor necrosis factor inhibitor (TNFi) in people with ankylosing spondylitis or psoriatic arthritis [37]. In patients with rheumatoid arthritis, the usage of TNFi was only associated with a reduction in risk for THR in those over 60 years old [38]. Therefore, there are still debates over the main cause of the decreased risk of THR/TKR in recent years.

5. Risk of Cervical Spine Surgery in Patients with Rheumatic Diseases

The risk of cervical spine surgery was only increased in patients with ankylosing spondylitis (aIRR = 2.36; 95% CI 1.55–3.59) (Table 3). When stratified by sex and age, only male (aIRR = 2.92; 95% CI 1.68–5.08) patients with ankylosing spondylitis showed an increased risk of receiving cervical spine surgery. Both the younger age group (aIRR = 5.75; 95% CI 2.08–15.86) and the middle age group (aIRR = 2.91; 95% CI 1.63–5.20) showed an increased risk of receiving cervical spine surgery in patients with ankylosing spondylitis. Although patients with rheumatoid arthritis are known to have cervical spine involvement, we did not find an increased risk of receiving cervical spine surgery in our cohort. A reason for this could be that the relative mean follow-up period was too short (only 6.0 years) in our patients with rheumatoid arthritis [39,40].

Table 3. A summary of the incidence rate ratio, 95% confidence interval, and p value of cervical spine surgery in patients with rheumatoid arthritis, ankylosing spondylitis, psoriasis, and systemic lupus erythematosus.

	Rheumatoid Arthritis [31] (n = 1287)	Ankylosing Spondylitis [30] (n = 3462)	Psoriasis (n = 10,677)	Systemic Lupus Erythematosus * (n = 471)
Overall	1.79 (0.68–4.71) 0.238	2.36 (1.55–3.59) <0.001	1.10 (0.74–1.65) 0.638	NA
Male	0.89 (0.11–7.44) 0.915	2.92 (1.68–5.08) <0.001	1.14 (0.71–1.84) 0.590	NA
Female	2.27 (0.74–6.98) 0.153	1.78 (0.92–3.44) 0.087	1.01 (0.47–2.16) 0.991	1.55 (0.31–7.78) 0.596
Age effect (only showed the significant age interval)	NS	20–39 years 5.75 (2.08–15.86) 0.001 40–59 years 2.91 (1.63–5.20) <0.001	NS	NS

Data were presented as an incidence rate ratio (IRR) and 95% confidence interval (CI), and p value; NA—not available; NS—no statistically significant association; * For systemic lupus erythematosus, only female patients were analyzed.

6. Risk of Lumbar Spine Surgery in Patients with Rheumatic Diseases

Both the patients with rheumatoid arthritis (aIRR = 2.14; 95% CI 1.46–3.15) and ankylosing spondylitis (aIRR = 2.33; 95% CI 1.85–2.93) showed an increased risk of lumbar spine surgery (Table 4). When stratified by sex, only female (aIRR = 2.44; 95% CI 1.61–3.69) patients with rheumatoid arthritis showed an increased risk of receiving lumbar spine surgery. Both male (aIRR = 2.13; 95% CI 1.53–2.96) and female (aIRR = 2.53; 95% CI 1.84–3.49) patients with ankylosing spondylitis showed an increased risk of receiving lumbar spine surgery.

When stratified by age, patients with rheumatoid arthritis in the middle (45–59 years) (aIRR = 2.32 95% CI 1.30–4.13) and old age group (59–80) (aIRR = 1.90; 95% CI 1.10–3.29) showed a higher risk of receiving lumbar spine surgery. On the other hand, in patients with ankylosing spondylitis, all three age groups showed an increased risk of receiving lumbar spine surgery (20–39 years: aIRR = 3.14; 95% CI 1.91–5.18; 40–59 years: aIRR = 2.43; 95% CI 1.72–3.43); 60–80 years: aIRR = 1.75; 95% CI 1.18–2.59). Generally, male patients with ankylosing spondylitis have more severe radiographic changes in the spine [41]. However, our study also showed an increased risk of lumbar spine surgery in female patients with ankylosing spondylitis. Therefore, clinicians should also be vigilant for the possibility of lumbar spine disorder in female patients with ankylosing spondylitis. The cause of increased risk for spinal surgery in patients with ankylosing spondylitis might be related to the disease manifestation itself.

Table 4. A summary of the incidence rate ratio, 95% confidence interval, and p value of lumbar spine surgery in patients with rheumatoid arthritis, ankylosing spondylitis, psoriasis, and systemic lupus erythematosus.

	Rheumatoid Rthritis [31] (n = 1287)	Ankylosing Spondylitis [30] (n = 3462)	Psoriasis (n = 10,677)	Systemic Lupus Erythematosus * (n = 471)
Overall	2.14 (1.46–3.15) <0.001	2.33 (1.85–2.93) <0.001	1.09 (0.89–1.34) 0.393	NA
Male	0.99 (0.32–3.05) 0.989	2.13 (1.53–2.96) <0.001	1.05 (0.80–1.38) 0.710	NA
Female	2.44 (1.61–3.69) <0.001	2.53 (1.84–3.49) <0.001	1.16 (0.85–1.58) 0.351	0.27 (0.04–1.99) 0.197
Age effect (only showed the significant age interval)	45–59 years 2.32 (1.30–4.13) 0.004 59–80 years 1.90 (1.10–3.29) 0.022	20–39 years 3.14 (1.91–5.18) <0.001 40–59 years 2.43 (1.72–3.43) <0.001 60–80 years 1.75 (1.18–2.59) 0.005	NS	NS

Data were presented as IRR (95% CI) and p value; NA—not available; NS—no statistically significant association; * In patients with SLE, we only included female patients.

7. Summary

The risk of receiving TKR was increased in patients with rheumatoid arthritis, psoriasis, and male patients with ankylosing spondylitis. On the other hand, the risk of receiving THR was increased in patients with rheumatoid arthritis, ankylosing spondylitis, and women with SLE. Patients with ankylosing spondylitis also showed a higher risk of cervical and lumbar spine surgery because of the nature of the disease itself. Moreover, patients with rheumatoid arthritis showed an increased risk of receiving lumbar spine surgery. Recent studies suggested that the trend for orthopedic surgery has declined in TKR and THR in rheumatoid arthritis, as well as in THR among patients with ankylosing spondylitis. The use of biologics for treating rheumatic diseases has been considered a key factor in reducing the risk of orthopedic surgery. However, direct evidence is still lacking. Physicians should be aware of the possibility of the knee, hip, and spinal destruction in patients with rheumatic diseases. Action should be taken to reduce the increased risk of receiving TKR in young patients with rheumatoid arthritis, receiving THR in patients with ankylosing spondylitis and female patients with SLE, and receiving cervical spine surgery in young patients with ankylosing spondylitis.

Author Contributions: Conceptualization, M.-C.H., C.-W.H., M.K. and M.-C.L.; methodology, M.K., M.-C.H. and C.-W.H.; software, M.K., M.-C.H. and C.-W.H.; validation, M.-C.H., C.-W.H. and M.-C.L.; formal analysis, C.-W.H.; investigation, M.-C.H., C.-W.H. and M.-C.L.; resources, M.-C.L.; data curation, M.-C.L.; writing—original draft preparation, M.-C.H. and C.-W.H.; writing—review and editing, M.K. and M.-C.L.; visualization, M.-C.L.; supervision, M.K. and M.-C.L.; project administration, M.-C.L.; funding acquisition, M.-C.L. All authors have read and agreed to the published version of the manuscript.

Funding: This work was supported by grants from Buddhist Tzu Chi Medical Foundation, Taiwan (No: TCMF-A 108-05).

Institutional Review Board Statement: Not applicable.

Informed Consent Statement: Not applicable.

Data Availability Statement: Not applicable.

Conflicts of Interest: The authors declare no conflict of interest.

References

1. Sebbag, E.; Felten, R.; Sagez, F.; Sibilia, J.; Devilliers, H.; Arnaud, L. The world-wide burden of musculoskeletal diseases: A systematic analysis of the World Health Organization Burden of Diseases Database. *Ann. Rheum. Dis.* **2019**, *78*, 844–848. [CrossRef]
2. Rubbert-Roth, A.; Jacobs, J.W.G.; Bijlsma, J.W.J.; Welsing, P.M.J. A disconnect between disease activity and functional ability already in patients with early rheumatoid arthritis, depending on large joint involvement. *Ann. Rheum. Dis.* **2018**, *77*, 1085–1086. [CrossRef]
3. Tago, M.; Sawada, T.; Nishiyama, S.; Tahara, K.; Kato, E.; Hayashi, H.; Mori, H.; Nishino, J.; Matsui, T.; Tohma, S. Influence of large joint involvement on patient-physician discordance in global assessment of rheumatoid arthritis disease activity analyzed by a novel joint index. *Int. J. Rheum. Dis.* **2018**, *21*, 1237–1245. [CrossRef]
4. Hagege, B.; Tubach, F.; Alfaiate, T.; Forien, M.; Dieudé, P.; Ottaviani, S. Increased rate of lumbar spondylolisthesis in rheumatoid arthritis: A case-control study. *Eur. J. Clin. Investig.* **2018**, *48*, e12991. [CrossRef]
5. Shlobin, N.A.; Dahdaleh, N.S. Cervical spine manifestations of rheumatoid arthritis: A review. *Neurosurg. Rev.* **2021**, *44*, 1957–1965. [CrossRef]
6. Scott, D.L.; Wolfe, F.; Huizinga, T.W. Rheumatoid arthritis. *Lancet* **2010**, *376*, 1094–1108. [CrossRef]
7. Chou, C.T.; Pei, L.; Chang, D.M.; Lee, C.F.; Schumacher, H.R.; Liang, M.H. Prevalence of rheumatic diseases in Taiwan: A population study of urban, suburban, rural differences. *J. Rheumatol.* **1994**, *21*, 302–306.
8. Kuo, C.F.; Luo, S.F.; See, L.C.; Chou, I.J.; Chang, H.C.; Yu, K.H. Rheumatoid arthritis prevalence, incidence, and mortality rates: A nationwide population study in Taiwan. *Rheumatol. Int.* **2013**, *33*, 355–360. [CrossRef]
9. Wang, S.; Tsou, H.K.; Chiou, J.Y.; Wang, Y.H.; Zhang, Z.; Wei, J.C. Increased risk of inflammatory bowel disease among patients with ankylosing spondylitis: A 13-year population-based cohort study. *Front. Immunol.* **2020**, *11*, 578732. [CrossRef]
10. Taurog, J.D.; Chhabra, A.; Colbert, R.A. Ankylosing spondylitis and axial spondyloarthritis. *N. Engl. J. Med.* **2016**, *374*, 2563–2574. [CrossRef]
11. Boehncke, W.H.; Schön, M.P. Psoriasis. *Lancet* **2015**, *386*, 983–994. [CrossRef]
12. Chang, Y.T.; Chen, T.J.; Liu, P.C.; Chen, Y.C.; Chen, Y.J.; Huang, Y.L.; Jih, J.S.; Chen, C.C.; Lee, D.D.; Wang, W.J.; et al. Epidemiological study of psoriasis in the national health insurance database in Taiwan. *Acta Derm. Venereol.* **2009**, *89*, 262–266. [CrossRef]
13. Alinaghi, F.; Calov, M.; Kristensen, L.E.; Gladman, D.D.; Coates, L.C.; Jullien, D.; Gottlieb, A.B.; Gisondi, P.; Wu, J.J.; Thyssen, J.P.; et al. Prevalence of psoriatic arthritis in patients with psoriasis: A systematic review and meta-analysis of observational and clinical studies. *J. Am. Acad. Dermatol.* **2019**, *80*, 251–265. [CrossRef]
14. Day, M.S.; Nam, D.; Goodman, S.; Su, E.P.; Figgie, M. Psoriatic arthritis. *J. Am. Acad. Orthop. Surg.* **2012**, *20*, 28–37. [CrossRef]
15. Dai, Y.X.; Hsu, M.C.; Hu, H.Y.; Chang, Y.T.; Chen, T.J.; Li, C.P.; Wu, C.Y. The risk of mortality among psoriatic patients with varying severity: A nationwide population-based cohort study in Taiwan. *Int. J. Environ. Res. Public Health* **2018**, *15*, 2622. [CrossRef]
16. Gottlieb, A.B.; Merola, J.F. Axial psoriatic arthritis: An update for dermatologists. *J. Am. Acad. Dermatol.* **2021**, *84*, 92–101. [CrossRef]
17. Lisnevskaia, L.; Murphy, G.; Isenberg, D. Systemic lupus erythematosus. *Lancet* **2014**, *384*, 1878–1888. [CrossRef]
18. Leong, P.Y.; Huang, J.Y.; Chiou, J.Y.; Bai, Y.C.; Wei, J.C. The prevalence and incidence of systemic lupus erythematosus in Taiwan: A nationwide population-based study. *Sci. Rep.* **2021**, *11*, 5631. [CrossRef]
19. Piga, M.; Saba, L.; Gabba, A.; Congia, M.; Balestrieri, A.; Mathieu, A.; Cauli, A. Ultrasonographic assessment of bone erosions in the different subtypes of systemic lupus erythematosus arthritis: Comparison with computed tomography. *Arthritis Res. Ther.* **2016**, *18*, 222. [CrossRef]
20. Mahmoud, K.; Zayat, A.; Vital, E.M. Musculoskeletal manifestations of systemic lupus erythematosus. *Curr. Opin. Rheumatol.* **2017**, *29*, 486–492. [CrossRef]
21. Mertelsmann-Voss, C.; Lyman, S.; Pan, T.J.; Goodman, S.; Figgie, M.P.; Mandl, L.A. Arthroplasty rates are increased among US patients with systemic lupus erythematosus: 1991–2005. *J. Rheumatol.* **2014**, *41*, 867–874. [CrossRef]
22. Ferguson, R.J.; Palmer, A.J.; Taylor, A.; Porter, M.L.; Malchau, H.; Glyn-Jones, S. Hip replacement. *Lancet* **2018**, *392*, 1662–1671. [CrossRef]
23. Price, A.J.; Alvand, A.; Troelsen, A.; Katz, J.N.; Hooper, G.; Gray, A.; Carr, A.; Beard, D. Knee replacement. *Lancet* **2018**, *392*, 1672–1682. [CrossRef]
24. Kumar, A.; Tsai, W.C.; Tan, T.S.; Kung, P.T.; Chiu, L.T.; Ku, M.C. Temporal trends in primary and revision total knee and hip replacement in Taiwan. *J. Chin. Med. Assoc.* **2015**, *78*, 538–544. [CrossRef]
25. Huang, Y.C.; Chang, C.H.; Lin, C.L.; Wang, L.J.; Hsu, C.W.; Su, Y.F.; Lo, Y.C.; Hung, C.F.; Hsieh, Y.Y.; Chen, C.S. Prevalence and outcomes of major psychiatric disorders preceding index surgery for degenerative thoracic/lumbar spine disease. *Int. J. Environ. Res. Public Health* **2021**, *18*, 5391. [CrossRef]

26. Lin, J.H.; Chien, L.N.; Tsai, W.L.; Chen, L.Y.; Hsieh, Y.C.; Chiang, Y.H. Reoperation rates of anterior cervical discectomy and fusion versus posterior laminoplasty for multilevel cervical degenerative diseases: A population-based cohort study in Taiwan. *Spine J.* **2016**, *16*, 1428–1436. [CrossRef]
27. Lu, M.C.; Fan, K.S.; Hsu, C.W.; Koo, M.; Lai, N.S. Increased incidence of total knee replacement surgery in patients with psoriasis: A secondary cohort analysis of a nationwide, population-based health claims database. *Front. Med.* **2021**, *8*, 666802. [CrossRef]
28. Lu, M.C.; Tung, C.H.; Yang, C.C.; Wang, C.L.; Huang, K.Y.; Koo, M.; Lai, N.S. Incident osteoarthritis and osteoarthritis-related joint replacement surgery in patients with ankylosing spondylitis: A secondary cohort analysis of a nationwide, population-based health claims database. *PLoS ONE* **2017**, *12*, e0187594. [CrossRef]
29. Chen, C.H.; Hsu, C.W.; Lu, M.C. Risk of joint replacement surgery in Taiwanese female adults with systemic lupus erythematosus: A population-based cohort study. *BMC Musculoskelet. Disord.* **2019**, *20*, 314. [CrossRef]
30. Lu, M.C.; Koo, M.; Lai, N.S. Incident spine surgery in patients with ankylosing spondylitis: A secondary cohort analysis of a nationwide, population-based health claims database. *Arthritis Care Res.* **2018**, *70*, 1416–1420. [CrossRef]
31. Chen, C.H.; Hsu, C.W.; Lu, M.C. Risk of spine surgery in patients with rheumatoid arthritis: A secondary cohort analysis of a nationwide, population-based health claim database. *Medicina* **2022**, *58*, 777. [CrossRef]
32. Lee, Y.H.; Ko, P.Y.; Kao, S.L.; Lin, M.C.; Cheng-Chung, W.J. Risk of total knee and hip arthroplasty in patients with rheumatoid arthritis: A 12-year retrospective cohort study of 65,898 patients. *J. Arthroplasty* **2020**, *35*, 3517–3523. [CrossRef]
33. Zhou, V.Y.; Lacaille, D.; Lu, N.; Kopec, J.A.; Garbuz, D.S.; Qian, Y.; Aviña-Zubieta, J.A.; Esdaile, J.M.; Xie, H. Has the incidence of total joint arthroplasty in rheumatoid arthritis decreased in the era of biologics use? A population-based cohort study. *Rheumatology* **2022**, *61*, 1819–1830. [CrossRef]
34. Asai, S.; Takahashi, N.; Asai, N.; Yamashita, S.; Terabe, K.; Matsumoto, T.; Sobue, Y.; Nishiume, T.; Suzuki, M.; Ishiguro, N.; et al. Characteristics of patients with rheumatoid arthritis undergoing primary total joint replacement: A 14-year trend analysis (2004–2017). *Mod. Rheumatol.* **2020**, *30*, 657–663. [CrossRef]
35. Nystad, T.W.; Furnes, O.; Havelin, L.I.; Skredderstuen, A.K.; Lie, S.A.; Fevang, B.T. Hip replacement surgery in patients with ankylosing spondylitis. *Ann. Rheum. Dis.* **2014**, *73*, 1194–1197. [CrossRef]
36. Mazzucchelli, R.; Almodóvar, R.; Turrado-Crespí, P.; Crespí-Villarías, N.; Pérez-Fernández, E.; García-Zamora, E.; García-Vadillo, A. Trends in orthopaedic surgery for spondyloarthritis: Outcomes from a National Hospitalised Patient Registry (MBDS) over a 17-year period (1999–2015).TREND-EspA study. *RMD Open* **2022**, *8*, e002107. [CrossRef]
37. Stovall, R.; Peloquin, C.; Felson, D.; Neogi, T.; Dubreuil, M. Relation of NSAIDs, DMARDs, and TNF inhibitors for ankylosing spondylitis and psoriatic arthritis to risk of total hip and knee arthroplasty. *J. Rheumatol.* **2021**, *48*, 1007–1013. [CrossRef]
38. Hawley, S.; Ali, M.S.; Cordtz, R.; Dreyer, L.; Edwards, C.J.; Arden, N.K.; Cooper, C.; Judge, A.; Hyrich, K.; Prieto-Alhambra, D. Impact of TNF inhibitor therapy on joint replacement rates in rheumatoid arthritis: A matched cohort analysis of BSRBR-RA UK registry data. *Rheumatology* **2019**, *58*, 1168–1175. [CrossRef]
39. Del Grande, M.; Del Grande, F.; Carrino, J.; Bingham, C.O., 3rd; Louie, G.H. Cervical spine involvement early in the course of rheumatoid arthritis. *Semin. Arthritis Rheum.* **2014**, *43*, 738–744. [CrossRef]
40. Zhu, S.; Xu, W.; Luo, Y.; Zhao, Y.; Liu, Y. Cervical spine involvement risk factors in rheumatoid arthritis: A meta-analysis. *Int. J. Rheum. Dis.* **2017**, *20*, 541–549. [CrossRef]
41. Lee, W.; Reveille, J.D.; Davis, J.C., Jr.; Learch, T.J.; Ward, M.M.; Weisman, M.H. Are there gender differences in severity of ankylosing spondylitis? Results from the PSOAS cohort. *Ann. Rheum. Dis.* **2007**, *66*, 633–638. [CrossRef]

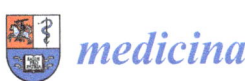

Article

How Did the Two Years of the COVID-19 Pandemic Affect the Outcomes of the Patients with Inflammatory Rheumatic Diseases in Lithuania?

Jolanta Dadonienė [1,2], Gabija Jasionytė [3], Julija Mironova [3], Karolina Staškuvienė [3] and Dalia Miltinienė [1,3,*]

1. State Research Institute Centre for Innovative Medicine, LT-08406 Vilnius, Lithuania
2. Department of Public Health, Institute of Health Sciences, Faculty of Medicine, Vilnius University, LT-03101 Vilnius, Lithuania
3. Clinic of Rheumatology, Orthopedics Traumatology and Reconstructive Surgery, Institute of Clinical Medicine, Faculty of Medicine, Vilnius University, LT-03101 Vilnius, Lithuania
* Correspondence: dalia.miltiniene@santa.lt; Tel.: +370-5-2365-301

Abstract: *Background and objectives*: the COVID-19 pandemic globally caused more than 18 million deaths over the period of 2020–2021. Although inflammatory rheumatic diseases (RD) are generally associated with premature mortality, it is not yet clear whether RD patients are at a greater risk for COVID-19-related mortality. The aim of our study was to evaluate mortality and causes of death in a retrospective inflammatory RD patient cohort during the COVID-19 pandemic years. *Methods*: We identified patients with a first-time diagnosis of inflammatory RD and followed them up during the pandemic years of 2020–2021. Death rates, and sex- and age-standardized mortality ratios (SMRs) were calculated for the prepandemic and pandemic periods. *Results*: We obtained data from 11,636 patients that had been newly diagnosed with inflammatory RD and followed up until the end of 2021 or their death. The mean duration of the follow-up was 5.5 years. In total, 1531 deaths occurred between 2013 and 2021. The prevailing causes of death in the prepandemic period were cardiovascular diseases, neoplasms, and diseases of the respiratory system. In the pandemic years, cardiovascular diseases and neoplasms remained the two most common causes of death, with COVID-19 in third place. The SMR of the total RD cohort was 0.83. This trend was observed in rheumatoid arthritis and spondyloarthropathy patients. The SMR in the group of connective-tissue diseases and vasculitis was higher at 0.93, but did not differ from that of the general population. The excess of deaths in the RD cohort during the pandemic period was negative (−27.2%), meaning that RD patients endured the pandemic period better than the general population did. *Conclusions*: The COVID-19 pandemic did not influence the mortality of RD patients. Strict lockdown measures, social distancing, and early vaccination were the main factors that resulted in reduced mortality in this cohort during the pandemic years.

Keywords: rheumatic diseases; standardized mortality ratio; COVID-19; excess mortality

1. Introduction

Inflammatory rheumatic diseases (RDs) are generally associated with premature mortality, mainly due to infections, premature atherosclerosis and subsequent cardiovascular complications, and major organ damage as a result of the RDs themselves [1–6].

Epidemiologic studies conducted before 2020 calculated that patients with inflammatory RD had up to 425% higher risk of death than that of the age- and sex-matched general population. The highest mortality was observed in patients with systemic connective-tissue diseases (CTDs; systemic sclerosis, systemic lupus erythematosus), systemic vasculitis, and myositis. The lowest mortality, comparable to the general population results, was observed in rheumatoid arthritis (RA), spondyloarthropathy (SPA), Sjogren's syndrome, and polymyalgia rheumatica patient groups [7]. The greatest decrease in life expectancy at the time of birth in comparison with the general population was estimated in systemic sclerosis patients and is up to 34 years of life [1,8–10].

At the end of 2019, coronavirus disease 2019 (COVID-19), caused by the SARS-CoV-2 virus, emerged and spread fulminantly worldwide as a severe pandemic that was responsible for increased global mortality. According to the World Health Organization (WHO), COVID-19 has already caused over 6.67 million deaths [11]. However, the full weight of the COVID-19 pandemic is much greater than what is indicated only by reported deaths due to COVID-19. The full impact of the pandemic is assessed by calculating excess mortality, which is defined as the increase in all-cause mortality over the expected mortality rates. It is estimated that more than 18 million people died globally because of the COVID-19 pandemic (as measured via excess mortality) over the period between 1 January 2020 and 31 December 2021 [12]. The extent of excess mortality varied significantly between countries. The highest excess mortality rate due to COVID-19 was observed in Bolivia, which reached 734.9 deaths per 100,000 individuals. Negative excess-mortality rates (pandemic mortality was lower than that in the prepandemic period) were estimated in Iceland, Australia, Singapore, New Zealand, and Taiwan [12,13]. Older age and concomitant diseases such as dementia, chronic kidney disease, severe mental illness, cardiovascular disease, diabetes, chronic obstructive pulmonary disease, and cancer are predictors for severity and death related to COVID-19 [14]. However, it is still unclear whether patients with inflammatory RD are at a greater risk of COVID-19-related mortality.

The objective of our study was to assess mortality and causes of death in a retrospective cohort of patients with inflammatory RD during the COVID-19 pandemic, in particular during 2020–2021, and to compare them with those of the general population of Lithuania and the results of the same cohort during the prepandemic years [7].

2. Materials and Methods

2.1. Data Sources

The retrospective cohort study was performed with data retrieved from Lithuanian compulsory health insurance information system database SVEIDRA. This is a population-based database that has been running since 1995 and registers all patients' visits to healthcare institutions, the established diagnoses, and the prescriptions of state-reimbursed medications to all residents of Lithuania. The Vilnius Regional Bioethics Committee approved assessing these data and conducting the study (approval number: 158200-17-958-462, approval date: 7 November 2017).

Information about all patients who had been newly diagnosed with inflammatory RD during the period between 1 January 2012 and 31 December 2019 was obtained from SVEIDRA. Patients with RA, SPA (psoriatic arthritis (PsA), ankylosing spondylitis, and undifferentiated SPA), systemic CTD, and vasculitis were included. Information about the prescription of state-reimbursed medication such as glucocorticoids, conventional synthetic disease-modifying antirheumatic drugs (csDMARDs) (hydrochloroquine, sulfasalazine, methotrexate, azathioprine, leflunomide), or biological disease-modifying antirheumatic drugs (bDMARDs) (etanercept, adalimumab, infliximab, tocilizumab or rituximab with available biosimilars) was used for the verification of RD cases.

A total of 95,289 RD cases with a first-time diagnosis of inflammatory RD established between 2012 and 2019 were selected. A case was considered first-time-diagnosed if the patient had had at least 1 year of no previous RD record in the database. As no data preceding 2012 were available, we excluded 22,526 first-time diagnoses in 2012 from the total cohort, as it was not possible to verify their RD diagnosis prior to the index date.

We excluded 2251 cases from the cohort because they were younger than 18 years old at the time of diagnosis, and 10 because of an unidentifiable identification code. To verify the cases, we excluded 58,866 patients with no records of at least one prescription of state-reimbursed medications for RD (glucocorticoids, csDMARDs, or bDMARDs).

The final 11,636 cases were cross-checked with the death registry of the health Information center at the Institute of Hygiene, and the date and cause of death were obtained if the death had occurred between 2013 and 2021. The cases were cross-checked using personal identification codes. The principal causes of death were compared between the prepandemic and pandemic time periods, and grouped under the following categories: deaths because of cardiovascular and circulatory causes, malignancies, infections, respiratory causes, musculoskeletal diseases, external causes of death, and unspecified causes of death. COVID-19, as a recorded cause of death, was only calculated in the pandemic period.

The final dataset used for analysis included sex, age, the ICD-10 code of RD, the date of RD diagnosis, the date and cause of death if applicable, and information about the prescription of state-reimbursed drugs.

For the comparison with the general population of Lithuania, information on the adult population census in 2013–2021 was obtained from Statistics Lithuania (www.stat.gov.lt, accessed on 27 November 2022).

2.2. Statistical Methods

Sex- and age-standardized mortality ratios (SMRs) were calculated by dividing the observed number of deaths in the RD patients' cohort by the expected number of deaths, calculated using the national rates from the Lithuanian Department of Statistics' official statistics website; 95% confidence intervals (CIs) for the SMRs were calculated.

All statistical analyses were performed using Microsoft Excel (2016) by the Microsoft Corporation.

3. Results

3.1. Demographic Characteristics of the RD Cohort

During the period of 2013–2019, 11,636 patients with newly diagnosed RD were identified comprising 6008 patients with RA, 3289 with SPA, and 2339 with systemic CTD and vasculitis. The cohort was further followed up during the COVID-19 pandemic years (2020–2021); the mean duration of total follow-up was 5.49 (standard deviation 2.22) years. The mean age of the patients at the time of RD diagnosis was 57 years (range, 18–97). 52% of the total cohort were RA patients. The majority of the cohort patients were women (70%), particularly in the RA and systemic CTD groups (77% and 76%, respectively). In SPA, the group gender distribution was equal (52% of women and 48% of men).

3.2. Death Cases and Leading Causes of Death

At a total follow-up of 63,901.16 person-years, 950 death cases had occurred in 2013–2019, and 581 death cases in 2020–2021. The demographic data of the death cases are presented in Table 1. Around 60% of the death cases were women in both periods of time. The majority of the death cases were observed in the RA group during both periods (54% in the 2013–2019 period and 55% in the period of 2020–2021). Age at the time of death in the RD cohort was higher in the pandemic period (76.42 years) compared with 73.5 years during the 2013–2019 period. SPA patients were the youngest at the time of death, around 67 years in both the analyzed periods of time, whereas the RA and CTD groups did not differ much from the average in either time period.

Table 1. Demographic characteristics of rheumatic-disease patient cohort's death cases in the prepandemic and pandemic periods.

Deaths/Periods	Prepandemic Period (2013–2019)	Pandemic Period (2020–2021)
Total number of deaths	950	581
Female (%)	562 (59.16)	358 (61.62)
Male (%)	388 (40.84)	223 (38.38)

Table 1. *Cont.*

Deaths/Periods	Prepandemic Period (2013–2019)	Pandemic Period (2020–2021)
Number of deaths in different disease groups:		
RA group (%) *	509 (53.58)	321 (55.25)
SPA group (%) **	142 (14.95)	81 (13.94)
CTD and vasculitis group (%) ***	299 (30.63)	179 (30.81)
Age at the time of death:		
Mean total-cohort age (SD ****)	73.50 (12.33)	76.42 (11.35)
Mean RA group age (SD)	74.95 (11.45)	77.64 (9.95)
Mean SPA group age (SD)	67.34 (13.45)	67.96 (14.75)
Mean CTD and vasculitis group age (SD)	73.98 (12.37)	78.04 (10.22)

* RA—rheumatoid arthritis, ** SPA—spondyloarthropathy, *** CTD—connective-tissue disease, **** SD—standard deviation.

We compared the main causes of death between the prepandemic and pandemic cohorts of patients. Despite the COVID-19 pandemic and deaths occurring because of this disease, the predominant causes of death for both cohorts were cardiovascular diseases and neoplasms. However, the reported COVID-19 disease was the third most common direct cause of death in the pandemic cohort. We present the proportions of the main causes of death in both cohorts in Table 2.

Table 2. Main causes of death in patients with rheumatic diseases in the prepandemic and pandemic cohorts.

Causes of Death	Prepandemic Cohort (2013–2019) $n = 950$	Pandemic Cohort (2020–2021) $n = 581$
Cardiovascular diseases (%)	**450 (47.4)** *	**266 (45.8)**
Neoplasms including lymphopoietic system (%)	**220 (23.2)**	**103 (17.7)**
Diseases of the respiratory system (%)	57 (6.0)	15 (2.6)
Diseases of the musculoskeletal system (%)	48 (5.1)	15 (2.6)
External causes of death (%)	38 (4.0)	15 (2.6)
Other causes of death (%)	**137 (14.4)**	81 (13.9)
COVID-19 (%)	0	**86 (14.8)**

* The three most common causes of death are represented by numbers in bold.

3.3. Death Rates and Standardized Mortality Ratios

Death rates that were adjusted to the general population were separately calculated in the RD cohort for the prepandemic and pandemic periods and compared to the national death rates. In the prepandemic period of 2013–2019, the adjusted death rate observed in the RD group was higher than that of the general population of Lithuania (2239.00 per 100,000 patient years and 1702.97 per 100,000 inhabitants per year, respectively). The excess of deaths of almost 16% was obvious for the general Lithuanian population during the pandemic period (the death rate in the period of 2020–2021 was 1973.39 per 100,000 inhabitants per year), while it was not the case for the adjusted RD cohort (excess of deaths in pandemic period, −27.2%), meaning that RD patients endured the pandemic period better than the general population did. Death rates are presented in Table 3.

Table 3. Death rates and excess of deaths observed in the general population of Lithuania and the cohort of rheumatic diseases during the prepandemic and pandemic periods.

	Prepandemic Period (2013–2019)	Pandemic Period (2020–2021)	Excess of Deaths
General population of Lithuania (average number of deaths per 100,000 inhabitants per year)	1702.97	1973.39	15.9%
RD * cohort (death rate, standardized according to age and sex, 95% CI)	2239 (2099;2386)	1630 (1500;1768)	−27.2%

* RD—rheumatic diseases.

The age- and sex-adjusted SMRs were calculated for the RD cohort for both periods of time. RD mortality was higher than that in the general population in the prepandemic years (the total SMR of the cohort was 1.32 (95% CI 1.23;1.40)), but in the pandemic years, RD mortality was significantly lower than that in the general population (the SMR of the total RD cohort was 0.83 (95% CI 0.76;0.90)). This trend was observed in RA and SPA patients except for the CTD and vasculitis group. The SMR in the CTD and vasculitis group did not differ from that of the general population, at 0.93 (95% CI 080; 1.07)). The SMRs of the total RD cohort and different RDs are presented in Table 4.

Table 4. Standardized mortality ratios in the RD cohort during the prepandemic and pandemic periods.

	Standardized Mortality Ratios in Prepandemic Period (95% CI)	Standardized Mortality Ratios in Pandemic Period (95% CI)
Total:	1.32 (1.23;1.40)	0.83 (0.76;0.90)
Women	1.31 (1.21;1.42)	0.79 (0.71;0.87)
Men	1.32 (1.19;1.46)	0.90 (0.78;1.02)
RA *	1.25 (1.14;1.36)	0.83 (0.74;0.92)
SPA **	1.16 (0.98;1.37)	0.67 (0.53;0.83)
CTD and vasculitis ***	1.55 (1.38;1.73)	0.93 (0.80;1.07)

* RA—rheumatoid arthritis, ** SPA—spondyloarthropathy, *** CTD—connective tissue diseases.

4. Discussion

In this article, we describe the mortality results of the follow-up of a large Lithuanian RD patient cohort starting from the diagnoses and following to the end of 2021. We found that the COVID-19 pandemic did not influence the mortality of the cohort. On the contrary, RD patients survived the pandemic period better than the general Lithuanian population did. The age- and sex-adjusted SMR of the total RD cohort was 0.83 (compared to an SMR of 1.32 in the prepandemic years). This trend was observed in the RA and SPA patient groups. Only mortality in the CTD and vasculitis group was a little higher, but did not differ from that of the general population, with an SMR of 0.93 (95% CI 0.80; 1.07).

The COVID-19 pandemic has been generally linked to an increased global mortality and excess of deaths. At the very beginning of the pandemic, patients diagnosed with cardiovascular disease (CVD), diabetes, chronic respiratory disease, hypertension, cancer, and older age had an increased mortality risk [15]. In 2021, Dessie et al. performed a systematic review and meta-analysis of the risk factors of COVID-19-related mortality. The meta-analysis of more than 400,000 cases of COVID-19 concluded that the male sex, older age, current smoking status, obesity, increased D-dimer level, and comorbidities such as acute kidney injury, chronic obstructive pulmonary disease, diabetes, hypertension, CVD, and malignancy determined a higher risk of death [16]. Predictors of the increase in all-cause mortality during the COVID-19 pandemic were also analyzed, revealing that people who were aged 65–79 years, single, and had elementary-school education (or below) were at higher risk for excess death from any cause [17]. In addition, a study from the USA revealed racial and ethnic disparities, reporting a twice higher rate of excess deaths in Black, American Indian/Alaska Native, and Latino males and females compared with White and Asian people [18]. Carey et al. reported that not only older age (>80 years) and non-White ethnicity are risk factors for excess mortality, but also a high body mass index (>40), dementia, learning disabilities, severe mental illnesses, and the specific place of residence (care home, most deprived) [19].

There are global data that the COVID-19 pandemic had a definite effect on different aspects of inflammatory RDs due to the challenges to healthcare systems, shortages of resources, limitations in performing routine care, possible delays in diagnosis, and even, in some cases, supply gaps of some medications, such as hydroxychloroquine [20]. Although it seems that there is no evidence that rheumatic patients are at higher risk of contracting SARS-CoV-2 [21], it is yet not clear whether patients with inflammatory RD are at a greater risk of COVID-19-related mortality. A number of studies have addressed this problem so far. A study conducted in South Korea examined data from 8297 patients diagnosed with inflammatory RD and reported an increased mortality rate among the aforementioned patients during the pandemic. They also found that taking ≥10 mg of systemic glucocorticosteroids was associated with a higher risk of testing positive for COVID-19, developing severe illness, and COVID-19-related death [22]. A Greek study that covered 12-month data derived from electronic databases of around 11 million Greek residents indicated that mortality due to COVID-19 was higher in patients with systemic sclerosis and RA in comparison to that of the general population, while the mortality rates in ankylosing spondylitis, systemic lupus erythematosus, and PsA were equal to those of the comparators [23]. A Swedish nationwide study also demonstrated that mortality rates differed among different types of arthritis. For example, RA has higher mortality rates; in the SPA group, mortality levels matched those of the general population [24]. A nationwide cohort study from Denmark also matched the Swedish data: patients diagnosed with RA were more likely to have a severe outcome (intensive care unit admission, acute distress syndrome, or death) of COVID-19 [25]. However, data throughout the literature are inconsistent. For example, an American multicenter study demonstrated that mortality rates in the general population and in patients with inflammatory RD were equal [26].

There is a discussion regarding which factors could have added to excess mortality during the COVID-19 pandemic. Apart from the lethal outcomes directly caused by COVID-19 infection, deaths caused by the collapse or overstretching of medical systems due to the COVID-19 pandemic may have also added to the excess deaths [27,28] There is recorded evidence about the higher rates of anxiety and depression during the pandemic period, which might have led to an increase in deaths from suicide, as was estimated in Japan [29–31].

There are also generally accepted factors that lowered excess mortality. Isolation requirements and other pandemic restrictions might have decreased the incidence of some conditions and injuries, such as traffic accidents, thereby resulting in a decrease in death rates due to these causes [32,33]. The lower rate of deaths from chronic respiratory conditions could have been influenced by the reduction in air pollution [34]. There was also noted decrease in deaths from chronic conditions such as ischemic heart disease or chronic respiratory disease, probably because these frail individuals were at higher risk to die from COVID-19 rather than from these chronic conditions in the pandemic period [35]. However, the most likely reason for the non-COVID-19 mortality to have decreased is the lower incidence of influenza and other infectious respiratory diseases during the COVID-19 pandemic—a decrease in cases of 80% or more was reported by the WHO. It was estimated that the decrease in influenza incidence alone could have led to a decrease in total annual mortality of 3–6% [13]. The main reasons for the decrease in the rate of respiratory infections are behavioral factors—mask use, reduced mobility, social distancing, and lockdown measures, which were really strict in Lithuania during the most severe pandemic periods. Lastly, the use of SARS-COV-2 vaccines has indisputably considerably lowered mortality rates among people who contracted the virus and among the general population. Inflammatory RD patients were among those who were the first to be vaccinated in Lithuania—as a group at higher risk, their vaccination began as early as April 2021. The strict lockdown measures and social distancing imposed by the state authorities, and by the conscious decision of immunocompromised patients themselves, as well as early vaccination were the main factors that resulted in the reduced mortality in the Lithuanian RD cohort during the pandemic years.

The main asset of our study is the populational coverage. We obtained data on the patients with RD and their death cases from the entire Lithuanian population from official state-run sources. No death case could have been omitted due to this.

The main limitation of the study is the possible exclusion of some RD cases if they had not been treated with the medications reimbursed by the state, as this was one of the exclusion criteria for the verification of the cases. This could have resulted in the exclusion of mild cases, and especially SPA patients, because the treatment of SPA is currently poorly reimbursed in Lithuania. Another limitation is that we followed up the cohort of the patients first diagnosed with RD during the period of 2013–2019 and did not include newly diagnosed RD cases during the pandemic years. COVID-19 infection itself could be a trigger of RD. A notable proportion of patients with COVID-19 present with fatigue, muscle pain, and other rheumatic manifestations, such as arthralgia, vasculitis, and chilblains, and up to 49% of COVID-19 patients present with different autoantibodies (antinuclear, antiphospholipid) [36,37]. However, it is not clear whether these antibodies show a temporary immune dysregulation or whether SARS-CoV-2 is capable of causing RD [38–40]. A number of new-onset rheumatic autoimmune diseases following SARS-CoV-2 infection were reported, with the most common being systemic vasculitis and inflammatory arthritis [41]. A few cases of inflammatory myopathies [42], systemic lupus erythematosus [43], and systemic sclerosis [44], during or after COVID-19, were also reported. However, it is unclear whether SARS-CoV-2 infection uncovers and accelerates previously subclinical rheumatic illness or induces de novo disease, since no direct causal relationship has been proven. On the other hand, an immense study in the USA demonstrated only a small rate of new-onset RD in patients with a positive polymerase chain reaction (PCR) test for the detection of SARS-CoV-2 (6 incident cases among over 15,200 patients), which was similar to the rate among the matched controls with a negative PCR test (five incident cases) [45]. However, this frequency might have been lower due to steroid therapy in COVID-19 pneumonia [46]. Other authors found that post-COVID-19 was strongly associated with the erythrocyte sedimentation rate and C-reactive protein, but not autoantibodies, which suggested an inflammatory rather than autoimmune mechanism of arthritis [47]. This could also explain the significantly increased number of new Kawasaki disease cases during the COVID-19 pandemic [48]. Derksen et al. compared the clinical phenotype and autoantibody patterns in patients with polyarthritis after COVID-19 and in RA patients, and concluded that RA following COVID-19 was seemingly a coincidence [49]. Taking the aforementioned into account, evidence on the role of SARS-CoV-2 in inducing RD is currently unclear, and large-sample studies with an adequate follow-up are still needed.

5. Conclusions

In conclusion, the data from existing studies referring to the mortality of patients with RD are inconsistent, and our study added new evidence that the RD patient mortality rate was less than that of the general population. We speculate that the proper management of the pandemic in the country and in the RD patient group resulted in a lower mortality rate than what was expected. The relation between COVID-19 and new occurrences of RD in Lithuanian cohort needs to be explored case by case and in a longer follow-up.

Author Contributions: Conceptualization, J.D.; methodology, J.D. and D.M.; software, J.D.; validation, J.D. and D.M.; formal analysis, J.D. and DM.; investigation, J.D., D.M., G.J., J.M. and K.S.; resources, J.D. and D.M.; data curation, J.D. and D.M.; writing—original draft preparation, D.M, J.M, G.J. and K.S.; writing—review and editing, J.D.; visualization, D.M.; supervision, J.D.; project administration, J.D.; funding acquisition, J.D. All authors have read and agreed to the published version of the manuscript.

Funding: This research received no external funding.

Institutional Review Board Statement: The study was conducted according to the guidelines of the Declaration of Helsinki and approved by the Vilnius Regional Bioethics Committee (approval number 158200-17-958-462, approval date 7 November 2017).

Informed Consent Statement: Patient consent was waived because data were obtained from national registries and official state run sources collected for the purposes of the management of health statistics, and due to the very high number of participants.

Data Availability Statement: The data presented in this study are available on request from the corresponding author. The data are not publicly available because they contain the personal identification codes of patients included in this study; therefore, they are sensitive personal data that are strictly protected by local ethical restrictions and the rules of personal data safety in Lithuania.

Conflicts of Interest: The authors declare no conflict of interest.

References

1. Mok, C.C.; Kwok, C.L.; Ho, L.Y.; Chan, P.T.; Yip, S.F. Life Expectancy, Standardized Mortality Ratios, and Causes of Death in Six Rheumatic Diseases in Hong Kong, China. *Arthritis Rheum.* **2011**, *63*, 1182–1189. [CrossRef] [PubMed]
2. Rho, Y.H.; Chung, C.P.; Oeser, A.; Solus, J.; Asanuma, Y.; Sokka, T.; Pincus, T.; Raggi, P.; Gebretsadik, T.; Shintani, A.; et al. Inflammatory Mediators and Premature Coronary Atherosclerosis in Rheumatoid Arthritis. *Arthritis Rheum.* **2009**, *61*, 1580–1585. [CrossRef] [PubMed]
3. Meune, C.; Touzé, E.; Trinquart, L.; Allanore, Y. High Risk of Clinical Cardiovascular Events in Rheumatoid Arthritis: Levels of Associations of Myocardial Infarction and Stroke through a Systematic Review and Meta-Analysis. *Arch. Cardiovasc. Dis.* **2010**, *103*, 253–261. [CrossRef] [PubMed]
4. Han, C.; Robinson, D.W.; Hackett, M.V.; Paramore, L.C.; Fraeman, K.H.; Bala, M.V. Cardiovascular Disease and Risk Factors in Patients with Rheumatoid Arthritis, Psoriatic Arthritis, and Ankylosing Spondylitis. *J. Rheumatol.* **2006**, *33*, 2167–2172. [PubMed]
5. Mok, C.C.; Ho, L.Y.; To, C.H. Annual Incidence and Standardized Incidence Ratio of Cerebrovascular Accidents in Patients with Systemic Lupus Erythematosus. *Scand. J. Rheumatol.* **2009**, *38*, 362–368. [CrossRef]
6. Gladman, D.D.; Ang, M.; Su, L.; Tom, B.D.M.; Schentag, C.T.; Farewell, V.T. Cardiovascular Morbidity in Psoriatic Arthritis. *Ann. Rheum. Dis.* **2009**, *68*, 1131–1135. [CrossRef]
7. Dadonienė, J.; Charukevič, G.; Jasionytė, G.; Staškuvienė, K.; Miltinienė, D. Mortality in Inflammatory Rheumatic Diseases: Lithuanian National Registry Data and Systematic Review. *Int. J. Environ. Res. Public Health* **2021**, *18*, 12338. [CrossRef]
8. Gabriel, S.E.; Michaud, K. Epidemiological Studies in Incidence, Prevalence, Mortality, and Comorbidity of the Rheumatic Diseases. *Arthritis Res. Ther.* **2009**, *11*, 229. [CrossRef]
9. Yurkovich, M.; Vostretsova, K.; Chen, W.; Aviña-Zubieta, J.A. Overall and Cause-Specific Mortality in Patients with Systemic Lupus Erythematosus: A Meta-Analysis of Observational Studies. *Arthritis Care Res.* **2014**, *66*, 608–616. [CrossRef]
10. Toledano, E.; Candelas, G.; Rosales, Z.; Martínez Prada, C.; León, L.; Abásolo, L.; Loza, E.; Carmona, L.; Tobías, A.; Jover, J.Á. A Meta-Analysis of Mortality in Rheumatic Diseases. *Reumatol. Clin.* **2012**, *8*, 334–341. [CrossRef]
11. WHO Coronavirus (COVID-19) Dashboard. Available online: https://covid19.who.int (accessed on 11 December 2022).
12. COVID-19 Excess Mortality Collaborators. Estimating Excess Mortality Due to the COVID-19 Pandemic: A Systematic Analysis of COVID-19-Related Mortality, 2020–2021. *Lancet* **2022**, *399*, 1513–1536. [CrossRef]
13. Karlinsky, A.; Kobak, D. Tracking Excess Mortality across Countries during the COVID-19 Pandemic with the World Mortality Dataset. *eLife* **2021**, *10*, e69336. [CrossRef]
14. Ge, E.; Li, Y.; Wu, S.; Candido, E.; Wei, X. Association of Pre-Existing Comorbidities with Mortality and Disease Severity among 167,500 Individuals with COVID-19 in Canada: A Population-Based Cohort Study. *PLoS ONE* **2021**, *16*, e0258154. [CrossRef]
15. Wu, Z.; McGoogan, J.M. Characteristics of and Important Lessons from the Coronavirus Disease 2019 (COVID-19) Outbreak in China: Summary of a Report of 72 314 Cases from the Chinese Center for Disease Control and Prevention. *JAMA* **2020**, *323*, 1239–1242. [CrossRef]
16. Dessie, Z.G.; Zewotir, T. Mortality-Related Risk Factors of COVID-19: A Systematic Review and Meta-Analysis of 42 Studies and 423,117 Patients. *BMC Infect. Dis.* **2021**, *21*, 855. [CrossRef]
17. Oh, J.; Min, J.; Kang, C.; Kim, E.; Lee, J.P.; Kim, H.; Lee, W. Excess Mortality and the COVID-19 Pandemic: Causes of Death and Social Inequalities. *BMC Public Health* **2022**, *22*, 2293. [CrossRef]

18. Shiels, M.S.; Haque, A.T.; Haozous, E.A.; Albert, P.S.; Almeida, J.S.; García-Closas, M.; Nápoles, A.M.; Pérez-Stable, E.J.; Freedman, N.D.; Berrington de González, A. Racial and Ethnic Disparities in Excess Deaths during the COVID-19 Pandemic, March to December 2020. *Ann. Intern. Med.* **2021**, *174*, 1693–1699. [CrossRef]
19. Carey, I.M.; Cook, D.G.; Harris, T.; DeWilde, S.; Chaudhry, U.A.R.; Strachan, D.P. Risk Factors for Excess All-Cause Mortality during the First Wave of the COVID-19 Pandemic in England: A Retrospective Cohort Study of Primary Care Data. *PLoS ONE* **2021**, *16*, e0260381. [CrossRef]
20. Talarico, R.; Aguilera, S.; Alexander, T.; Amoura, Z.; Antunes, A.M.; Arnaud, L.; Avcin, T.; Beretta, L.; Bombardieri, S.; Burmester, G.R.; et al. The impact of COVID-19 on rare and complex connective tissue diseases: The experience of ERN ReCONNET. *Nat. Rev. Rheumatol.* **2021**, *17*, 177–184. [CrossRef]
21. Landewe, R.B.; Machado, P.M.; Kroon, F.; Bijlsma, H.W.; Burmester, G.R.; Carmona, L.; Combe, B.; Galli, M.; Gossec, L.; Iagnocco, A.; et al. EULAR provisional recommendations for the management of rheumatic and musculoskeletal diseases in the context of SARS-CoV-2. *Ann. Rheum. Dis.* **2020**, *79*, 851–858. [CrossRef]
22. Shin, Y.H.; Shin, J.I.; Moon, S.Y.; Jin, H.Y.; Kim, S.Y.; Yang, J.M.; Cho, S.H.; Kim, S.; Lee, M.; Park, Y.; et al. Autoimmune Inflammatory Rheumatic Diseases and COVID-19 Outcomes in South Korea: A Nationwide Cohort Study. *Lancet Rheumatol.* **2021**, *3*, e698–e706. [CrossRef] [PubMed]
23. Fragoulis, G.E.; Bournia, V.-K.; Sfikakis, P.P. Different Systemic Rheumatic Diseases as Risk Factors for COVID-19-Related Mortality. *Clin. Rheumatol.* **2022**, *41*, 1919–1923. [CrossRef]
24. Bower, H.; Frisell, T.; Di Giuseppe, D.; Delcoigne, B.; Ahlenius, G.-M.; Baecklund, E.; Chatzidionysiou, K.; Feltelius, N.; Forsblad-d'Elia, H.; Kastbom, A.; et al. Impact of the COVID-19 Pandemic on Morbidity and Mortality in Patients with Inflammatory Joint Diseases and in the General Population: A Nationwide Swedish Cohort Study. *Ann. Rheum. Dis.* **2021**, *80*, 1086–1093. [CrossRef] [PubMed]
25. Cordtz, R.; Lindhardsen, J.; Soussi, B.G.; Vela, J.; Uhrenholt, L.; Westermann, R.; Kristensen, S.; Nielsen, H.; Torp-Pedersen, C.; Dreyer, L. Incidence and Severeness of COVID-19 Hospitalization in Patients with Inflammatory Rheumatic Disease: A Nationwide Cohort Study from Denmark. *Rheumatology* **2021**, *60*, SI59–SI67. [CrossRef] [PubMed]
26. D'Silva, K.M.; Jorge, A.; Cohen, A.; McCormick, N.; Zhang, Y.; Wallace, Z.S.; Choi, H.K. COVID-19 Outcomes in Patients with Systemic Autoimmune Rheumatic Diseases Compared to the General Population: A US Multicenter, Comparative Cohort Study. *Arthritis Rheumatol.* **2021**, *73*, 914–920. [CrossRef]
27. Zubiri, L.; Rosovsky, R.P.; Mooradian, M.J.; Piper-Vallillo, A.J.; Gainor, J.F.; Sullivan, R.J.; Marte, D.; Boland, G.M.; Gao, X.; Hochberg, E.P.; et al. Temporal Trends in Inpatient Oncology Census before and during the COVID-19 Pandemic and Rates of Nosocomial COVID-19 among Patients with Cancer at a Large Academic Center. *Oncologist* **2021**, *26*, e1427–e1433. [CrossRef]
28. Folino, A.F.; Zorzi, A.; Cernetti, C.; Marchese, D.; Pasquetto, G.; Roncon, L.; Saccà, S.; Themistoclakis, S.; Turiano, G.; Verlato, R.; et al. Impact of COVID-19 Epidemic on Coronary Care Unit Accesses for Acute Coronary Syndrome in Veneto Region, Italy. *Am. Heart J.* **2020**, *226*, 26–28. [CrossRef]
29. Gunnell, D.; Appleby, L.; Arensman, E.; Hawton, K.; John, A.; Kapur, N.; Khan, M.; O'Connor, R.C.; Pirkis, J. COVID-19 Suicide Prevention Research Collaboration Suicide Risk and Prevention during the COVID-19 Pandemic. *Lancet Psychiatry* **2020**, *7*, 468–471. [CrossRef]
30. John, A.; Pirkis, J.; Gunnell, D.; Appleby, L.; Morrissey, J. Trends in Suicide during the Covid-19 Pandemic. *BMJ* **2020**, *371*, m4352. [CrossRef]
31. Sakamoto, H.; Ishikane, M.; Ghaznavi, C.; Ueda, P. Assessment of Suicide in Japan during the COVID-19 Pandemic vs Previous Years. *JAMA Netw. Open* **2021**, *4*, e2037378. [CrossRef]
32. Rozenfeld, M.; Peleg, K.; Givon, A.; Bala, M.; Shaked, G.; Bahouth, H.; Bodas, M. COVID-19 Changed the Injury Patterns of Hospitalized Patients. *Prehospital Disaster Med.* **2021**, *36*, 251–259. [CrossRef]
33. Salottolo, K.; Caiafa, R.; Mueller, J.; Tanner, A.; Carrick, M.M.; Lieser, M.; Berg, G.; Bar-Or, D. Multicenter Study of US Trauma Centers Examining the Effect of the COVID-19 Pandemic on Injury Causes, Diagnoses and Procedures. *Trauma Surg. Acute Care Open* **2021**, *6*, e000655. [CrossRef]
34. Bourzac, K. COVID-19 Lockdowns Had Strange Effects on Air Pollution across the Globe. Available online: https://cen.acs.org/environment/atmospheric-chemistry/COVID-19-lockdowns-had-strange-effects-on-air-pollution-across-the-globe/98/i37 (accessed on 18 December 2022).
35. Schwarz, V.; Mahfoud, F.; Lauder, L.; Reith, W.; Behnke, S.; Smola, S.; Rissland, J.; Pfuhl, T.; Scheller, B.; Böhm, M.; et al. Decline of Emergency Admissions for Cardiovascular and Cerebrovascular Events after the Outbreak of COVID-19. *Clin. Res. Cardiol.* **2020**, *109*, 1500–1506. [CrossRef]
36. Ciaffi, J.; Meliconi, R.; Ruscitti, P.; Berardicurti, O.; Giacomelli, R.; Ursini, F. Rheumatic Manifestations of COVID-19: A Systematic Review and Meta-Analysis. *BMC Rheumatol.* **2020**, *4*, 65. [CrossRef]
37. Chang, S.E.; Feng, A.; Meng, W.; Apostolidis, S.A.; Mack, E.; Artandi, M.; Barman, L.; Bennett, K.; Chakraborty, S.; Chang, I.; et al. New-Onset IgG Autoantibodies in Hospitalized Patients with COVID-19. *Nat. Commun.* **2021**, *12*, 5417. [CrossRef]
38. Caso, F.; Costa, L.; Ruscitti, P.; Navarini, L.; Del Puente, A.; Giacomelli, R.; Scarpa, R. Could Sars-Coronavirus-2 Trigger Autoimmune and/or Autoinflammatory Mechanisms in Genetically Predisposed Subjects? *Autoimmun. Rev.* **2020**, *19*, 102524. [CrossRef] [PubMed]

39. Shah, S.; Danda, D.; Kavadichanda, C.; Das, S.; Adarsh, M.B.; Negi, V.S. Autoimmune and Rheumatic Musculoskeletal Diseases as a Consequence of SARS-CoV-2 Infection and Its Treatment. *Rheumatol. Int.* **2020**, *40*, 1539–1554. [CrossRef] [PubMed]
40. Ahmed, S.; Zimba, O.; Gasparyan, A.Y. COVID-19 and the Clinical Course of Rheumatic Manifestations. *Clin. Rheumatol.* **2021**, *40*, 2611–2619. [CrossRef] [PubMed]
41. Gracia-Ramos, A.E.; Martin-Nares, E.; Hernández-Molina, G. New Onset of Autoimmune Diseases following COVID-19 Diagnosis. *Cells* **2021**, *10*, 3592. [CrossRef]
42. Beydon, M.; Chevalier, K.; Al Tabaa, O.; Hamroun, S.; Delettre, A.-S.; Thomas, M.; Herrou, J.; Riviere, E.; Mariette, X. Myositis as a Manifestation of SARS-CoV-2. *Ann. Rheum. Dis.* **2021**, *80*, e42. [CrossRef]
43. Mantovani Cardoso, E.; Hundal, J.; Feterman, D.; Magaldi, J. Concomitant New Diagnosis of Systemic Lupus Erythematosus and COVID-19 with Possible Antiphospholipid Syndrome. Just a Coincidence? A Case Report and Review of Intertwining Pathophysiology. *Clin. Rheumatol.* **2020**, *39*, 2811–2815. [CrossRef]
44. Fineschi, S. Case Report: Systemic Sclerosis after COVID-19 Infection. *Front. Immunol.* **2021**, *12*, 686699. [CrossRef]
45. Hsu, T.Y.-T.; D'Silva, K.M.; Patel, N.J.; Fu, X.; Wallace, Z.S.; Sparks, J.A. Incident Systemic Rheumatic Disease following COVID-19. *Lancet Rheumatol.* **2021**, *3*, e402–e404. [CrossRef]
46. Zacharias, H.; Dubey, S.; Koduri, G.; D'Cruz, D. Rheumatological Complications of Covid 19. *Autoimmun. Rev.* **2021**, *20*, 102883. [CrossRef]
47. Taha, S.I.; Samaan, S.F.; Ibrahim, R.A.; El-Sehsah, E.M.; Youssef, M.K. Post-COVID-19 Arthritis: Is It Hyperinflammation or Autoimmunity? *Eur. Cytokine Netw.* **2021**, *32*, 83–88. [CrossRef]
48. Ouldali, N.; Pouletty, M.; Mariani, P.; Beyler, C.; Blachier, A.; Bonacorsi, S.; Danis, K.; Chomton, M.; Maurice, L.; Bourgeois, F.L.; et al. Emergence of Kawasaki Disease Related to SARS-CoV-2 Infection in an Epicentre of the French COVID-19 Epidemic: A Time-Series Analysis. *Lancet Child Adolesc. Health* **2020**, *4*, 662–668. [CrossRef]
49. Derksen, V.F.A.M.; Kissel, T.; Lamers-Karnebeek, F.B.G.; van der Bijl, A.E.; Venhuizen, A.C.; Huizinga, T.W.J.; Toes, R.E.M.; Roukens, A.H.E.; van der Woude, D. Onset of Rheumatoid Arthritis after COVID-19: Coincidence or Connected? *Ann. Rheum. Dis.* **2021**, *80*, 1096–1098. [CrossRef]

Disclaimer/Publisher's Note: The statements, opinions and data contained in all publications are solely those of the individual author(s) and contributor(s) and not of MDPI and/or the editor(s). MDPI and/or the editor(s) disclaim responsibility for any injury to people or property resulting from any ideas, methods, instructions or products referred to in the content.

MDPI
St. Alban-Anlage 66
4052 Basel
Switzerland
www.mdpi.com

Medicina Editorial Office
E-mail: medicina@mdpi.com
www.mdpi.com/journal/medicina

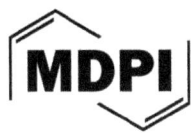

Disclaimer/Publisher's Note: The statements, opinions and data contained in all publications are solely those of the individual author(s) and contributor(s) and not of MDPI and/or the editor(s). MDPI and/or the editor(s) disclaim responsibility for any injury to people or property resulting from any ideas, methods, instructions or products referred to in the content.

www.ingramcontent.com/pod-product-compliance
Lightning Source LLC
LaVergne TN
LVHW070635100526
838202LV00012B/814